Dimensions of Cancer

Books in the Wadsworth Biology Series

DIMENSIONS OF CANCER

CHARLES E. KUPCHELLA
Western Kentucky University

with a chapter on cancer treatment by

SALVATORE J. BERTOLONE
University of Louisville School of Medicine

Wadsworth Publishing Company
Belmont, California
A Division of Wadsworth, Inc.

Biology Editor: Jack Carey

Production Editor: Harold Humphrey

Managing Designer: MaryEllen Podgorski

Print Buyer: Karen Hunt

Art Editor: Marta Kongsle

Text and Cover Designer: Detta Penna

Copy Editor: Linda Purrington

Illustrator: Barbara Barnett

Compositor: Thompson Type

Cover Photograph: Light micrograph of blood smear,

leukemia, 87500×. Peter Arnold, Inc.

Printed in the United States of America

1 2 3 4 5 6 7 8 9 10——91 90 89 88 87

Library of Congress Cataloging-in-Publication Data

Kupchella, Charles E.
    Dimensions of cancer.

    (Wadsworth biology series)
    Includes bibliographies and index.
    1. Cancer—Popular works. I. Bertolone,
Salvatore J. II. Title. III. Series. [DNLM:
1. Medical Oncology—popular works. QZ 201 K958d]
RC263.K85   1987   616.99′4   86-23435
ISBN 0-534-06900-2

To Condict Moore

---

and to the memories of
Eugenia Buoite, Dina Woodling, Alan Kiel,
Louis Krumholz, and Jack Yankeelov.

BRIEF CONTENTS

DETAILED CONTENTS

PREFACE

The reasons for public interest in cancer are obvious. Nearly all of us have been touched by cancer in a profound way—or we know that we likely will be. Most of us know that we have a one-in-three chance of getting cancer ourselves. Beyond personal interest, cancer fascinates in the same way that tornados, electrical storms, poisonous snakes, and all things that blend danger and mystery fascinate. Cancer is perhaps the most feared cause of death in the Western world. Cancer also fascinates because it is an elusive biological mystery made even more intriguing because it is in the process of being solved. Solving puzzles—even hearing about puzzles being solved—is exciting.

Cancer is science in action. There has been a great increase in the number of courses about cancer being taught at the undergraduate level in colleges and universities. The reason for this is that students learn a lot about science by studying cancer. Cancer has elements of physics, chemistry, biology, psychology, geography, and sociology, and it offers a vehicle by which these sciences can be shown in their relationship to one another and to the very real world. Science educators have been quick to realize that cancer offers a powerful means of illuminating science for what it is: namely, a dynamic, action-packed approach to the unknown—a way of getting at the truth, a way of discovering generalizations by making generalizations and then seeing if they stand up to challenges designed to disprove them.

Readers who have had only one or a few introductory science courses, and who may have come to think of the sciences as carefully honed collections of immutable facts and long lists of names and labels to memorize, may be in for an attitude adjustment here. Such readers should be prepared for accounts without closure, for words and phrases such as "perhaps," "possibly," "one possibility," "hypothesis," "it is not yet clear," and "we don't know." There are many such phrases throughout this book because we will be dealing with science at its most rapidly moving edges—where explanations are taking shape.

This book was written expressly in response to the need for an up-to-date, comprehensive text to support cancer courses aimed at both science and nonscience students at the beginning undergraduate level. *Dimensions of Cancer* will also be useful to many others, including people not even taking courses. It should serve as a good resource for people who simply want to know more about cancer for whatever reason. The book assumes only a limited science background on the part of its readers. *Dimensions of Cancer* was designed to blend the biology of cancer with clinical cancer and includes descriptions of all of the most common cancers and a special chapter on the psychosocial aspects of cancer.

Some of the other important features of this book are as follows.

Organization

The book has five parts. Cancer in all of its dimensions is introduced in the first chapter. The remainder of Part I is devoted to a background description of normal cells, normal tissue organization, and several key physiological concepts. Part II presents the essence of cancer at the cellular level. Chapter topics include the structural and functional characteristics of the cancer cell, the classification of cancer types, and the dynamics of invasion and metastasis. Part III describes and relates the causes of cancer; separate chapters are devoted to oncogenes, chemicals, viruses, radiation, and genetics. An epilog to Part III explores the relative importance of genetics and the environment in the causation of cancer. Part IV looks at the impact of cancer, first on individuals and then on populations. A separate chapter is devoted to the methods of epidemiology. "Cancer and the Immune System" was a difficult topic to place; it comes at

the end of Part IV because cancer has an impact on the immune system, but the immune system is also relevant to cancer detection, diagnosis, and treatment, covered in Part V. Part V, entitled "Dealing with Cancer," has separate chapters on cancer prevention, detection/diagnosis, and treatment, plus a synopsis of the most common types of human cancer and a review of the psychosocial impacts of cancer on cancer patients and their families.

The book is designed to be flexible, with many cross references. The chapters can be taught or read in almost any order.

Illustrations

We have set a new standard in illustrations for books of this type. *Dimensions of Cancer* contains more than 130 illustrations, including many detailed line drawings and a superb collection of photographs provided by cancer researchers throughout the country. The text is also full of data-rich tables and charts.

References

Original sources of research findings are cited throughout the text, and many sources of additional information are provided at the end of each chapter. The end-of chapter bibliographies are gateways to the great wealth of cancer literature, guides to who's who doing what, and identifiers of the best ongoing sources of information. Most "further-reading" entries were chosen for their accessibility. Where possible I identified sources likely to be found in nearly every college library; public libraries in major cities will have many of the sources, and librarians will be able to get others via inter-library loans quite easily. Many of the items in the bibliography can be obtained free by writing or calling the American Cancer Society, the National Cancer Institute, and other organizations and simply asking for them. There are enough readable items in every end-of-chapter bibliography to permit the nonspecialist to follow particular topics in more depth quite easily.

Definitions

All key terms are printed in **boldface** the first time they are used in the text in a context that defines the term. The index doubles as a glossary by indicating the pages on which key terms are defined.

Acknowledgments

I have many people to thank. The members of my family provided indispensable support and encouragement; I worked on this project mostly on their time. I must also acknowledge the generous help, support, encouragement, and stimulus I received from the administration, faculty, staff, and students at Murray State University and Western Kentucky University, particularly Louis Beyer, Gary Boggess, Velvet Dowdy, Marti Erwin, Robert Etherton, Karla Guess, Tom Hejkal, Wayne Higgins, Adele (Kiel) Kupchella, Kelley Larson, Oliver Muscio, Charles Smith, James Stuart, and Vaughn Vandegrift, all of whom reviewed parts of the manuscript. I would also like to thank reviewers Jane Bramham, Walter Kuebler, Larry Kupchella, and Elizabeth Westbrook.

I would not have been able to write this book without the unique opportunity I have had to interact with friends and colleagues in nearly all walks of cancer research and clinical cancer. I am particularly grateful for the education I received through my teaching and research interaction with colleagues at the University of Louisville—Condict Moore, Bob Burton, Sal Bertolone (the author of Chapter 17), Ralph Scott, Curt Sigdestad, John Mansfield, William Christopherson, Don Kemetz, Norbert Burzinski, Per Carstens, John Wallace, Gerry Sonnenfield, Daniele Turns, Young Liu, Lung Yam, Stan Lowenbraun, Jerry Hoffman, Ron Doyle, Uldis Streips, Carlo Tamburro, Tom Day, Dick Greenberg, John Creech, Hans Eickenberg, Jim Whittliff, John Wong, Grant Taylor, Bill Waddell, and Enrique Espinosa—to name just a few. Many of these individuals also served as reviewers of the text as it was developed—as did many other specialists (see below). I deeply appreciate the effort made by editors Jean-Francois Villain and Jack Carey to engage a very capable group of expert reviewers; they were somehow able to get this group of very busy individuals to provide me with timely, detailed, extremely helpful criticism and suggestions.

I thank those scientists who provided me with many of the most striking and instructive photographs sprinkled throughout the text. I would specifically like to thank J. Carl Barrett, Bruce Wetzel, Peter A. Netland, Garth L. Nicolson, Jerry A. Shields, Lloyd J. Old, and especially Per H.B. Carstens.

Writing this book was also made much easier by the help I received from unusually capable typists. Most of the typing was done by Susan Vance and Donna Marine; other contributors included Jean Lynch, Vera Howerton, Sally Feeney, Pat Thomas, Gail Raspberry, Debbie Lynn, and Helga Keller.

Lastly, and by no means least, I acknowledge the very capable assistance of the library staffs at the University of Louisville Health Sciences Center, Murray State University, and Western Kentucky University. I particularly wish to thank Jean Almand of Western Kentucky University's Science Library, who cheerfully verified and helped complete hundreds of reference citations.

Review and Text Development

In this age of specialization, no one individual could write a book about cancer without the help of many different kinds of experts. The people listed below reviewed various parts of the book during its development and gave me invaluable suggestions, pointed out potentially misleading sentences, called my attention to new information, identified misspelled words and extraneous or missing commas, and otherwise made significant contributions to the accuracy and usefulness of this book. Some of the reviewers were chosen by the editor because they were teaching the kinds of cancer courses this book is intended to support; their job was to help make sure the book would be useful. Others were chosen because of their subject matter expertise; their job was to help make doubly sure the book was accurate. The arrangement with reviewers was such that they had no control over the final outcome. The responsibility for any errors that may remain is mine.

Per H.B. Carstens, University of Louisville

William Christopherson, University of Louisville.

Wayne E. Criss, Concord College

Richard S. Demaree, Jr., California State University, Chico

Ronald Doyle, University of Louisville

Judah Folkman, Harvard University

Melvin H. Green, University of California, San Diego

Richard A. Greenberg, University of Louisville

M. Ward Hinds, Kentucky Cabinet for Human Resources

Ronald Hybertson, Mankato State University

Yosh Maruyama, University of Kentucky

Lois Matsuoka, Southern Illinois University

John P. Minton, Ohio State University

Edwin A. Mirand, Roswell Park Memorial Institute

Condict Moore, University of Louisville

Wiltraud Pfeiffer, University of California, Davis

Albey M. Reiner, University of Massachusetts, Amherst

Curtis P. Sigdestad, University of Louisville

Saul Slapikoff, Tufts University

Gerald Sonnenfeld, University of Louisville

Uldis N. Streips, University of Louisville

Len Troncale, California State Polytechnic University, Pomona

John Wallace, University of Louisville

Jacobo Wortsman, Southern Illinois University

David S. Yohn, Ohio State University

Bruce S. Zwilling, Ohio State University

Dimensions of Cancer

PART ONE
SOME BACKGROUND

The first section of this book introduces cancer and provides some background to allow cancer to be better appreciated as a cellular/biochemical phenomenon that affects whole organisms. Every cell of the human body is made up of chemicals behaving in accordance with physical laws. Normally, trillions of cells—organized into tissues, organs, and organ systems—interact with other cells in a highly orderly fashion. If we are to appreciate the difference between normal cells and cancer cells, and the effects cancer has on the human body, we must know something about normal cells and the chemical basis of coordinated cellular behavior. Chapter 1 provides an overview summarizing the many dimensions of cancer. Chapter 2 describes the biology of normal cells. Chapter 3 discusses some basic human anatomy and physiology.

1

The Many Faces of Cancer

Somewhere, in what had been up until then a near perfectly harmonious community of some one hundred trillion cells, a normal cell becomes a cancer cell.

There is no sharp jab of pain to mark the event. There is no "festering" at the site of the transformation. There is no rallying of the immune system.

The body accepts the cell as if it were one of its own (which it is), still under the control of the collective whole (which it is not).

For a long time, maybe twenty or thirty years, the cancer cell divides again and again. Even when its descendants number in the billions, the body exhibits no readily apparent sign or symptom of what has by then become a semi-independent mass with its own blood supply. By this time some tiny "gangs" of cancer cells have broken away from the original mass and have started thriving colonies in the brain and in the lungs, places to which the "colonists" were carried by the bloodstream.

About the time the original mass reaches the ten-billion cell size, the body notices a lump.

There is a hasty visit to a doctor.

An anesthesiologist puts the body to sleep, and a surgeon cuts a small piece of the tumor off and gives it to a pathologist, who looks at it under a microscope and says the tumor is malignant. An examination of adjacent lymph nodes, chest X-rays, and brain scans indicate that the cancer has spread; the case is declared "advanced." The surgeon tells the family that not all the cancer was removed. A medical oncologist is called in. There are regular trips to the outpatient clinic, but in this case, the body dies.

Death comes only after a long period in which the victim slowly and progressively deteriorates. When it is finally over, the survivors are glad; some had even prayed for an early end, and now some of them feel guilty. There are large medical bills to be paid.

In the most fundamental sense, cancer is a family of diseases in which cells divide, move around the body, and secrete things as if the rest of the organism had no control over them. But cancer has other faces.

For two-thirds of its victims, cancer is a thing that ends life; for the other one-third, cancer is a thing that changes life. To its victims and

```
┌─────────────────────────────────────────────┐
│                                               │
│   The Seven Warning Signs of Cancer           │
│   ─────────────────────────────────────       │
│                                               │
│   1.  A sore that does not heal               │
│                                               │
│   2.  A change in bowel or bladder habits or  │
│       function                                │
│                                               │
│   3.  Abnormal bleeding or bloody discharge   │
│                                               │
│   4.  Indigestion or difficulty swallowing    │
│                                               │
│   5.  Persistent cough or hoarseness          │
│                                               │
│   6.  A change in a wart or mole              │
│                                               │
│   7.  A lump or thickening                    │
│                                               │
└─────────────────────────────────────────────┘
```

their friends, it is an arbitrary affliction. "Why me?" "Why him? Why her?"

To its victims and those who care about them, cancer is numbing despair punctuated by surges of hope and rushes of anxiety. Cancer is often a painful emotional and financial burden. It makes family members feel helpless, inadequate, powerless.

Men worry mainly about lung cancer; women worry about breast cancer.

To physicians, cancer is a frustrating mixture of too few successes and too many quiet conversations that end with an often unspoken, "There's nothing more we can do."

To smokers, it's something not to think about. They do anyway.

To epidemiologists, environmentalists, and public health professionals, cancer is an epidemic with a bewildering array of causes and possible causes. They worry about chemicals with long names measured in parts per billion, some of which may or may not cause cancer. Some of the worriers smoke.

To life insurance underwriters, a history of cancer means risk. Smoking means higher premiums.

To cancer researchers, cancer is a fascinating biological phenomenon. They endure long periods with little progress and take great satisfaction in advances in understanding—even small

advances, detached as they are in their work from the real thing. Working with cancer cells in plastic flasks creates the illusion of being immune from cancer, perhaps even of being in control of cancer—safe.

To sociologists, cancer is a social disease of tremendous impact. It is the "wages" of our modern lifestyle. When medical costs are added to the costs of lost productivity and other less direct costs, the impact of cancer runs into many billions of dollars each year.

Cancer has many dimensions, all of them bad.

While everybody has to die of something, most of us would prefer to die of something less insidious, less painful, less costly, less arbitrary, and less wasting-away and lingering than cancer. As each of us gradually gives up the inborn certainty of our physical immortality, we hope to die of very old age quickly and in full control of our faculties up to the last minute. "Let it be anything but cancer."

Perhaps you already know that you have one chance in three of getting cancer yourself. Perhaps, like me, you have, or have had, friends or family members with cancer. Perhaps you had cancer once. Perhaps you have it now.

This year, cancer will kill almost a half-million Americans; it is second only to heart disease as a cause of death in the United States (Table 1.1). If the impact of disease is measured in terms of its effect on shortening life, cancer is actually ahead of heart disease (Cairns, 1975).

Table 1.2 illustrates the impact of cancer on hypothetical, present-day American cities of different sizes. One in three Americans will develop cancer, and one in five will die of it (Seidman, Mushinski, et al., 1985)—if present trends continue. Not shown in Table 1.2 is the unknown but undoubtedly significant impact of cancer-induced fear and anxiety.

The magnitude of the cancer problem is determined by a complex interplay of many different *kinds* of factors: the number of carcinogenic agents in the environment, our ability to identify them, and our ability to do something about

The Impact of Cancer in the United States: Incidence, Prevalence, Mortality and Other Impacts

Some general facts about the impact of cancer:

Cancer kills more children aged 3 to 14 than any other disease.

Nearly 71 million Americans now living will get cancer eventually.

During the 1970s, 3.5 million people died of cancer; 6.5 million learned that they had it.

In 1985 alone, 910,000 people learned that they had cancer; only about 340,000 of these people will likely be alive in 1990.

Approximately 462,000 Americans died of cancer in 1985.

Cancer kills 1,266 Americans every day.

Smoking accounts for about 85 percent of the lung cancer in men; 75 percent in women; it accounts for about 30 percent of cancer deaths overall.

For every 46 women that die of cancer, 54 men suffer the same fate.

One out of every five deaths in America is a cancer death.

The total direct medical cost of cancer is in the neighborhood of $10 billion per year; counting indirect costs such as lost wages, the total is around $50 billion.

Sources: American Cancer Society, 1985, and various National Cancer Institute publications.

Table 1.1   Mortality for Leading Causes of Death, United States—1983

Rank	Cause of Death	Number of Deaths	Death Rate per 100,000 Population	Percent of Total Deaths
	All Causes	*2,019,201*	*743.4*	*100.0*
1.	Heart diseases	770,345	276.2	38.2
2.	Cancer	442,986	169.0	21.9
3.	Cerebrovascular diseases	155,598	54.1	7.7
4.	Accidents	92,488	36.5	4.6
5.	Pneumonia and influenza	55,854	19.2	2.8
6.	Chronic obstructive lung diseases	45,814	16.8	2.3
7.	*Diabetes mellitus*	36,246	13.4	1.8
8.	Suicide	28,295	11.0	1.4
9.	Cirrhosis of liver	27,266	11.1	1.4
10.	Arteriosclerosis	26,371	8.6	1.3
11.	Homicide	20,191	7.8	1.0
12.	Diseases of infancy	19,310	9.0	1.0

Adapted courtesy of the American Cancer Society from Silverberg, 1986. Used by permission.

Table 1.2 The Impact of Cancer on Various-Sized Cities

Community Population	Estimated No. Who Are Alive, Saved from Cancer	Estimated No. Cancer Cases under Medical Care in 1985	Estimated No. Who Will Die of Cancer in 1985	Estimated No. of New Cases in 1985	Estimated No. Who Will Be Saved from Cancer in 1985	Estimated No. Who Will Eventually Develop Cancer	Estimated No. Who Will Die of Cancer if Present Rates Continue
2,000	20	11	4	7	3	560	360
5,000	50	26	9	16	6	1,400	900
10,000	100	52	18	33	12	2,800	1,800
25,000	250	131	45	79	30	7,000	4,500
100,000	1,000	525	180	325	122	28,000	18,000
500,000	5,000	2,625	900	1,575	590	140,000	90,000

Note: The figures can only be the roughest approximation of actual data for your community and should be used with caution.

Adapted from American Cancer Society, 1985. Used by permission.

them after they have been identified; our ability to detect cancers, and our willingness to avail ourselves of methods of detection and to seek help at the first sign of a problem; our ability to cure cancer; and our ability to minimize the side effects of therapy. Improvements in any of these factors favorably changes the outcome of the cancer equation.

Causes of Cancer

Cancer is apparently the result of one or more cellular mutations or other persistent changes in the control of genetic expression. This is the only way to explain why, when a cancer cell divides, the result is two cancer cells. Also, the things that are known to be able to cause cancer—radiation, chemicals, and viruses—are all capable of interacting with genetic material.

Carcinogens (cancer-causing agents) are found in the environment in ever-increasing amounts. We breathe them, we eat them, and we come into contact with them in other ways. A small fraction of cancers may arise as a result of spontaneous mistakes but the majority are

caused by environmental factors such as sunlight and cigarette smoke (Fig. 1.1).

Recent evidence suggests that some carcinogens may work by activating previously dormant genes called *oncogenes*, found in all normal cells. Oncogene products then somehow change normal cells into cancer cells (see Chapter 7).

That most carcinogens come from the environment is deduced from (1) consistent associations between certain cancers and certain environmental factors (Fig. 1.1), (2) the great differences seen in patterns of cancer mortality worldwide, and (3) from the fact that when people migrate from one place to another, they and their descendants tend to adopt the cancer death patterns of their new country. There are even great differences in cancer death rates seen in different parts of the same country. The exact reasons for such patterns are not known, although the underlying causes are believed to be predominantly environmental factors and different lifestyles, as opposed to genetic differences.

Based on the belief that geographic differences in the occurrence of different kinds of cancer are really environmental differences, it has been estimated that up to 90 percent of all cancer is caused by factors in the environment—cigarette smoke and sunlight included. If this is true, and if it is possible to find all these factors and to eliminate them (obviously no small assumption), the impact of cancer could theoretically be reduced to one-tenth of what it is now.

Some Definitions

In the following discussions about patterns and trends, you will need to understand these terms and the differences among them:

Cancer death rate   The number of people who die (of cancer) per year per unit number of people who are alive and who could die; usually expressed as the number of deaths per 100,000 people per year.

Cancer incidence   The number of people who contract cancer per 100,000 per year, without regard to whether or not they die of it.

Mortality rate   A synonym for *death rate*.

Age-specific death rate   The number of people per 100,000 who die in a year in some particular age category.

Cancer prevalence   The number of people per 100,000 who *have* cancer at a particular point in time or who have it for any part of a particular span of time. In arriving at a prevalence rate for a particular year, let's say, a person would be counted even if he or she died on January 1 or was diagnosed as having cancer on December 31.

Cancer survival rates   Such rates measure the fraction or percentage of people remaining alive for some number of years after the diagnosis of cancer. By convention, we speak of the percentage of survivors after a certain number of years. Also by convention, those who survive 5 years are considered cured, although this is not strictly true—roughly 85 percent of those alive after 5 years will be alive after 10 years. A distinction is made between "**observed survival**

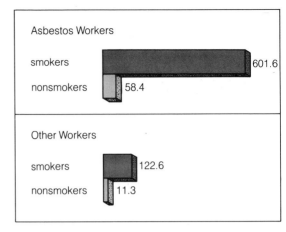

Figure 1.1 Lung cancer death rates for workers in contact with asbestos versus all other workers (deaths per 100,000 man-years, standardized for age). (*Source:* National Cancer Institute, 1981)

rates" and "**relative survival rates.**" Today, three of eight patients are expected to be alive 5 years hence. Thus, the "observed" survival rate is expected to be 39 percent. If normal life expectancy is taken into account (if an adjustment is made for those deaths expected to occur from causes other than cancer during that 5-year period), however, the relative survival rate is expected to be 49 percent.

Age-adjusted mortality rates   Sometimes when two or more groups are to be compared, it is necessary to adjust the statistics for any differences in the age profiles of the groups—to correct for the fact that cancer is more likely in older age groups. After such corrections are applied, the resultant rates are said to be "age-adjusted."

Patterns

In terms of the numbers of different tissues of different organs from which it can arise, more than a hundred different kinds of cancer exist. This statement is not just a matter of hairsplitting distinctions. Each kind of cancer seems

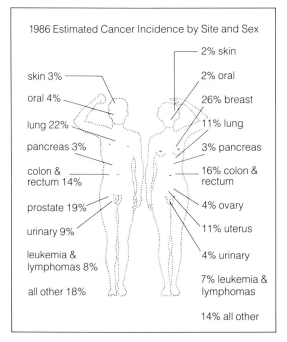

1986 Estimated Cancer Incidence by Site and Sex

2% skin

skin 3%
oral 4%
lung 22%
pancreas 3%
colon &
rectum 14%
prostate 19%
urinary 9%
leukemia &
lymphomas 8%
all other 18%

2% oral
26% breast
11% lung
3% pancreas
16% colon &
rectum
4% ovary
11% uterus
4% urinary
7% leukemia &
lymphomas
14% all other

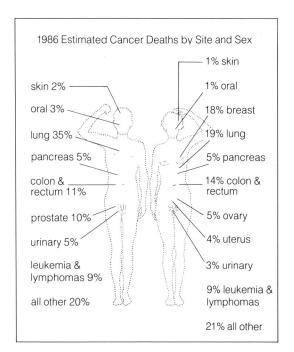

1986 Estimated Cancer Deaths by Site and Sex

1% skin

skin 2%
oral 3%
lung 35%
pancreas 5%
colon &
rectum 11%
prostate 10%
urinary 5%
leukemia &
lymphomas 9%
all other 20%

1% oral
18% breast
19% lung
5% pancreas
14% colon &
rectum
5% ovary
4% uterus
3% urinary
9% leukemia &
lymphomas
21% all other

Figure 1.2 Cancer statistics, estimates of incidence based on the National Cancer Institute's Surveillance, Epidemiology, and End Results (SEER) program (1977–1981). Nonmelanoma skin cancer and carcinoma *in situ* have not been included. (Adapted courtesy of the American Cancer Society, Inc., from Silverberg, 1986)

also to have its unique arrays of causes, behavioral features, likelihoods of occurring, likelihoods of causing death, and degrees of responsiveness to therapy (see Chapter 17).

Consider the following facts: about half of all cancer deaths are the result of malignancies of lung, breast, and large intestine (Fig. 1.2). Figure 1.2 also shows that patterns of cancer death are somewhat different in men and women—and the differences go beyond the obvious differences in anatomy. The differences between incidence percentages and death percentages in both men and women (Fig. 1.2) indicate the degree to which some cancers are deadlier than others. When ethnic groups are compared in the same way, the similarities are striking, but so are the differences.

In men, lung and prostate gland cancer predominate in white and black Americans but the incidence rates differ significantly. In women,

breast cancer predominates in both groups but the relative importance of cervical, stomach, and other cancers differ. Cancer incidence is higher for blacks than for whites in general, and this difference is believed to be related to economic, environmental, and social factors rather than to genetic differences. Childhood cancer patterns are different from adult cancer patterns, and the patterns of cancer death change throughout life.

Some kinds of cancer are much more likely to have already spread when detected than others (Fig. 1.3), and this fact manifests itself in differential five-year survival rates (see Chapter 16).

Cancer is basically a disease of the old (Fig. 1.4). A 20-year-old can die of colon cancer, but the risk of such a death is 1,000 times greater in an 80-year-old (Cairns, 1975). What we know about cancer suggests two reasons for the age connection. First, it takes time to accumulate the

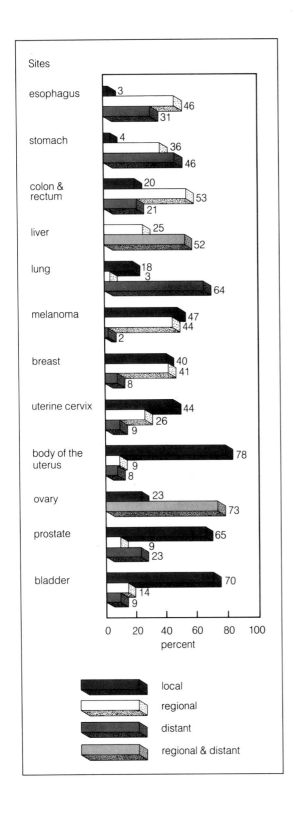

Sites

esophagus — 3, 46, 31

stomach — 4, 36, 46

colon & rectum — 20, 53, 21

liver — 25, 52

lung — 18, 3, 64

melanoma — 47, 44, 2

breast — 40, 41, 8

uterine cervix — 44, 26, 9

body of the uterus — 78, 9, 8

ovary — 23, 73

prostate — 65, 9, 23

bladder — 70, 14, 9

0   20   40   60   80   100
percent

■ local
□ regional
■ distant
■ regional & distant

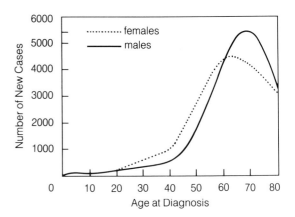

········· females
——— males

Number of New Cases: 1000, 2000, 3000, 4000, 5000, 6000

0 10 20 30 40 50 60 70 80
Age at Diagnosis

Figure 1.4 Cancer is a disease of the old—as illustrated by the absolute numbers of new cases in 1978. (*Source:* National Cancer Institute, SEER program)

necessary genetic insults. Secondly, it takes a while for cancer to reveal itself after it begins— sometimes two, three, or even four decades. Circumstantial evidence indicates that for the U.S. population as a whole, the "lag" between the induction of lung cancer by cigarette smoking and lung cancer death, appears to be about 20 years (see Cairns, 1975).

Another dimension of cancer patterns, already mentioned, has to do with geography. Cancer of the stomach is about six times more common in Japan than in the United States, but the Japanese get less breast cancer and less prostatic cancer. Within the United States, skin cancer death rates are much higher in the Sunbelt states, cervical cancer death rates are significantly higher than average in many counties of Appalachia, and breast cancer death rates are significantly elevated in many northeastern states.

Figure 1.3 Percent of cancer cases by site, by stage (localized disease, disease spread regionally, and disease widely spread) at which the cancer was diagnosed 1977–1982. (*Source:* National Cancer Institute data, adapted courtesy of the American Cancer Society, Inc., from Silverberg, 1986)

Trends

Except possibly for "lag," the patterns we have just discussed are not static. Indeed, these patterns have changed quite dramatically even in the last few decades. Let's look at some major trends in the way cancer has afflicted human beings, particularly in the United States.

First of all, from the very broad biological and historical perspective, cancer is neither new nor unique to humans or even to mammals. The fossil record indicates that more than 100 million years ago, dinosaurs got cancer and that plants had it before that (Moodie, 1918, 1923). The earliest known human cancer was diagnosed in an Egyptian mummy dated from 3,000 B.C. (Mettle and Cecilia, 1947). Still, cancer, like heart disease, is a modern disease. It has emerged as a leading killer only within the last 50 to 100 years. A century ago, most Americans died of infectious diseases like typhoid, influenza, cholera, diptheria, and pneumonia. Improved sanitation, and then antibiotics, made a great impact on these diseases, and very few Americans die of them today. Heart disease and cancer are the principal death-dealing diseases in industrialized nations today.

In very recent times, while heart disease has been declining as a cause of death, cancer death has continued to increase at a rate of about 1 percent per year since the turn of the century. An interesting thing about this trend is that lung cancer is almost solely responsible. If lung cancer is disregarded, cancer death rates have remained about the same for the last fifty years or longer—and have actually fallen in very recent years. Lung cancer is only part of the changing story; stomach cancer incidence rates have inexplicably fallen almost as far and as fast as lung cancer has risen. In general, Americans have been dying of somewhat different kinds of cancer over the years; mortality rates for some forms of cancer have gone up, while rates for other kinds have gone down (see Fig. 1.5).

Some particularly interesting features of cancer trends in the United States are as follows:

The rate of new cancer cases is going down in women, up in men.

The overall cancer death rate for those younger than age 45 has been falling for more than a decade.

Stomach cancer has declined eight-fold in the last half century. Nobody knows why.

If the cancer death rate is age-adjusted, the trend since 1930 has been as follows: 1930, 143/100,000; 1940s, 152; 1950s, 158; 1960s, 162; 1970s, 169 (American Cancer Society, 1985).

When changes in the size of the American population and its age composition are factored in, cancer death rates have actually risen only slightly for men since about 1937; death rates have declined for women.

As for trends in detecting cancer and in treating cancer—the good news has been considerable.

Progress

Ironically, the fact that cancer is such a major problem is, itself, a result of progress. It is a result of progress in that modern technologies and lifestyles have brought new and more plentiful carcinogens into our lives. But it is also a result of new technologies that keep people from dying of infectious disease and starvation—allowing us to live long enough to die of cancer. Nonetheless, progress has been, and is being, made all across the broad front of detection, diagnosis, therapy, rehabilitation, and prevention of cancer.

Earlier detection, improved surgical procedures, better anticancer drugs, and better supportive care for cancer patients have all contributed to the fact that treatment now saves three times as many lives as it did before World War II. Hidden within this fact is the reality that while dramatic progress has been made with some kinds of cancer, such as Hodgkin's disease and testicular cancer, cure rates have not really

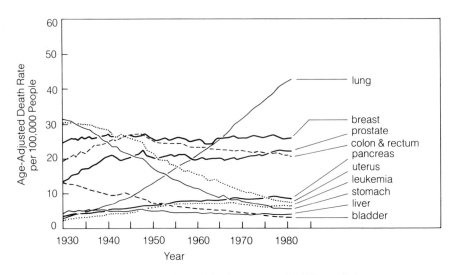

Figure 1.5 Cancer trends: age-adjusted death rates per 100,000 people for selected cancers in the United States from 1930 to 1982. (*Source:* U.S. National Center for Health Statistics. Adapted courtesy of the American Cancer Society, Inc., from Silverberg, 1986. Used by permission.)

Table 1.3   Trends in Survival for Selected Cancer Sites:
Cases Diagnosed in 1960−63, 1970−73, 1973−75, and 1976−81

Site	Relative 5-Year Survival Rate (Percent)			
	1960−1963	*1970−1973*	*1973−1975*	*1976−1981*
Colon	43	49	49	53
Rectum	38	45	47	49
Lung and bronchus	8	10	12	13
Melanoma of skin	60	68	76	80
Breast	63	68	74	75
Uterine cervix	58	64	68	67
Ovary	32	36	36	37
Prostate	50	63	65	71
Testis	63	72	76	87
Bladder	53	61	73	74
Hodgkin's disease	40	67	67	74
Leukemia	14	22	33	33

Note: Survival rates for samples of white Americans from various hospital and population-based registries.

Original data from Biometry Branch, National Cancer Institute. Table adapted courtesy American Cancer Society, Inc., from Silverberg, 1985, p. 35. Used by permission.

improved much for some of the most common solid tumors—colon cancer and lung cancer, for example (Table 1.3).

Improved treatment, mainly in the form of chemotherapy, has brought some dramatic improvements in survival for many kinds of cancer, including acute lymphocytic leukemia, certain adult leukemias, Burkitt's lymphoma, Hodgkin's disease and other lymphomas, testicular cancer, ovarian cancer, and childhood kidney and bone cancers (Fig. 1.6).

Less than a decade ago, very few children survived acute leukemia. Today, 90 percent respond to chemotherapy, and more than half are alive and well after five years. Figures given in the National Cancer Institute Directors Annual Report (1982) compare five-year survival rates for patients diagnosed from 1960 to 1963, with those diagnosed from 1970 to 1973. While five-year survival for breast cancer and pancreatic cancer rose only 5 and 2 percent respectively, the five-year survival for white males with leukemia rose from 4 to 23 percent and from 3 to 29 percent for white females. Hodgkin's disease (almost surely fatal just three decades ago) five-year survival jumped from 34 to 66 percent in males and from 48 to 69 percent in females. More such data are given in later chapters (see also Moore, 1985).

Some very recent therapeutic advances that have not yet had much of a chance to influence five-year survival rates include (1) the use of ultra high voltage linear accelerators capable of delivering radiation therapy to "deep" cancers with pinpoint precision, (2) the development of some new and promising anticancer drugs (Chapter 17), including some that stimulate the body's own immune system to attack cancer (Chapter 14), and (3) the identification of common denominator "oncogenes" (Chapter 7) in many kinds of cancer, raising the possibility that common gene products may serve as common immunotherapeutic and/or chemotherapeutic targets for many kinds of cancer.

Advances in other areas of cancer include the discovery of the anticancer activity of interferon and the development of monoclonal antibodies. Interferon has failed to live up to its initial promise but it may still prove useful in treating slow-growing cancers (see Chapter 17). Monoclonal antibodies appear to have a very bright future. The ability to make large amounts of antibodies to proteins associated with cancer cells (see Chapter 14) means that antibodies can be used to find occult tumors—by affixing radioactive tags to the antibodies and then determining where they go, using radiation detection equipment. It means that antibodies can be used to deliver toxic anticancer drugs right to cancer cells, like letter bombs or guided missiles (Chapter 17).

Gene splicing and other new genetic engineering technologies have opened up a whole new dimension of progress and potential progress in cancer research. By inserting the right gene into bacteria, genetic engineers have created interferon "factories," which, in turn, have provided amounts of interferon that have made possible its full testing. Genetic engineering has also yielded the "hybridomas" that produce monoclonal antibodies.

Recent advances in detection and diagnosis of cancer include the use of ultrasound, nuclear magnetic resonance imaging, and CAT scans (Chapter 16). Since the advent and widespread use of the Pap smear in detecting cancer of the uterine cervix, the death rate for this form of cancer has declined drastically (Fig. 1.5).

Also in the area of detection, heightened awareness of breast cancer, the increasing use of the breast self-examination, and the use of mammography (Chapter 16) are all apparently resulting in much earlier detection of breast cancers. Many are being found at stages in which they are highly curable.

There has also been some significant progress in cancer prevention. According to the American Cancer Society, 33 million Americans have quit smoking; only 15 percent of all medical doctors smoke today—over half did in the 1950s, when so many TV commercials made it seem like such a good idea. In 1985, the incidence of lung cancer in white males decreased significantly (3.4 percent) for the first time in half

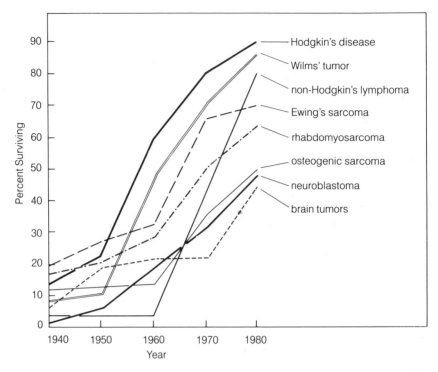

Figure 1.6 Proportion of children with solid tumors surviving two years from diagnosis. (*Source:* National Cancer Institute, 1981).

a century—following, by two decades, a decline in smoking by white males.

We should not end this section without mentioning that a particularly important mark of progress against cancer is that the medical profession now generally recognizes oncology as a legitimate subspecialty. Today there are perhaps a hundred times more board-certified cancer specialists (oncologists) in pediatrics, internal medicine, surgery, radiation therapy, and in gynecology than there were as recently as 1970.

Present Situation

The story "at the front" in our battle with cancer is optimistic but is still not good. As stated earlier, of every eight people who are diagnosed as having cancer, only three are saved. Another person could also be saved if he or she brought overt symptoms to a doctor sooner. But there is nothing that modern medicine can do for the rest save prolong life a little and improve its quality somewhat. Why? Because we simply don't know enough about the basic biology of cancer.

We have learned a lot but we still have much to learn. At least part of the problem is that we do not seem to put all of what we *do* know to work. According to various sources, cigarette smoking is probably the cause of 30 to 40 percent of the cancer in American men—perhaps half the cancers in men in England (Cairns, 1975). Genetic inheritance, something we can do very little about, probably accounts for maybe 5 percent. Perhaps we should redirect the money being spent to identify cancer-causing substances, to research into human motivation.

Still, we need to know cancer very much better than we do if major new advances are to be made. The very most fundamental problem is that cancer cells are simply too much like normal cells and therefore do not have obvious exploitable differences from normal cells. Infectious disease is a much simpler problem than cancer chiefly because there the enemy are clearly different life forms: viruses and bacteria. Penicillin takes advantage of a very basic difference between human cells and bacterial cells: bacterial cells have cell walls and human cells do not; penicillin interferes with the construction of cell walls. We have yet to find the equivalent of the bacterial cell wall (some key exploitable difference) in cancer cells. To quote Walt Kelly's Pogo completely out of context, the problem with cancer is that "the enemy is us." The enemy is us in two senses of the word *us*. We are our own enemy in the sense that we expose ourselves to carcinogens; and the enemy is our own cells gone wrong somehow.

The task of finding "the" cure will be much more difficult than finding pesticides that kill only one kind of living organism and harm no other. Someone once said that expecting to find a drug that kills cancer cells but harms no other is like expecting to be able to concoct something that if taken by mouth will destroy one ear and leave the other unscathed. An exaggeration? Yes, but it helps put the fight against cancer into perspective.

Perhaps we should put much more of our resources into prevention.

There are many things we have to put into more complete perspective, and so we had better get on with it. Let us begin by looking at normal cells and how they work together as part of a smoothly functioning whole organism—before we look at cancer cells and how they do not.

References and Further Reading

American Cancer Society. 1985. *Cancer Facts and Figures: 1985*. New York: American Cancer Society.

Becker, F. 1975–1977. *Cancer: A Comprehensive Treatise* (6 vols.). New York: Plenum.

Cairns, J. 1975. The Cancer Problem. *Scientific American*. 233:64–79.

Cutler, Sidney J., and Young, John L., Jr. 1975. *Third National Cancer Survey: Incidence Data*. National Cancer Institute Monograph 41. NIH Publication No. 75-787. Bethesda, Md.: NCI.

Enstrom, J. E., and Austin, D. F. 1977. Interpreting Cancer Survival Rates. *Science*. 195:847–51.

Gold, M. 1983. Cancer: When the Chromosome Breaks. *Science 83*. September, pp. 16–17.

Mason, T., Hoover, R., Blot, W., and Fraumeni, J. 1977. *Atlas of Cancer Mortality for U.S. Counties: 1950–1969*. Washington, D.C.: U.S. Department of Health, Education, and Welfare.

Mettle, R., and Cecilia, C. 1947. *History of Medicine*. Philadelphia: Blakeston.

Meyers, M. H., and Hankey, B. F. 1980. *Cancer Patient Survival Experience*. National Institutes of Health Publication No. 80–2148. Bethesda, Md.: NIH.

Miller, D. G. 1980. On the Nature of Susceptibility to Cancer. (Presidential Address, American Society of Clinical Oncology, 1979). *Cancer*. 46(6):1307–18.

Moodie, R. L. 1918. Pathologic Lesions Among Extinct Animals. *Surg. Clin. Chicago*. 2:319–31.

Moodie, R. L. 1923. *Antiquity of Disease*. Chicago: University of Chicago Press.

Moore, C. 1985. Multidisciplinary Pretreatment Cancer Planning. *J. Surg. Oncology*. 28:79–86.

National Cancer Institute. 1981. *Decade of Discovery: Advances in Cancer Research 1971–1981*. U.S. Department of Health and Human Services, Public Health Service, National Institutes of Health, National Cancer Institute. NIH Publication No. 81–2323.

National Cancer Institute. 1982. *National Cancer Program: 1981 Director's Report and Annual Plan FY 1983–1987*. U.S. Department of Health and Human Services Public Health Service. NIH Publication 82-2449.

Seidman, H., Mushinski, M., et al. 1985. Probabilities of Eventually Developing or Dying of Cancer—United States, 1985. *Ca-A Cancer Journal for Clinicians*. 35:36–56.

Shimkin, M. B. 1977. *Contrary to Nature*. U.S. Department of Health, Education, and Welfare Publication No. (NIH) 76-720. Washington, D.C.: U.S. Government Printing Office.

Silverberg, E. 1985. Cancer Statistics. *Ca-A Cancer Journal for Clinicians.* 35(1): 19–35.

Silverberg, E. 1986. Cancer Statistics, 1986. *Ca-A Cancer Journal for Clinicians.* 36:9–25.

Weinhouse, S., and Klein, G., eds. 1983. *Advances in Cancer Research,* Vol. 38. New York: Academic Press.

Note: Many additional sources of related information are given in later chapters, particularly the last four.

If we are to appreciate the abnormalities of cancer cells, we should see them in light of how normal cells are organized and how their parts interact. Our purpose in Chapter 2 will be to review the *general* structure of normal cells and the basic functions of the various parts of cells, paying particular attention to those cell features that seem to be different in cancer cells.

The Parts of a Cell

Robert Hooke (1627–1703) was apparently the first to use the term *cell*. He was looking at the microscopic structure of cork at the time, and what he saw reminded him of the "cells" or rooms found in the monasteries of that day. It doesn't matter that Hooke was looking at cell walls and that he didn't actually see cells at all; the term stuck anyway. Even if he had actually been looking at real cells, Hooke could not have seen much detail. His microscopes and even modern light microscopes simply do not have enough resolving power to reveal much of the detail of subcellular structure. Only since the advent of the electron microscope* have we been able to discern the fine structure described throughout the rest of this chapter.

There are many different kinds of cells, so it is with considerable poetic license that we now describe some of the features of the "typical" animal cell. The parts of a typical animal cell

2

General Features of the Structure, Function, and Reproduction of Normal Cells

*The limit of resolution of the light microscope is set by the wavelengths of the visible light spectrum. The limit is such that it doesn't do any good to magnify something more than 1,000 times as long as visible light is the source of illumination. In the electron microscope, the "illumination" is provided by a beam of electrons—focused with magnets. Since the wavelengths of the electromagnetic radiation in such a stream are much smaller than those in the visible part of the spectrum, resolution is better—up to 1,000 times better than with a light microscope. We can't look directly into an electron microscope, of course; our eyes aren't able to perceive wavelengths outside the "visible range." So we focus the images carried by electron beams on phosphor screens and look at the resultant "television" picture.

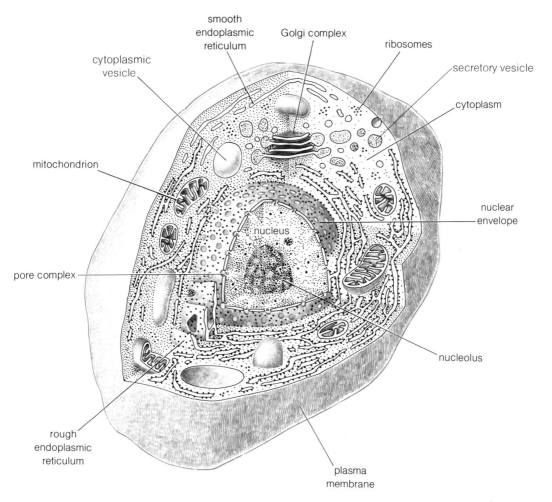

cytoplasmic
vesicle

mitochondrion

pore complex

rough
endoplasmic
reticulum

smooth
endoplasmic
reticulum

Golgi complex

ribosomes

secretory vesicle

cytoplasm

nucleus

nuclear
envelope

nucleolus

plasma
membrane

Figure 2.1 The parts of a "typical" animal cell

are shown in Figure 2.1; the functions of each are listed in Table 2.1. We begin with the cell membrane.

The Cell Membrane

The boundary that truly separates the inside of a cell from the outside is the cell membrane. The cell membrane is found in *all* cells and should not be confused with the cell wall, which is found only in plant cells. Whereas cell walls give plant cells their shape and rigid support,

cell membranes control what goes into and out of the cell—they can even "pump" certain things from one side to the other.

Cell membranes bear protein-carbohydrate and lipid-carbohydrate complexes (see Fig. 2.2) that serve as a means by which cells can receive messages from other cells. Such complexes, mostly glycoproteins, function as molecular "antennae" capable of receiving chemical and other signals from other cells. When these "antennae" receive (bind) hormones, for example, the combination in turn elicits some kind of response (see Fig. 2.3) inside the cell. The re-

Table 2.1 The Parts of a Cell

Structure or Organelle	Function
Cell coat	Protecting and recognizing
Cell membrane	Regulating transport and recognizing other cells and specific signals
Lysosomes	Containing digestive enzymes
Golgi bodies	Refining and packaging cell products
Mitochondria	Performing aerobic respiration
Ribosomes	Serving as site of protein synthesis
Nucleus	Containing genetic material
Nuclear envelope	Defining the nucleus and containing nuclear material.
Nucleoli	Preparing ribosomes
Endoplasmic reticulum	Providing internal structure and transport
Microtubules	Moving
Microfilaments	Moving
Flagella and/or cilia	Moving
Extracellular matrix	Giving structural support

sponse might be to increase protein synthesis, to increase the oxidation of glucose, to divide, not to divide, or whatever the cell is "programmed" to do in response to the presence of that particular hormone. Depending on the cell, there may be thousands of receptor molecules on the surface.

Cell membranes also bear recognition groups by which cells can recognize *other* cells and be recognized by them. It is these "signatures" by which cells "know" other cells that are part of the same organism and by which cells of the immune system recognize and initiate the destruction of invading microorganisms and tissue transplanted from another organism. Cell-cell recognition based on cell membrane chemistry is also the basis by which cells move around to find their *places* in a developing embryo.

The cell surface is obviously an important means by which cells function as components of multicellular organisms.

As for the membrane's role in determining what goes in or out: if a particular chemical compound, element, or ion is able to pass through the cell membrane, diffusion will continue as long as there is a **gradient** (more on one side of the membrane than on the other). Some things can move across cell membranes, and others cannot. Permeability is selective.

Some chemical substances can move across the cell membrane only with help. Such help is called **facilitated diffusion**. Facilitated diffusion is in the direction of the gradient—from high to low—but a carrier molecule is needed to get the substance through the membrane. There is also energy-consuming or **active transport**. Active transport is transport across the cell membrane *against* a concentration gradient. Active transport requires energy.

Other mechanisms by which things can enter or leave a cell through the cell membrane are endocytosis (in) and exocytosis (out). Certain cells of the immune system deal with an invading bacterium by engulfing it, internalizing it, and ultimately digesting it. The internalization of particles in this way is called **phagocytosis**.

Table 2.2 Some Important Types of Molecules Found in Cells

Class	Basic Subunits*	Function
Proteins	Amino acids; *short* chains of amino acids are called peptides.	Serve as structural components, e.g. collagen; as enzymes, e.g. trypsin; as hormones, e.g. insulin; and in other ways, e.g. hemoglobin.
Polysaccharides	Simple sugars.	Energy storage and transfer; some polysaccharides have structural roles.
Lipids Fats	Fatty acids and glycerol in a 3 to 1 ratio.	Long-term energy storage.
Phospholipids	Fats with a phosphate group (PO_4) attached.	Serve as basic components of cell membranes among other functions.
Nucleic Acids Deoxyribonucleic acid (DNA) Ribonucleic acid (RNA)	Nucleotide bases plus ribose-sugar, and phosphate. DNA contains these bases: adenine, guanine, cytosine, and thymine; in RNA, thymine is replaced by uracil. DNA is double stranded; RNA is single stranded.	Serve as the molecular essence of heredity; i.e., are the means by which genetic information is transmitted from generation to generation and by which protein synthesis is specified and controlled.
Nucleotides		In addition to serving as subunits of nucleic acids, nucleotides also serve other important functions in the cell.
Adenosine triphosphate (ATP)		Mediate energy transfer—from energy-yielding reactions to energy-requiring reactions.
Cyclic adenosine monophosphate (cyclic AMP)		Signal molecules within the cytoplasm controlling the rate of various chemical reactions.
Cyclic guanosine monophosphate (cyclic GMP)		"Signal" molecule within cells.
Glycoproteins	Protein/sugar complexes.	Membrane receptors, membrane recognition groups, etc.
Glycolipids e.g., Gangliosides	Sugar/fat complexes.	Cell membrane components—they may serve as receptors.
Steroids	These are small molecules (not polymers).	Function as hormones (e.g., estrogen, testosterone, cortisone) and serve various other functions.

*Cellular macromolecules are made up of smaller subunits strung together as polymers; proteins are chains of amino acids, polysaccharides are "poly"mers of simple sugars, etc.

Phagocytosis is a form of endocytosis. Generally speaking, **endocytosis** is the surrounding of some external material by the cell membrane and the budding off of the membrane-surrounded material *internally.* In **exocytosis**, a membrane-bound vacuole (Fig. 2.1) *inside* the cell fuses with the cell membrane and the contents are *ejected* into the cell's environment.

Chemistry of the Cell Membrane When Schleiden and Schwann realized that they could safely say (in 1839) that all living things are made of cells, it was already recognized that there must be some kind of boundary that defined each cell. It wasn't until the very *late* 1800s, however, that the chemistry of the cell membrane began to receive much attention.

Table 2.2 *(continued)*

*The Nucleotide Base
Cytosine*

*A Simple
Sugar, Ribose*

A "Typical" Phospholipid

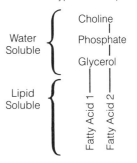

Water
Soluble }

Choline
|
Phosphate
|
Glycerol

Lipid
Soluble }

Fatty Acid 1   Fatty Acid 2

*The Amino Acid
Alanine*

*General Structure
of Amino Acids*

*The General Structure
of Steroids, e.g., cholesterol,
estrogen, testosterone, cortisone*

R = Radical; each amino
acid has a different
characteristic R. For
alanine, R = CH₃.

Chain of
variable length
attached here

Adenosine Triphosphate (ATP)

*Cyclic Adenosine Monophosphate
(cyclic AMP)*

Overton suggested in 1895 that the membrane must contain lipid, and electrical-resistance studies in the early 1900s confirmed that the cell membrane must be made of insulating material, like lipid.

In the 1920s, Gorter and Grendel determined that the amount of lipid extractable from a red blood cell would just about provide two layers of lipid molecules over the entire red blood cell surface. This was the beginning of the *lipid bilayer* model of the cell membrane.

Just before World War II, Danielli and Davson presented a generalized theory of cell membrane structure. According to the model, cell membranes had a lipoid core bordered by two layers of phospholipid molecules, each with

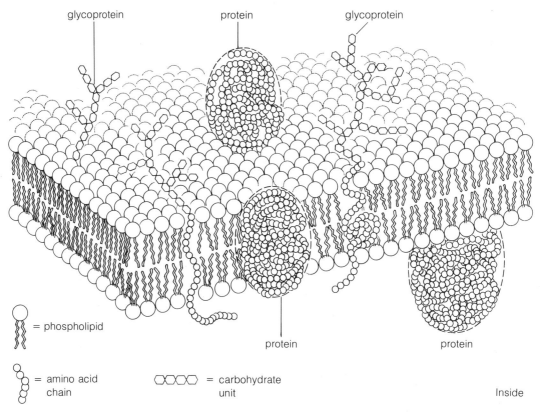

glycoprotein   protein   glycoprotein

= phospholipid

= amino acid
  chain

= carbohydrate
  unit

protein   protein

Inside

Figure 2.2 The fluid mosaic model of the cell membrane. Integral proteins form part of the membrane, being deeply imbedded in the lipid bilayer. Other proteins, called *peripheral proteins*, are more loosely bound to the outer or inner membrane surfaces.

their hydrophobic tails projecting into the lipoid core and with their polar heads oriented outward (Fig. 2.2).

With the advent of the electron microscope used in conjunction with special stains, it became clear that the outer surface of the membrane was different from the inner surface. Staining properties of the outer surface indicated that the cell membrane was carbohydrate-coated. For a period of 15 to 20 years, the commonly held view was that *all* cellular membranes consisted of the same kind of lipid bilayer with outer surfaces covered by nonlipid materials, largely carbohydrate.

In the early 1970s, Nicholson and Singer proposed a more elaborate, "fluid mosaic" model of the cell membrane. A key difference in this model from earlier models was the notion that large protein molecules floated in the lipid bilayer like icebergs. Some of the protein actually extended from the outer to the inner surface, providing a nonlipid passage through the membrane (see Fig. 2.2). An important feature of this model is that all the proteins are free to move laterally within the membrane. It is now generally believed that all membranes contain both integral and peripheral protein. **Integral proteins** are tightly bonded to the membrane

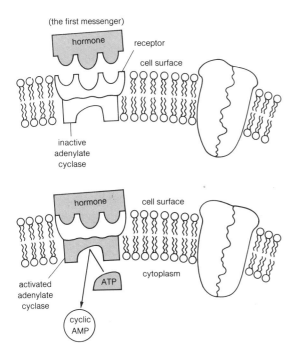

(the first messenger)

hormone

receptor

cell surface

inactive
adenylate
cyclase

hormone

cell surface

activated
adenylate
cyclase

ATP

cytoplasm

cyclic
AMP

Figure 2.3 One mechanism by which cell membranes are involved in the receiving of messages by the cell. A "primary messenger," such as a hormone, combines with a specific "receptor" on the outer cell surface. This "binding," in turn, causes the activation of an enzyme called *adenylate cyclase*, which then converts adenosine triphosphate or "ATP" into cyclic adenosine monophosphate or "cyclic AMP." Cyclic AMP then acts as a specific signal or "second messenger" within the cytoplasm.

through hydrophobic (lipid to lipid) association. **Peripheral proteins** are those stuck to the inside or outside surface of the membrane and are relatively easily "washed off."

Microtubules and Microfilaments

Microtubules are hollow rods of protein. They are the main structural components of cilia, flagella (see below), and an organelle called the *centriole*. Microtubules are also the main structural members of the spindle apparatus that pulls chromosomes apart during cell division.

Recent work suggests that the microtubules are important in moving and locking into place the proteins of the cell membrane.

Microfilaments are made of actin, the same fibrous protein that is found in, and is partly responsible for the contraction of, muscle. Contractions of microfilaments are the basis of amoeboid cell movement and for changes in the shape of cells.

Endoplasmic Reticulum

There are membranes inside the cell, too! Since there could be hundreds of different chemical reactions going on inside a cell at any one time and since the product(s) of one reaction may well be the starting material of the "next" reaction in a sequential biochemical pathway, we should expect to find a high degree of spatial organization inside the cell. Another way of saying this is that the things that go on in cells are too complex to be served by a protoplasm that is a homogeneous "soup" of molecules. Intuition tells us that the insides of cells must be at least as highly organized as the insides of factories. The electron microscope has revealed that the insides of cells are highly ordered indeed: there are extensive networks of membranes, and numerous experiments have shown that particular chemical reactions are associated with different parts of this intracellular membranous network in highly ordered ways.

Endoplasmic reticulum (ER) is the name given to the general network of membranes found throughout the cell. Electron micrographs suggest that the ER is continuous with the outer membrane of the nuclear envelope.

Functionally the ER is like the floors of a multistory factory. It even has "machines" attached to it. In certain regions, the ER looks "rough" under the electron microscope because of the numerous ribosomes associated with it. Ribosomes (as we will see in a later section) are the "workbenches" upon which proteins are

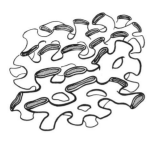

smooth ER

a

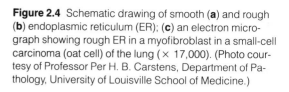

Figure 2.4 Schematic drawing of smooth (**a**) and rough (**b**) endoplasmic reticulum (ER); (**c**) an electron micrograph showing rough ER in a myofibroblast in a small-cell carcinoma (oat cell) of the lung (× 17,000). (Photo courtesy of Professor Per H. B. Carstens, Department of Pathology, University of Louisville School of Medicine.)

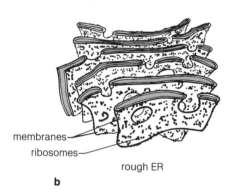

membranes
ribosomes

rough ER

b

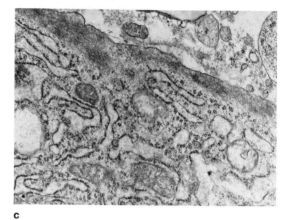

c

manufactured. Parts of the ER with lots of ribosomes attached are called **rough endoplasmic reticulum** or rough ER. Regions of the ER without ribosomes are called **smooth endoplasmic reticulum** (Fig. 2.4).

Enzymes bound to the *smooth* ER catalyze a variety of chemical reactions. Among these are various steps leading to the synthesis of lipids and certain modifications of the proteins made elsewhere on ribosomes. Enzymes of the smooth ER of liver cells are known to be involved in detoxification—breaking down drugs such as barbiturates. Of particular relevance to the cancer problem is that these detoxification enzymes sometimes inadvertently convert toxic chemicals and even some otherwise harmless chemicals into carcinogens (Chapter 8).

The amount of ER and the relative number of associated ribosomes in a cell is highly variable and proportional to how busy the cell happens to be. A cell making large amounts of protein, for example, would have a much more extensive and rougher ER than a cell simply serving as a storage depot for fat.

Ribosomes

Sprinkled throughout the typical cell are thousands and thousands of ribosomes. Some are attached to the ER as just described, and some occur free in the cytosol. It is in association with the surfaces of the ribosomes that proteins are made. Later we summarize just how this is done; for now it will be enough to appreciate (1) that ribosomes are themselves made of RNA and protein; (2) that there are many or few of them, depending upon how active the cell happens to be; and (3) that proteins to be *kept* by the cell are made on free-floating ribosomes, while those to be *exported* tend to be made on ribosomes attached to the ER.

Golgi Apparatus

Around the turn of the century, an Italian scientist named Golgi reported that he had observed a new cellular organelle—but that he couldn't always find it. Not until the electron microscope clearly revealed what Golgi had described, was the structure generally acknowledged to exist.

We know now that the Golgi apparatus is a packaging and finishing device. Apparently the Golgi apparatus assembles proteins and other chemical components made by other machinery in the cell and puts them together—much like the way that a bicycle is assembled from parts on Christmas morning. The Golgi is where sugars are affixed to proteins to make certain glycoproteins, for example. Also, the Golgi takes proteins and protein complexes and wraps them in a membrane forming a vesicle that is either released into the cytoplasm as a lysosome or is extruded from the cell via exocytosis (see Fig. 2.5). The packing serves to isolate the product from the interior of the cell.

Lysosomes

Lysosomes belong to the group of organelles called **vacuoles**. All vacuoles are membranous bags. They may contain stored food—fat for example, stored waste on its way to being dumped, cell products on their way to being exported, or just plain water. The latter are called **contractile vacuoles** because they appear to eject water from the cell by contracting when they get to the cell surface. Such water vacuoles form un-

der circumstances wherein cells take on too much water.

Lysosomes are vacuoles that contain enzymes—sometimes a very powerful array of 40 or so different enzymes capable of digesting virtually every kind of biochemical in the cell—making the benefit of their being isolated in a package more or less obvious. Lysosomes have at least four functions:

1. They release their contents when the cell is damaged and serve to finish the job of breaking the cell up for removal.

2. The contents of lysosomes are programmed for release to digest tissue when, for instance, it is time for a tadpole's tail to disintegrate as the tadpole becomes a frog or when, in a human fetus, it is time for the webbing between fingers to disintegrate, leaving individual fingers.

3. Lysosomes can combine with food vacuoles—the result being the digestion of the food, subsequent absorption of breakdown products by the cell, and the ejection of residual waste by exocytosis.

4. Phagocytic cells such as macrophages (Chapter 14) ingest bacteria and other foreign substances, which are then combined with lysosomal contents intracellularly to be digested and destroyed.

It is conceivable (there is even some evidence) that *in*appropriate release of lysosomal proteases or other enzymes could alter the outer surface of a cell or the immediate extracellular matrix, in effect making cells act like cancer cells. More on this in Chapter 4.

Mitochondria

Power is provided to cellular factories by **mitochondria** (the singlar is *mitochondrion*). Mitochondria average 1 micrometer in diameter and 2 to 8 micrometers in length. If they were larger,

Figure 2.5 The Golgi apparatus: (**a**) four different Golgi zones in a cell from a carcinoid tumor of the lung (× 14,000). (Photo courtesy of Professor Per H. B. Carstens, Department of Pathology, University of Louisville School of Medicine); (**b**) schematic showing the roles of both the rough endoplasmic reticulum and the Golgi complex in the process of secretion.

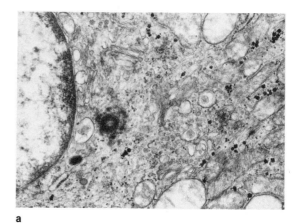

a

proteins for export
amino acids
free ribosomes
proteins, polysaccharides, etc.
attached ribosomes
rough endoplasmic reticulum
proteins used inside cell
enzymes for assembly of fats
secretion vesicles
smooth endoplasmic reticulum
Golgi complex
enzymes for assembly of polysaccharides
plasma membrane

b

they would look like cucumbers (see Fig. 2.1 and Fig. 2.6), except that mitochondria continuously change their shape.

Cells are designed to run on chemical energy in the form of an energy-rich chemical, **adenosine triphosphate** or **ATP**. It is the job of the mitochondria to convert the chemical energy derived from various other energy-rich molecules into chemical energy in the form of ATP. Mitochondria are ATP factories. Inside each mitochondrion is a convoluted membrane bearing highly structured arrays of energy-stripping and energy-transferring enzymes (see pages 27 and 28).

Different kinds of cells have different numbers of mitochondria; generally there are several thousand per cell.

The Nucleus

If the cell is a factory, then the nucleus is the main office—where the president, plant manager, and board of directors stay. The nucleus is also where the plans for the factory are kept—in fact, a set of developmental, structural, operational, and maintenance plans (genes) can be

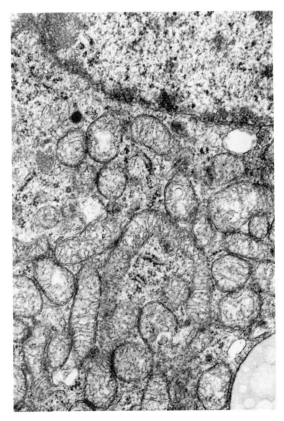

Figure 2.6 A large group of mitochondria from an oncocytoma of the pituitary. Part of the nucleus is shown at the top (× 19,000). Photo courtesy of Professor Per H. B. Carstens, Department of Pathology, University of Louisville School of Medicine)

Chromosomes contain rather precise amounts and kinds of DNA molecules such that each species of living beings has a characteristic number of chromosomes in each cell. Human beings have 46 chromosomes in every body cell.

Nuclei have one or more dense regions called **nucleoli**, which consist of RNA molecules in compact association. Nucleoli are sites where the components of ribosomes are assembled. A little later in this section, we will review just how the nucleus directs the fabrication of proteins.

Cilia and Flagella

Some cells have hairlike, long projections called *flagella*; others have short projections called *cilia*. Single-celled organisms use cilia and flagella to propel themselves through liquid environments. Other single-celled creatures use their cilia to move water past them so that they can take food or oxygen or both from the water. Higher organisms have *special* cells with cilia or flagella. The cells that make up the surface of the human bronchial tract are ciliated. Coordinated movement of these cilia serves to sweep debris out of the respiratory tract. Cigarette smoke paralyzes the cilia, depriving the respiratory tract of one of its main lines of defense.

We will have much more to say about cigarettes as we go on.

The Extracellular Matrix

The extracellular matrix (ECM) is a yet incompletely defined assortment of macromolecules that serves as a structural framework upon which the cells hang like individual rooms in a steel-framed high-rise. It is believed that the molecules of the ECM play important roles in influencing growth and differentiation. A collection of recent reports on some of the work now going on can be found in the volume edited by Hawkes and Wang (1982) cited at the end of this chapter (see also Hay, 1981).

found there for all the different kinds of factories that make up a body.

It seems fitting that the nucleus has its own *double* membrane. This envelope has holes through which message-bearing molecules come in and important instructions go out to the cytoplasm. Inside the nuclear envelope and suspended in a fluid called **nucleoplasm** is chromatin. **Chromatin** is a material made from DNA and protein. When the cell is not dividing, chromatin is diffusely scattered throughout the nucleoplasm. During cell division, chromatin condenses into structures called **chromosomes**.

The Activities of Cells: Metabolism

Other than move a little and occasionally change shape, cells do mostly chemical things. Animal cells basically spend their time making new large molecules from the small molecules and the energy they get by tearing down large molecules (seems rather pointless, doesn't it?). We use the term **metabolism** to mean *all* the chemical activities of cells; the term **catabolism** encompasses all tearing-down kinds of reactions and the term **anabolism** is used for all the "constructive," or bio*synthetic* activities.

Cellular Respiration

Most of the energy that cells get comes from the oxidation of sugar by a process called *cellular respiration*, summarized as follows:

$$C_6H_{12}O_6 + 6O_2 \rightarrow 6CO_2 + 6H_2O + 38ATP$$

Essentially, cellular respiration is the "controlled burning" or "oxidation" of glucose in an enzymatically catalyzed (see box), stepwise, series of reactions through which the cell gets 38 ATP molecules instead of a lot of heat and smoke. As mentioned earlier, ATP molecules are "energy-rich" molecules by which cells can transfer the energy derived from energy-yielding reactions to those requiring a net input of energy.

The first stage of cellular respiration is called **glycolysis** (sugar-splitting). In this stage, one six-carbon sugar molecule is converted into two three-carbon molecules (pyruvic acid), two hydrogen atoms are affixed to a carrier molecule, and the cell gets two energized ATP molecules (see Fig. 2.8).

Glycolysis takes place even in the absence of oxygen. In fermentation, yeast carry out an-

---

Enzymes: The Cancer Connection

In order for chemical reactions to take place, some energy must usually be added to get things started—even if the reaction is ultimately an energy-yielding reaction. A spark that ignites an explosive reaction of gasoline and oxygen is perhaps a familiar example. The energy required initially is called the **energy of activation**. A **catalyst** is a substance that doesn't enter into a reaction directly or become changed by the reaction, but somehow lowers the energy of activation needed to cause a reaction to proceed—and thus speeds the reaction up. **Enzymes** are proteins that act as catalysts.

Enzymes tend to be named for the substrate (starting material that interacts with the enzyme) and/or for the nature of the reaction catalyzed—both of which are *usually* specific for each enzyme. The enzyme named *maltase*, for example, splits maltose into its constituent monosaccharides. Nearly every reaction in a living cell requires a specific enzyme to catalyze it. Enzymes can be converted from inactive forms to active forms or

vice versa through chemical reactions—reactions that thus serve regulatory functions. Enzymes must have a particular shape in order to function as a catalyst. Chemicals that react with enzymes may change their shape such that they may be made more, or less, effective as catalysts. Such modifications of enzymes amount to one of the ways in which the activity of cells is regulated (later in this chapter, we will see that another way is to regulate the *supply* of enzymes).

Kinases are enzymes that add phosphate groups to proteins and other substances that are then said to be *phosphorylated*; tyrosine kinases put the phosphate group specifically on tyrosine, which is one of the amino acids that make up proteins. This positioning has much relevance to cancer now that the products of at least some "oncogenes" (see Chapter 7) are known to be tyrosine kinases, enzymes that activate other enzymes that may then somehow bring about the changes that characterize a cancer cell.

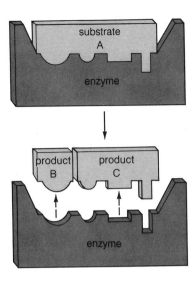

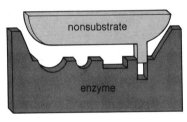

Figure 2.7 An enzyme is a large molecule, only part of which combines directly with the enzyme's substrate. The specific, particular location on the enzyme molecule where the substrate binds is called the *active site*. If another molecule combines with part of this site, it directly blocks the action of the enzyme. (Note: if a chemical combines with some other part of an enzyme molecule such that the active site is distorted, the result is indirect blockage. See Fig. 2.10.)

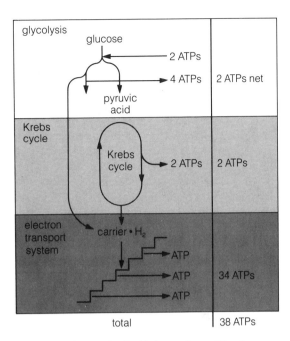

Figure 2.8 Glycolysis, the Krebs cycle, and the electron transport system and the balance sheet for ATP generation

aerobic respiration; the alcohol in wine is a result of the fact that the yeast cell is able to conclude respiration in the absence of oxygen by stripping a carbon dioxide molecule from pyruvic acid—the CO_2 is visible as bubbles in a fermentation vat—and it then transfers hydrogens from a carrier molecule to the two-carbon compound left when CO_2 is cleaved from pyruvic acid, to form ethyl alcohol. The yeast can continue to ferment until the buildup of alcohol in the vat kills them.

As suggested by the equation given earlier (see also later), if respiration is allowed to proceed through *all* the stages of respiration in the presence of oxygen, far more ATPs can be generated from a molecule of glucose than the two ATPs that an organism gets if it must stop after glycolysis. It seems that cancer cells have a tendency to lapse into anaerobic respiration and are better able to withstand low-oxygen conditions than normal cells. We will elaborate on this aspect of cancer cell metabolism in Chapter 4.

The Krebs Cycle

The **Krebs cycle** is the second stage of cellular respiration. The Krebs cycle and its connection to glycolysis are depicted in Figure 2.8.

For every *two* molecules of pyruvic acid that enter the Krebs cycle (for every molecule of glucose started through cellular respiration, in other words), six molecules of carbon dioxide, two molecules of energized ATP emerge, and all remaining hydrogen atoms end up associated with electron-hydrogen carrier molecules and enter the electron transport system.

The Electron Transport System

Actually, mitochondria bear two types of enzyme arrays. One type effectively converts pyruvic acid into carbon dioxide. The other—called the **electron transport system**—drops the electrons (and accompanying hydrogen ions) from the high-energy state they have when the carrier gets them to a lower-energy state in a stepwise fashion, forming energy-rich bonds in ATP along the way. The last step in the electron transport system adds electrons to oxygen, which then combines with accompanying hydrogen ions to form water. It is in the electron transport system that the bulk of the ATPs are generated in cellular respiration (see Fig. 2.8).

Respiration of Molecules Other Than Sugar

Chemicals other than sugars can be used as energy sources. The hydrolysis of fat yields three molecules of fatty acid and a molecule of glycerol. Glycerol can be converted into the very same three-carbon compound that results from the initial split of the six-carbon compound into the three-carbon compound in glycolysis (see Fig. 2.9). Respiration proceeds from that point just as if the three-carbon compound had come from sugar. Similarly, fatty acids can be, and are, broken up into two-carbon compounds that can enter the Krebs cycle directly (see Fig. 2.9). Fats broken up and fed into the respiratory scheme in this way actually generate nearly twice the ATPs pound for pound as does sugar.

Proteins can also serve as energy sources. In this case the protein must first be broken down into individual amino acids and the amino groups removed. Urea in urine is the disposal form of the amines stripped from amino acids in protein respiration. Free of its amine group, an amino acid becomes a **keto acid**—depending on *which* keto acid, it may enter the Krebs cycle at one of several points in the cycle.

Cellular Respiration Pathways as Metabolic Crossroads

As they are stripped of their energy via glycolysis and the Krebs cycle, energy-rich molecules go through many steps and are converted into other forms. While these different chemical forms represent entry points for different kinds of compounds being respired they can also serve as the starting points of bio*synthetic* pathways. The respiratory pathways represent so many pivotal points between catabolism and anabolism. Sugars being fed in can be stripped partially of energy and then the partially respired (oxidized) result used as a precursor in the synthesis of a particular amino acid, for example.

This description is greatly simplified. Cellular metabolism is far more complicated than what we have presented here.

Control of Metabolism

A cell's metabolism is all the cell's chemical reactions. Since biological reactions are catalyzed by enzymes, metabolism is what the enzymes *say* it is. If metabolism is to be regulated or controlled, we should expect this regulation would have to be done by controlling relevant enzymes. There are two fundamental ways to do so. One way is to structurally alter enzymes so as to influence their activity. The other way is to change the ratio of the rates of enzyme synthesis and enzyme degradation—to regulate the *number* of enzyme molecules, in other words.

Controlling Metabolism by Changing the Shape of Enzymes The configuration of enzymes and other protein molecules varies with the presence of chemicals able to combine chem-

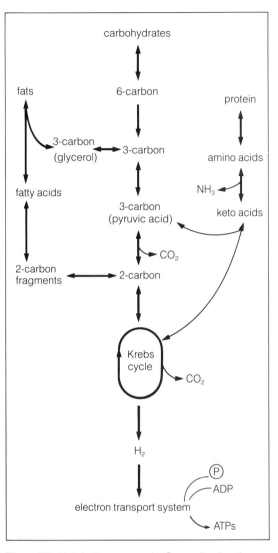

carbohydrates

fats

6-carbon

protein

3-carbon
(glycerol)

3-carbon

amino acids

fatty acids

NH_3

3-carbon
(pyruvic acid)

keto acids

CO_2

2-carbon
fragments

2-carbon

Krebs
cycle

CO_2

H_2

(P)
ADP

electron transport system

ATPs

Figure 2.9 Metabolic crossroads. Generalized pathways by which cells can get energy from carbohydrates, fats, or protein and by which fats, proteins, and carbohydrates are interconvertible.

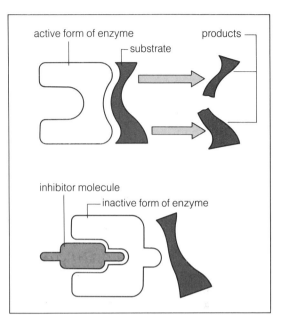

active form of enzyme

products

substrate

inhibitor molecule

inactive form of enzyme

Figure 2.10 How a regulator molecule might influence an enzyme to change its effectiveness as a catalyst

ically with protein. Since the active site of an enzyme must have a particular shape in order for the enzyme to function optimally, anything that influences the overall configuration of an enzyme can, by distorting the active site, directly or indirectly influence the ability of the enzyme to catalyze reactions. This phenomenon is the basis of a very important form of the chemical control of metabolism.

A schematic diagram of how a regulator molecule could, by combining with a portion of an enzyme remote from the active site, turn an enzyme off, is presented in Figure 2.10. Throughout the spectrum of metabolism are instances where, through similar kinds of influences, "regulator" molecules turn enzymes off, turn enzymes on, and enhance or diminish enzyme activity. What regulates the regulator molecules? This question can be answered using end product inhibition as an example.

End Product Inhibition   To appreciate just how end product inhibition works, picture metabolism as a series of branching and otherwise interconnecting pathways (see Fig. 2.11). At the tips of the branches is an end product generated by the action of a series of enzymes that serve to convert some *substrate* through one or more steps. In some cases, end products are able to

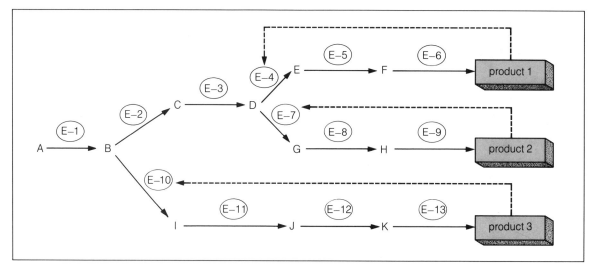

Figure 2.11 A hypothetical, branching, metabolic pathway. Enzymes are numbered E-1, E-2 . . .; the letters of the alphabet represent intermediate chemical forms of "A" as it is converted into three different products. Note that "product 3" influences the first enzyme specific to the pathway that produces it.

interact with the first enzyme in the pathway *committed* to that end product. The interaction renders the enzyme less effective, and the result is that when the levels of an end product rise "too high," the "extra" molecules interact with the enzyme at the very beginning of the pathway, and the pathway is "turned down."

When levels of the end product in question fall too low, there is not enough to cover all the regulatory enzymes. By default, the enzymes are again able to catalyze the initial step, and the pathway is turned back on. In control theory, this type of control is called *negative feedback control*. Thermostats by which furnaces are controlled also operate via negative feedback.

End products are not the only kinds of molecules that regulate metabolism by combining with enzymes altering their efficiency as catalysts. But the example should suffice to make the point that metabolism can in fact be controlled through chemical signals.

One point that we wish to make about metabolic control via regulation of enzyme shape is that it offers a very direct and very fast means of control. Another kind of metabolic control—a

slower, but over the long term a more efficient, form of control—is control of enzyme synthesis. Before we can consider this form, we must look at the general way in which proteins are made.

How DNA Is Involved in Making More DNA and in Making Proteins

A piece of DNA that has a particular function is called a **gene**. A **structural gene** is a piece of DNA that contains the information necessary to make a particular protein. There is another kind of gene—nonstructural genes that function in controlling the expression of the structural genes. In the following discussion, we talk about *both* kinds of genes.

The Duplication of DNA

The duplication of DNA begins when an enzyme unzips what we will call the *original* molecule, as shown in Figure 2.12. As the unzipping proceeds, new individual nucleotide bases are

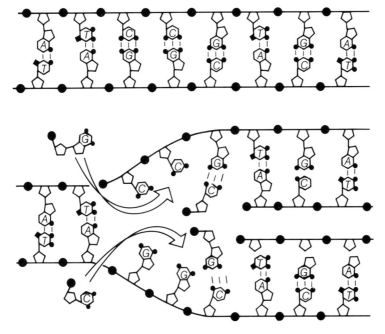

Figure 2.12 The nucleotide chains of the DNA double helix showing the complementary pairing of nucleotide bases (adenine, thymine, guanine, and cytosine). The bottom figure shows how DNA is replicated. Under the control of special enzymes, the double helix is "unzipped" and free nucleotides are added to each half so as to produce two identical double helices.

aligned to form complementary strands of bases as shown in Figure 2.12. The ultimate result of this process is that each half of the original molecule gets a new complementary strand, and the original molecule becomes two molecules exactly like the original. It should be obvious just why it is said that DNA serves as the "template" for the synthesis of new DNA.

One of the two copies of DNA ends up in each cell that results from cell division. Since effectively *all* of a cell's DNA is replicated in the same way (in preparation for division), the cells that result from cell division are genetically identical to each other and to the parent cell.

The Code for Making Proteins

The language of the genetic code is made up of words that are all three letters long. It takes a sequence of three nucleotide bases* to represent one amino acid. Three bases amount to one unit of code (called a **codon**). Since there are only four different nucleotide bases in DNA, there are only 64 words in the genetic code—only 64 different ways of arranging four bases in groups of three.

Since there are only *twenty* different amino acids, this arrangement allows a certain amount of redundancy. Six different sequences of three bases call out the amino acid lecuine. Four specify alanine. There is only one "word" for methionine. Although there may be more than one

---

*Since the sequence of bases in one strand is a function of the sequence in the other strand, no new information is available in the second strand. Double-strandedness has relevance in DNA replication; it has no relevance in the translation of the genetic code into protein; we can think of the second strand as a cover for the first.

code for any one amino acid, there is no ambiguity; every "triplet" of DNA bases has one meaning and one meaning only.

Of the 64 words in the DNA-amino acid dictionary, nearly all represent amino acids. Some serve as stop or start signals to the machinery stringing amino acids together.

Transcription and Translation

For our purposes here, we can think of DNA as being in the nucleus and of protein synthesis as taking place in the cytoplasm in association with the ribosomes. This arrangement requires some mechanism by which the code can be carried out of the nucleus to the ribosomes. RNA is an important part of that mechanism.

There are three different kinds of RNA. We have already talked about **ribosomal RNA** (rRNA), which helps make up the structure of ribosomes. Two other kinds of RNA are important in converting the genetic code into protein. **Messenger RNA** (mRNA) is the means by which the genetic code is transferred from the nucleus to the ribosomes; **transfer RNA** (tRNA) brings individual amino acids to the ribosomes.

Transcription Like DNA, RNA is a nucleic acid made from four different bases. A strand of RNA can carry encoded information, just as DNA can. Messenger RNA is made from a DNA template by an enzyme called *DNA-dependent RNA polymerase*. This enzyme reads one of the strands of DNA and assembles a complementary-strand of RNA (Fig. 2.13), which then amounts to a copy of the information in the DNA template.

Translation Messenger RNA leaves the nucleus and travels to a ribosome, where the strand is "read." By "reading," we mean that after the "initiator sequence" or start signal, every mRNA triplet calls in a particular amino-acid-tRNA complex. The mRNA codons match a complementary "anticodon" on the tRNA (see Fig. 2.13). Each tRNA is associated with a particular amino acid. As the tRNA-amino acid complex tumbles into position, the amino acids are "dropped off" by the tRNA and the amino acids joined to form a peptide chain.

Mutations: What Are They and What Do They Mean?

Mutations are permanent changes in the base sequences of DNA. Mutations can be brought about by reactions with chemical substances, by radiation of the right wavelength, or by certain biological agents. There is also a certain probability that a spontaneous mistake will be made as DNA is being replicated. Generally speaking, three kinds of mutations can occur in a molecule of DNA: (1) deletion of a base, (2) insertion of a base, and (3) substitution of a base. The first two are drastic changes because they amount to a *frame shift*. Following a deletion or substitution, everything from that point on in the molecule is read differently; the translation or replication enzymes blindly persist in reading the code in units of three bases. If a protein is made at all in such a case, it is almost certainly nonfunctional and the cell could very well die.

The consequences of a substitution, however, depend on the nature of the substitution. Three thymines (TTT) in DNA calls for the amino acid lysine. Two thymines and a cytosine (TTC) also code for lysine. A point mutation or simple substitution mutation in which the last T was substituted for C would therefore have no effect. But if the T were replaced by guanine (TTG), asparagine would be inserted into the protein instead of lysine. The consequences of this change *could* be disastrous. Arginine might work just as well or nearly as well, but more likely the protein would be nonfunctional. The only difference between normal hemoglobin and the hemoglobin of sickle-cell anemia is the substitution of valine for glutamic acid in one of its two kinds of peptide chains.

Almost as if nature anticipated problems in faithfully replicating DNA, there are cell en-

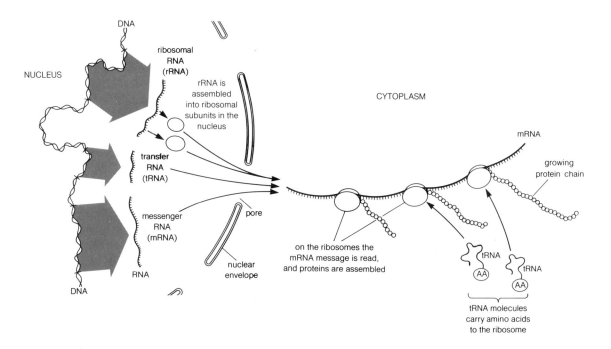

Figure 2.13 The synthesis of protein by the cell. The genetic code carried in the DNA of the nucleus is "transcribed" in the nucleus into messenger RNA (mRNA). Then mRNA moves to a ribosome in the cytoplasm where amino acids carried on transfer RNA (tRNA) molecules are bonded together to form proteins. The sequence of amino acids is determined by the sequence of nucleotide bases in the mRNA, each "triplet" calling for a matching tRNA molecule, each of which carries a specific amino acid.

zymes whose job it is to repair damaged DNA. We will consider this aspect of molecular biology in a later chapter.

Control of Metabolism at the Level of the Gene

The idea is basically simple: all metabolic reactions are catalyzed by enzymes, and enzymes are proteins transcribed from genes. Metabolism can, therefore, be controlled over the long term by controlling the *manufacture* of enzymes—controlling gene expression in other words. We say "over the long term" because it takes a while for

enzymes to "wear out." Normally, they would be replaced by newly made enzymes. Shutting down the gene would shut off replacement, and the pathway in question would more or less gradually grind to a halt as more and more of the production lines wore out and quit.

The example of genetic control found in nearly all general biology textbooks is that of the lac operon in *bacteria*. The adjective "lac" stands for *lactose*, and refers to the series of genes that specify the enzymes needed to take up and digest the sugar lactose. All the genes involved are found on a continuous stretch of DNA, together with a number of nonstructural control genes. Such a unit of related structural genes and control genes is called an **operon** (Fig. 2.14).

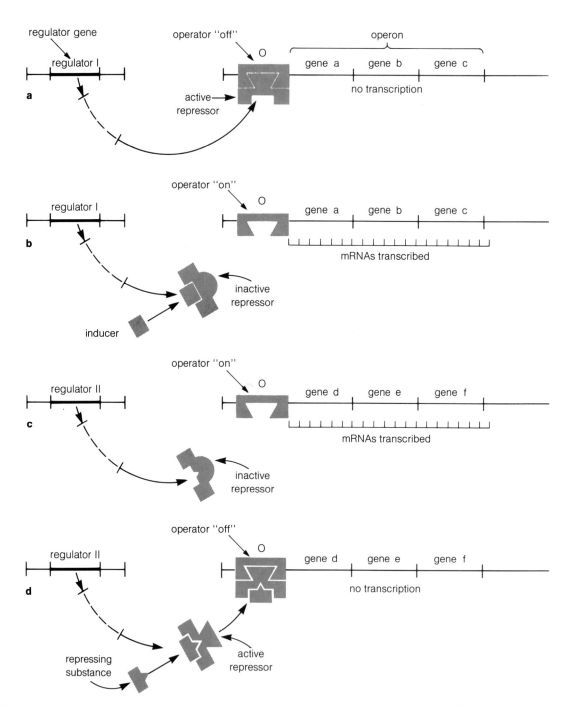

Figure 2.14 Regulation of transcription. In certain simple organisms, gene expression is regulated by the operon mechanism illustrated here. One kind of regulator produces an active repressor (**a**) that must be inactivated by an "inducer" substance before the operator can be switched "on" (**b**). In another kind of regulator system, the regulator gene produces an inactive repressor substance (**c**) that must be converted to the active form by a repressing substance if the operon is to be turned "off" (**d**).

The lac operon doesn't function—none of the enzymes are made—unless there is some lactose present. The system in effect says, "There is no point in making the enzymes needed to utilize lactose until lactose is available!"

One of the lac operon control genes called the "*promoter*," serves as a binding site for the enzyme RNA polymerase—the enzyme that makes messenger RNA—using DNA as a template. Unless RNA polymerase has a promoter gene it can attach to, the structural genes in the operon can't be transcribed. In fact, it is apparently the efficiency with which the promoter region is able to bind RNA polymerase that has most to do with how often the associated structural genes are transcribed.

Overlapping the *promoter* gene is a DNA sequence, called the "*operator*." The operator serves as a binding site for a protein molecule called a *repressor* protein. Whenever there is sufficient repressor present, the operator-repressor complex serves as a barrier to RNA polymerase. RNA polymerase simply cannot get to its binding site and thus to the structural genes that lie beyond. The result: no transcription!

The key to control is the fact that the repressor, being a protein, is subject to structural modification by chemical interaction. In the case of the lac operon, a derivative of lactose binds to the repressor, rendering it *in*effective in binding with the operator. With the repressor out of the way, RNA polymerase is able to make the mRNA that codes for the enzymes needed to use lactose. When the lactose is gone, the repressor molecules—which have been *reversibly* bound to the lactose derivative—again become *effective* repressors shutting down the system.

Systems such as the lac operon that are off until a substrate is present are called **inducible enzyme systems**; the substrate—lactose, in the case just cited—is called an *inducer*. Other systems, called **constitutive systems**, are "on" until turned off. In some such cases, there simply isn't any operator and transcription is simply a function of the rate at which the relevant promoter can bind RNA polymerase. In some oper-

ons, the repressor is in the inactive state until interaction with one or more regulatory molecules converts it into an *active* form. Such systems are called **repressible systems**.

Systems such as those just described could be called "negative" control systems since in each case, the *absence* of a repressor substance results in the activation of a gene or group of genes. There are also positive forms of control. It is known that in bacteria, for instance, "gene activator proteins" are able to change promoter sites with relatively weak affinities for RNA polymerase into those with stronger affinities. That the *position* of the binding site on DNA for activators and repressors may be most of, if not the whole, story is suggested by the observation that the same protein may serve as an activator for some genes and a repressor for others.

It is believed that positive and negative control by regulatory proteins such as described above operate in higher organisms as well as in bacteria where they were discovered. The facts that human cells have many tens of thousands of genes per cell (as opposed to relatively few in bacterial cells) and have hundreds of different kinds of cells, all somehow derived from a single fertilized egg, suggest that genetic control should be somewhat more complicated in human beings than it is in bacteria. Only about 7 percent of the genes in the "typical" cell in a higher organism are active at any one time. The rest amount to tens of thousands of genes turned off. It is unlikely that each of the "quiet" genes is shut off by a different regulatory protein. It is more likely that genes are controlled by combinations of relatively few regulatory proteins. During the development of the embryo, particular regulatory proteins probably appear that control the appearance of still other regulatory proteins in cells that result from later divisions. Since there could be more than a million combinations of just 20 different regulatory proteins, many different cell types could result from the sequential appearance of just a few regulatory proteins.

Activation of genes in higher organisms apparently also involves proteins able to "loosen-up" chromatin. In higher organisms, DNA is tightly associated with proteins in a structural aggregation called **chromatin**. This association is such that under unactivated conditions, RNA polymerase has no access to the DNA. There are apparently regulatory proteins somehow able to open up certain gene regions where the proteins recognize particular base sequences. Control of gene expression in higher organisms may therefore involve at least two distinct stages, or two different kinds of action: first the opening up of chromatin, then positive or negative control by activator or repressor proteins.

Actually, we know very little about the specific mechanisms by which the genes in cells are turned on and off during embryogenesis and under different circumstances in human cells. Indeed, if we did know, we might have by now solved the cancer problem. We do know something about the mechanisms that operate to control gene expression in simple organisms such as bacteria and fruit flies, and we suspect that similar mechanisms operate in higher organisms. To learn more about gene regulation is one of the key objectives of cancer research.

The foregoing are but a few of the kinds of ways in which the expression of genes is controlled. There are at least a few other possible ways of regulating gene expression: (1) increasing the number of genes or operons that carry the same information; (2) stabilizing or destabilizing mRNA—regulating how long it lasts, in other words; (3) speeding up translation at the ribosome level; and (4) stabilizing or destabilizing the enzymes themselves. Nature has apparently thought of, and uses, all these strategies in metabolic control. We discuss the specifics of some of these strategies in other chapters.

The Cell Cycle

The stages of cell division, as memorized by all biology students for the past three decades or so, are:

Prophase   Chromosomes become visible.

Metaphase   Chromosomes align in the center of the cell.

Anaphase   One chromosome from each duplicate pair (duplication of DNA has already taken place, and there are two identical sets of chromosomes when they become visible in prophase) begin to move toward opposite sides of the cell.

Telophase   The chromosomes reach opposite ends of the cell, and the cell divides into two cells, each with a complete set of chromosomes.

Interphase   No evidence of cell division. (It used to be said that the cell was at rest during interphase. We now know that this couldn't be further from the truth.)

The life of most cells is punctuated by division at both ends; cells originate with division, and each divides to give rise to two cells. In between, cells go through "the cell cycle" (Fig. 2.15).

On the average, cells in growing tissue take about 20 hours to go through a cycle; of this, only about one hour is needed for division. Interphase is 19 hours long. The cell cycle is a little shorter in some cells, longer in others.

DNA is replicated during interphase—this was found out by watching when cells took up artificially-made, radioactive nucleotide bases and made nucleic acids out of them. The period within interphase during which DNA was doubled was called the S phase (S for *synthesis*) by Howard and Pele in the early 1950s. Other phases of the cell cycle were named as follows:

M   Mitosis and cell division (time: 1 hour)

G-1   Growth phase 1 (time: 8 hours)

G-0   or "G-1 Arrest" (varies from "zero" time to lifetime, depending on the cell and the circumstance)

S   DNA synthesis–replication (time: 6 hours)

G-2   Growth phase 2 (time: 5 hours)

G-0 can be thought of as retirement from cell division. Some cells—nerve cells, for example—go into G-0 when they are fully differentiated, and never return. Liver cells go into G-0 when the liver reaches mature size, but they can be called back into the cycling when the liver is damaged. Cells in rapidly growing tissue do not go into G-0; instead, they move directly from one cycle to the next. Cancer cells fall into this category. They often don't divide any faster than other cells, they simply fail to stop dividing.

If only we knew more about why they do that.

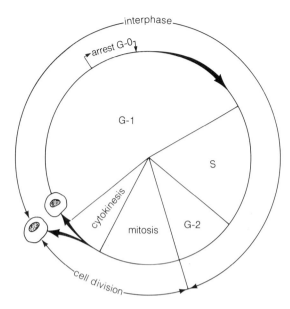

Figure 2.15 The cell cycle. The G-1 period of interphase is of variable length. During this phase the cell may go into an arrested state—a retirement from cell division sometimes called G-0—that may last a lifetime or a short time. There is a restriction point somewhere in G-1 after which the cell is committed to go through another cycle. The S, G-2, and division segments of the cycle are of relatively uniform duration.

Summary

Cells are the fundamental units of nearly all forms of life. The fact that this holds even for very large organisms consisting of hundreds of trillions of cells means that all such organisms have potential organizational and control problems. The amazing thing is that most multicellular organisms function very well most of the time; the sad thing is that there are failures. Cancer can be thought of as one category of organizational and/or control failure in multicellular organisms.

Normal cells are highly complex structures with many parts (Table 2.1) functioning in a highly integrated manner. The control of what goes on inside cells involves cell surface receptors, cell membrane permeability, the outside chemical environment, the intracellular chemical environment, primary messengers, secondary messengers, regulators of gene expression, regulators of enzymes activity, and so on. Somewhere in all the complexity of normal cells are the seeds that sometimes give rise to cancer cells. Cancer is still the problem that it is because we have yet to sort out the roots of cancer from all the many things that *could* be involved in the wayward behavior of cells.

References and Further Reading

Alberts, B., Bray, D., Lewis, J., Raff, M., Roberts, K., and Watson, J. 1983. *Molecular Biology of the Cell*. New York: Garland.

Curtis, H. 1983. *Biology*. 4th ed. New York: Worth.

Gurdon, J. 1978. *Gene Expression During Cell Differentiation*. Burlington, N.C.: Carolina Biological Supply.

Hawkes, S., and Wang, J. L., eds. 1982. *Extracellular Matrix*. New York: Academic Press.

Hay, E. 1981. *Cell Biology of Extracellular Matrix*. New York: Plenum Press.

Lucy, J. 1978. *The Plasma Membrane*. Burlington, N.C.: Carolina Biological Supply.

Mader, S. 1982. *Inquiry into Life*. Dubuque, Iowa: Brown.

Mazia, D. 1974. The Cell Cycle. *Scientific American*. 230(1): 54–64.

Porter, K. R., and Tucker, J. B. 1981. The Ground Substance of the Living Cell. *Scientific American*. 244(3): 56–67.

Purves, W. K., and Orians, G. H. 1983. *Life: The Science of Biology*. Sunderland, Mass.: Sinauer Associates.

Robertson, J. D. 1981. Membrane Structure. *J. Cell. Biol.* 91(3): 189–204.

Stein, G. S., Stein, J. S., and Kleinsmith, L. J. 1975. Chromosomal Proteins and Gene Regulation. *Scientific American*. 232(2): 46–57.

Travers, A. 1978. *Transcription of DNA*. Burlington, N.C.: Carolina Biological Supply.

Trelstad, R. 1984. *The Role of Extracellular Matrix in Development*. New York: Liss.

Tzagoloff, A. 1982. *Mitochondria*. Cellular Organelle Series. New York: Plenum Press.

We have already considered the cell. If we are to appreciate the impacts that cancer has on the whole body, we must know something of how cells are organized into tissue, tissue into organs, organs into organ systems, and organ systems into human organisms. This chapter will serve as background for our consideration of metastasis in Chapter 6, our consideration of the effects of cancer on the host in Chapter 12, and for our review of cancer of particular organ sites in the last section of the book.

Tissue: The First Order of Cellular Organization

Tissue is the level of biological organization just above that of the cell. **Tissue** is defined as a group of similar cells with a characteristic matrix or ground substance between them, all organized into a functional unit. Although there are some two hundred different kinds of cells that make up the body, they are organized into only four basic types of tissue: epithelial, connective, muscle, and nervous.

Epithelial Tissue

Epithelial tissue is found throughout the body. Functionally, it is the tissue that specializes in protection, absorption, and secretion. Epithelial tissue covers the body surface; it lines body cavities; it lines blood and lymph vessels; it lines the digestive, respiratory, and urinary tracts; and it forms glands. Epithelial cells tend to occur in sheets of cells attached to an underlying connective tissue by a highly permeable layer of material called the **basement membrane**, or **basal lamina**, because it is not really a membrane. Epithelial tissues contain no blood vessels; they receive nutrients and get rid of wastes through diffusion-driven exchange with capillaries on the opposite side of the basement membrane. Epithelial tissue characteristically has very little intercellular material.

3

An Outline of Anatomy and Physiology

With Emphasis on the Circulatory and the Immune Systems

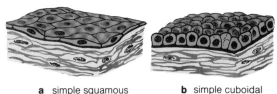

a simple squamous   **b** simple cuboidal

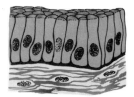

c simple columnar (nonciliated)

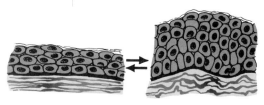

d transitional epithelium

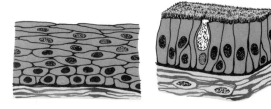

e stratified squamous   **f** pseudostratified columnar (ciliated)

Figure 3.1 Classification of epithelial tissue

The cells that make up epithelial tissue come in three basic shapes: squamous, cuboidal, and columnar. Squamous cells are flat (Fig. 3.1**a**), cuboidal cells are cube-shaped (Fig. 3.1**b**), and columnar cells are oblong (Fig. 3.1**c**). Transitional epithelial cells may be flat or cuboidal, depending on how much stress they are under and on the degree to which the tissue is stretched. Tran-

sitional epithelium lines the bladder and the ureters. When the bladder is empty, the epithelial cells are cuboidal; when it is distended, they look more like squamous cells (Fig. 3.1**d**). Epithelial tissue is subdivided into **stratified epithelium** (when it occurs in three or more layers of cells); **simple epithelium** (when there is only one layer); and **pseudostratified epithelium** (when there is a single layer that sometimes appears to be more than one layer).

Pathologists and anatomists use cell arrangement, shape, and embryonic origin* when describing tissue. Simple squamous epithelium (Fig. 3.1**a**) can be found lining the air sacs of the lung. The simple squamous epithelium lining the blood and lymph vessels is actually called *endo*thelium; these cells originate in embryonic mesodermal tissue, not in the ectoderm. The simple squamous epithelium lining the pericardium and the body cavity is called the *mesothelium* because it originates in the embryonic mesoderm. Stratified squamous epithelium is shown as it looks lining the mouth in Figure 3.1**e**; simple columnar epithelium as it looks lining the stomach is shown in Figure 3.1**c**; an example of pseudostratified columnar epithelium is shown in Figure 3.1**f**. Glandular epithelium makes up the secreting cells of the glands of the body.

Connective Tissue

The feature that all **connective tissue** has in common is a predominance of intercellular material—the so-called **matrix** or **ground substance**, and relatively *few* cells. Otherwise, connective tissue looks like a miscellaneous category. Blood, bone, cartilage, fat, and "ordinary," loose, or areolar connective tissue are all connective tissues. Connective tissues not only connect, they also support, transport, store, and defend.

---

*Three primary tissues are formed early during embryonic development: the ectoderm, the mesoderm, and the endoderm. These ultimately give rise to all the tissues of the body.

Ordinary, loose, or **areolar connective tissue** is a flexible filler material found throughout the body. Its matrix material consists mainly of the protein, collagen, and polymers of sugarlike molecules, e.g., *hyaluronic acid*. Fibroblasts and macrophages are the predominant cells. Fibroblasts synthesize the collagen and the hyaluronic acid of the ground substance; macrophages are part of the immune system.

Blood consists of different kinds of blood cells (Fig. 3.2) in a fluid matrix called *plasma*. We will have much more to say about blood, especially in the context of immune defense, later in the chapter.

Muscle and Nerve Tissue

Muscle cells are specialized for contraction and muscle tissue moves things around. Skeletal muscle moves arms, legs, and so forth; cardiac (heart) muscle drives blood through the circulatory system; and smooth muscle moves the internal organs "involuntarily"—for example, it is responsible for peristalsis and mixing movement within the gastrointestinal tract.

The cells that make up nervous tissue include neurons and cells that *support* neurons, the **neuroglia**. **Neurons** are cells specialized to receive stimuli and to transmit them to other neurons or to muscle cells or other "action" cells. The function of the nervous system is to coordinate the activities of all other organ systems as they deal collectively with the ups and downs of environmental and internal stimuli. The parts of the nervous system are the central nervous system including the brain and the spinal cord, the autonomic nervous system, and the peripheral nerves.

Some Organ Systems Particularly Relevant to Cancer

An **organ** is an *organization* of several different kinds of tissue that performs some special function. The large intestine is an organ made up of

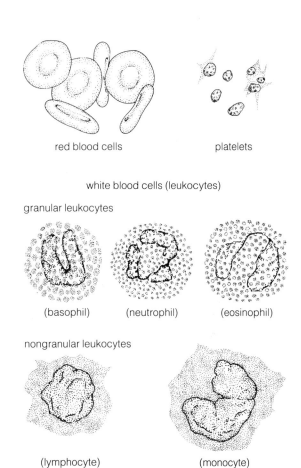

red blood cells

platelets

white blood cells (leukocytes)

granular leukocytes

(basophil)   (neutrophil)   (eosinophil)

nongranular leukocytes

(lymphocyte)   (monocyte)

Figure 3.2 Human blood cells.
White blood cells or "leukocytes" are differentiated by their morphology and by their staining properties. Each milliliter of blood contains 4.5 to 5.5 million red blood cells and an average of 7,500 white blood cells.

epithelial tissue, muscle tissue, nervous tissue, and connective tissue—some of each of the four major subgroups of tissue. The special function of the large intestine is to store waste and to absorb water from undigested, unabsorbed waste material. The large intestine is a component of the digestive system, an organ *system* whose job it is to digest, absorb, and process food.

An **organ system** can be defined as an organization of variable numbers of different organs that takes care of an important general task for the body. An organism is literally a collection of organ systems. The human organism has nine organ systems: the digestive, skeletal, endocrine, muscular, nervous, circulatory (including the heart, vascular system, and lymphatics), respiratory, urinary, and reproductive systems.

The Circulatory System

Since cancer can arise in practically any organ or tissue, all organ systems have some relationship to cancer. Beyond this broad generalization, however, the cancer relevance of each organ system is highly variable. Overall, the circulatory system is unquestionably the most important organ system relative to cancer.

The circulatory system consists of a pump, the heart; a network of vessels, including the arteries, veins, capillaries, and the lymph vessels with their associated "lymph nodes"; and circulating fluids, including both blood and lymph. The connections between the circulatory system and cancer are manifold.

Blood consists of cells some of which can become leukemia cells; lymphoid cells can become lymphomas. Cancer spreads throughout the body via the circulatory and lymphatic vascular systems. Capillary beds play a major role in arresting metastatic cancer cells. Cancer cells are somehow able to induce the growth and development of blood vessels (see Chapter 6) that nourish growing tumors. Hemorrhage and blood-clotting problems are often the ultimate causes of death in cancer patients.

The Blood Vessels The principal arteries of the body are shown in Figure 3.3. The arteries carry blood under high pressure to every tissue. As they branch throughout the body, they become smaller and smaller, blood pressure gets lower and lower, and flow becomes more even. The arteries end as **arterioles** (very small arteries) in very thin-walled, small-diameter vessels called **capillaries**.

In the capillaries, the circulatory system exchanges nutrients for wastes with the tissues.

Blood flows from the capillaries into the venous system, which takes the blood to the heart. From the heart, the blood is sent to the lungs via the pulmonary artery for gas exchange with the outside.

Functionally then, arteries carry blood *away* from the heart, veins bring it back, and the capillaries conduct the business of material exchange with tissue. Separate "plumbing" loops carry blood to the lungs for oxygenation and to the tissues to nourish and oxygenate cells (Fig. 3.3).

Every cell in the human body is within easy diffusion distance of a capillary. Fluid actually flows out of the capillaries and circulates around adjacent cells as tissue fluid, and most of it normally flows back into the capillaries further downstream. The remainder of the exudate enters the lymphatics and flows back to the heart via the lymphatic system. Although there is more to it (see Chapter 6), the capillary beds slow down metastatic cancer cells and help make it possible for secondary tumors to become established. Their extensive capillary beds are at least part of the explanation why cancer preferentially spreads to lung, brain, and bone.

The Blood Only about 40–45 percent of the blood is made up of formed elements; the rest consists of a straw-colored fluid called plasma. The formed elements of blood consist of red cells, white cells, and platelets. The red cells predominate; there are about 5 million of them in every cubic millimeter of blood (about 1/50th of a drop). Their principal function is to transport gases; in fact, it is the oxygen-carrying molecule, hemoglobin, that makes them look red. Red cells last about four months; 2 million new red cells are made by the bone marrow every second to replace those that wear out.

Platelets are actually cell fragments. Their role is principally blood coagulation. The chemistry of blood coagulation is complex and involves more than a dozen different coagulation factors. In essence, platelets adhere to jagged, damaged (wounded) areas and release factors that ultimately cause the conversion of the soluble plasma protein, fibrinogen, into its fibrous, clot-stabilizing form, called *fibrin*. The same kinds of factors are also released from tissue when it is damaged. The result in either case is a clot.

Platelets also release growth factors that speed cell division and healing. We will have much more to say about platelet-derived growth factors later in the book.

The delicacy of the balance between anticoagulation and procoagulation forces in the blood is such that many things can act to shift the balance one way or the other. If blood clots too easily, a "**thrombosis**" or internal clot can form that may then block off a part of the brain (stroke) or the heart (heart attack). If blood doesn't clot readily enough, the result can be blood loss to the extent of anemia and, if the hemorrhage is severe, to shock or even death.

There are almost a thousand times more red cells than white cells. The five different kinds of white cells found in blood are shown in Figure 3.2. They are distinguished by their appearance under the microscope after they have been subjected to a special stain.

The principal job of the white cells is defense. They deal with viruses, bacteria, and other foreign particles through a combination of phagocytosis and special secretions. They are part of the body's "police force," and as such they are able to leave the bloodstream to deal with infections and otherwise move to trouble spots under their own power. White cells do not always win. New white cells are formed in the bone marrow, spleen, and in other locations to replace the casualties. Later we'll look at the role of white cells in immunity.

The Lymphatic System   The lymphatic system is like a second venous system in that lymph vessels serve to return fluid to the heart. In this case, the fluid is **lymph**, a cell-free and largely protein-free ultrafiltrate of blood plasma (large molecules and blood cells normally can't get out of the capillaries). Fluid from the tissues flows

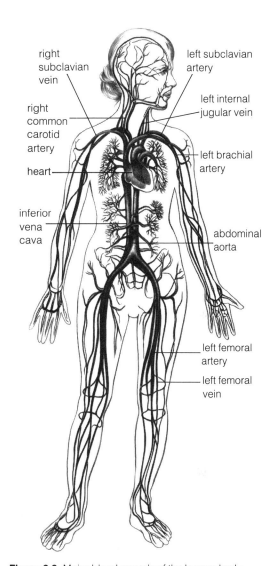

Figure 3.3 Major blood vessels of the human body

into lymphatic capillaries, from which it enters larger and larger lymph vessels. Ultimately it reenters the bloodstream at the veins in the upper chest (Fig. 3.4).

Lymph nodes—tiny masses of spongy tissue scattered throughout the lymphatic system (Fig. 3.4)—act as tiny filters that clean the lymph of cellular debris, bacterial cells, and other foreign particles. A second function of lymph

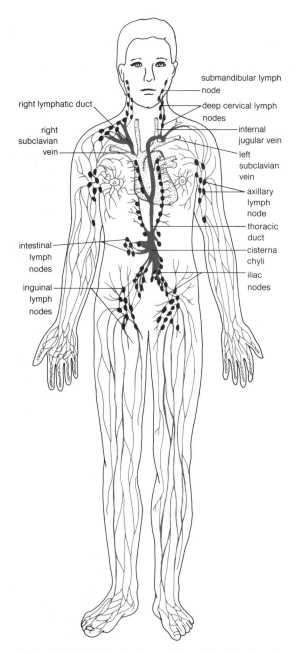

right lymphatic duct

right subclavian vein

submandibular lymph node

deep cervical lymph nodes

internal jugular vein

left subclavian vein

axillary lymph node

thoracic duct

intestinal lymph nodes

cisterna chyli

inguinal lymph nodes

iliac nodes

Figure 3.4 Major lymphatic vessels and lymph nodes of the human body

nodes is to serve as sites for the production of lymphocytes—white blood cells important in immunity. This "lymphoid" function of lymph nodes is shared by the spleen, the tonsils, the bone marrow, and the thymus gland. Lymph nodes are important in cancer because they are often the first place that cancer cells take up residence as a cancer spreads (Chapter 6).

The Immune System

The immune system is one of three lines of defense against invading bacteria and other foreign invaders. There is an outer line of defense that consists of the skin and mucous membranes. There is a backup inflammation response, chiefly effected by the phagocytic white cells. The inflammation response deals with local failures of the outer defenses. If all else fails, the body falls back on the immune system for defense.

The immune defense system differs from the other two defenses in that it is highly specific; it mounts unique immune responses for every kind of invader. The immune response also has a memory.

The first time a particular bacterium or virus invades an immune-competent organism, the immune system makes a primary response in which particular lymphocytes are stimulated to divide and then they deal with the invader. The initial attack primes the immune system so that it "remembers" that particular invader. If that particular invader enters the body again, it is attacked much more resoundingly and quickly. Often a second infection is prevented entirely, and so the body is said to be immune to that disease. Chicken pox and measles are examples of diseases for which this pattern holds true in humans.

To be vaccinated or immunized against a disease is to be given an artificial first "infection" or exposure. The **ideal vaccine** confers absolute immunity to a disease but does not, itself, produce any symptoms of that disease. Sometimes

The relationship between cancer and the immune system is one of the most important areas of cancer research today. The relationship has many aspects. First of all, both cancer itself as well as cancer treatment sometimes suppress the immune system. This effect is a major problem in caring for cancer patients. Secondly, the immune system is a potential defense against cancer. Much research is aimed at finding ways to cause the immune system to attack cancer more effectively. The immune system is also being used to detect and diagnose cancers by attaching tracer materials to antibodies, capitalizing on the affinity of antibodies for specific, cancer-associated "antigens." This very same affinity is also being exploited in attaching anticancer drugs to antibodies that then carry the drug to the cancer cells. All these topics are covered later, most notably in Chapters 12, 14, 16, and 17. A focused consideration of cancer and the immune system is presented in Chapter 14, after our consideration of the antigens associated with carcinogenic transformations (Part III), and after the general discussion of how cancer affects the human body (Chapter 12). You may want to skim Chapter 14 now, and then read it more thoroughly later, in the contexts of detection and treatment.

killed bacteria or viruses are used; it is also possible to vaccinate using live, but weakened organisms—organisms much less able to produce the disease or any of its symptoms while still eliciting a full immune response.

There are two ways in which the immune system deals with invaders. *Humoral immunity* is immunity in which cells of the immune system deal with foreign invaders indirectly, by producing **antibodies**—defense-related proteins carried in solution in the "humors" or fluids of the body. *Cell-mediated immunity* is immunity in which cells other than those that make antibodies deal directly with foreign invaders—by ingesting them or otherwise destroying them. We will give full consideration to the relationship between cancer and the immune system in a later chapter.

Homeostasis: Organ Systems in Concert

"Homeostasis" comes from two Greek words: *homeo*, meaning "similar" and *stasis*, which means "to stay." Homeostasis refers to the relative constancy of internal conditions in a living organism. Physiology is the branch of biology concerned with how the organs and organ systems of an organism maintain homeostasis in the face of changing internal and external environments. Each organ system can be thought of as a means by which particular features of the internal environment—such as temperature, dissolved oxygen, pH, water content, sodium ion concentrations, blood sugar levels, and so on—are monitored and readjusted to keep them within the limits suitable for cellular life.

Chapter 12 is devoted to the general effects that cancer has on the body. Ultimately, every dimension of the impact of cancer involves a "fall from homeostasis." Homeostasis is an important concept for us, then, and it will be worthwhile to consider a few examples, as follows.

Blood Sugar Levels

Practically every cell in the body needs sugar for its energy supply. Cells must rely on the circulatory system to keep the sugar coming, and this is done by a system that maintains blood sugar levels at a relatively constant 90 mg percent. The

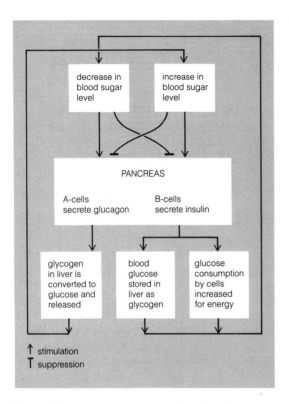

Figure 3.5 The role of glucagon and insulin in the regulation of blood sugar levels

throughout the body it stimulates cells throughout the body to increase their uptake of sugar. It stimulates muscle cells and particularly liver cells to take up glucose and store it as glycogen. Enhanced cellular uptake and storage have the effect of lowering blood sugar, and so it can be said that insulin serves to clear the blood of extra sugar.

Now imagine being lost in the woods and not eating for two days! This is where glucagon comes in. As body cells go on using sugar—even though no food is being consumed—the level of sugar in the blood tends to fall. Low blood sugar stimulates a different set of cells in the pancreas to secrete glucagon. Glucagon's principal effect is to cause the glycogen in the liver to be released as sugar into the blood—raising blood sugar levels.

The combined effect of the two hormone systems we have just described is to keep blood sugar levels in the normal range—not too high and not too low! The combined control system is depicted in Figure 3.5.

Body Temperature

The human body has a core (central region of the body) temperature of 98.6°F or 37°C. The 0.6 suggests precision—that the temperature is tightly controlled. Actually, body temperature fluctuates quite a bit around this figure—it can rise several degrees during a fast set of tennis, and it can fall a little during sleep. But the control system always works to bring it back. To see how this system works, let's imagine sitting in a hot sauna and then jumping into cold water.

There is a thermostat in the part of the brain called the *hypothalamus*. In a sauna, when body temperature begins to rise, the thermostat sends signals to a "heat-losing center" also located in the hypothalamus. The heat-losing center, in turn, (1) inhibits the heat-promoting center, (2) dilates the blood vessels of the skin so that heat can be radiated or conducted away more quickly, (3) induces sweating, and (4) depresses

control system that keeps blood sugar levels constant must compensate for the things that would tend to raise or lower blood sugar. It adjusts for highly variable sugar intake (banana splits, Christmas candy, diets) and for highly variable sugar consumption by cells under conditions ranging from strenuous physical exercise to sleep. Adjustments are made primarily through the actions of two pancreatic hormones, insulin and glucagon. Let's imagine eating a giant hot fudge sundae and then starving, to see how the system works.

As soon as a sundae hits the intestine, a surge of sugar enters the bloodstream and blood sugar levels rise. As the blood passes through the pancreas, the extra sugar serves as a stimulus to certain cells to secrete insulin. Insulin passes into the bloodstream, and as it travels

metabolism and thus reduces the generation of metabolic heat.

A jump into cold water will basically have the opposite effect. As body temperature starts to fall, the thermostat stimulates the "heat-promoting center," which (1) inhibits the heat-losing center, (2) constricts peripheral blood vessels, and (3) increases metabolism and causes involuntary muscle spasms (shivering). The thermostat in conjunction with the heat-promoting and heat-losing control centers amounts to a control system that keeps body temperature constant.

These two examples, blood sugar and temperature control, should help us to keep in mind the rest of the way through the book that the body is a collection of monitoring and control systems that serve to keep nearly every physical and chemical feature of the internal environment within narrow limits. This chapter explains why some problems associated with cancer have to do with the following cascade of facts: when cells go wrong, tissues go wrong; when tissues go wrong, organs go wrong; when organs go wrong, organ systems go wrong; when organ systems go wrong, the result is chaos. For any living thing, organizational chaos is synonymous with disease; in the extreme, with death.

Further Reading

Dozens of excellent anatomy and physiology textbooks provide extensive coverage of the material introduced in this chapter. Other sources include textbooks of histology, hematology, and immunology, and specialty books on single organ systems (for example, respiratory physiology, neuroanatomy, neurophysiology, and endocrinology).

PART TWO
CANCER AT THE LEVEL OF CELLS AND TISSUE

Part II deals with cancer cells, how they look, how they function, and how they behave relative to one another and relative to the host. Part III focuses on the causes of cancer. Logic might seem to demand that these parts be reversed. But there is also some logic in looking at the features of both normal cells and cancer cells before describing how the former are converted into the latter.

Although cancer has many dimensions, the key player in cancer is the cancer cell, and it's time we met the villain.

4

How Cancer Cells Are Different

The two deceptively simple-sounding *basic* aims of cancer research are (1) find out how cancer is *caused* and then use this information to *prevent* cancer; and (2) find out how cancer cells are *different* and exploit this information to *detect, control,* and/or *cure* cancer. We will consider the first objective in Part III; here we concern ourselves with the second objective.

The two aims are actually related to one another—through genes. Cancer is caused by things that alter genes or disturb genetic control. The products of the affected genes express themselves as the features of cancer cells. Put another way, the second objective can be expressed as a series of questions: "What do these genes do? What protein products do they speed up, slow down, establish, or fail to complete? What are the ultimate consequences in terms of cell structure and function, and what pathways connect them to the gene(s)?" If we could answer these questions, we would have ways to "get at" cancer even if we never did establish the *genetic* essence of cancer. Even if we couldn't get at the responsible genes, we *might* be able to get at the gene products, or at products of the products—or both. Obviously, we want the answers.

Maybe, in seeking the answers, we will find that one or a few gene products are the primary or principal expressions of malignancy; maybe few key gene products cause every other feature of cancer cells through some kind of "domino effect." If a way could be found to block or influence such a key product, the cancer problem would be a long way toward being solved.

As we will see throughout the remainder of this chapter, there are many differences between cancer cells and noncancer cells. Some of the differences are the same as those between dividing and nondividing normal cells. When we try to exploit these differences, normal dividing cells get "hit" along with cancer cells. Cancer patients lose their hair and have problems with their intestines because drugs designed to kill dividing cancer cells also kill dividing hair-producing cells and intestinal epithelial cells.

We need to continually find more fundamental and more cancer-specific differences to exploit.

Let's look at what has been found out thus far. We will begin with a brief description of difficulties in comparing cancer cells with normal cells.

Transformed Cells and Other Models

One problem that complicates the search for key differences between cancer and normal cells, is that there is no sure way of identifying the normal counterpart of a human cancer cell.

For most, if not all, human cancer, the normal precursors are unknown. All normal tissue from which tumors arise are made up of a variety of types of cells and cells in different stages of becoming what they will be. By the time human tumors are looked at, many have undergone considerable evolution. The historical connection to the original tissue may be far from obvious.

Liver tumors have been, are being, and no doubt will continue to be compared to normal liver tissue. We can learn from such comparisons. But comparing normal human tissue from which cancer arises, to cancer tissue itself may not be the same as comparing a cancer cell to the normal cell from which it came.

Because of this limitation, tumor biologists have tended to rely on cell culture models. They use stable cell lines derived from a variety of animal species as "normal" cells, and for "cancer" cells they use normal cell lines "transformed" by chemical carcinogens, radiation, or viruses. This approach solves the problem of not having a definitive "before" and "after," but problems still arise when we try to apply what we've learned to human cancer.

The unannounced shifts from "real" tumor cells to "transformed" cells in the following pages will imply that the two are one and the same. They are in fact *not* the same. We simply assume that transformed cells and *actual* cancer cells share many identical features, and that

things found out about transformed cells may well be applicable to "real" cancer. This presumption may *or may not* be confirmed by future experimentation.

Transformed Cell Lines

Transformed cells are cells derived from "normal" cell lines. **Cell lines** are cells that grow out of small pieces of normal tissue or embryonic tissue put into a cell culture flask under the "right" conditions. Such cells become permanent or **continuous cell lines** when they acquire the ability to be propagated indefinitely in tissue culture (see Fig. 4.1).

Normal cells can go through only about 50 divisions in cell culture before they die out. Arising spontaneously from such normal cell cultures—sometimes—are variants that do not die out but go right on dividing as long as they are fed, subcultured, and maintained properly. With qualification, they serve very nicely as models of normal cells. Except for their "immortality"—which disqualifies them from *absolute* "normalcy"—the cells of cell lines behave normally. The cells of cell lines can be **transformed**—converted to cells that behave like tumor cells in culture.

Although the ultimate test of a **transformed cell line** is its ability to develop into a malignant neoplasm when implanted into an appropriate host species, transformed cells can be recognized by other characteristics. Pitot (1978) and Ruddon (1981) list the most important criteria of "transformedness." These include altered antigenicity, diminished contact inhibition, reduced requirements for certain nutrients, and the ability to grow in suspension or otherwise unattached to a solid substratum. Not all transformed cell lines exhibit *all* the characteristics *generally* found in transformed cells.

Cell lines are transformed by the same kinds of agents that cause tumors to arise in animal tissue, namely viruses, chemical carcinogens, and radiation (see Part III).

The beauty of cell line and/or transformed

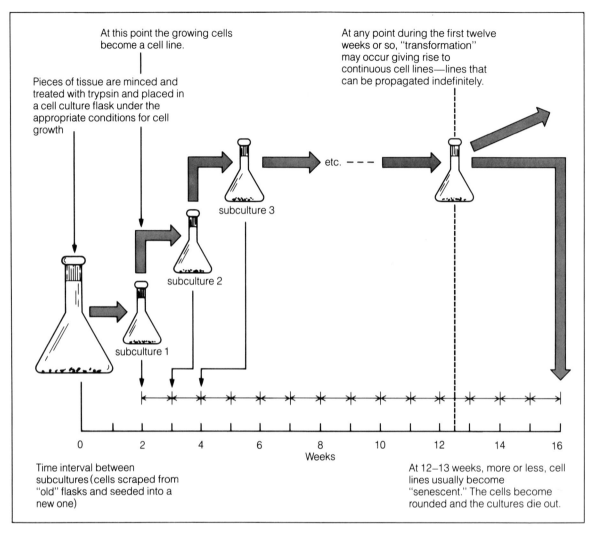

At this point the growing cells become a cell line.

Pieces of tissue are minced and treated with trypsin and placed in a cell culture flask under the appropriate conditions for cell growth

At any point during the first twelve weeks or so, "transformation" may occur giving rise to continuous cell lines—lines that can be propagated indefinitely.

subculture 1

subculture 2

subculture 3

etc.

Weeks

Time interval between subcultures (cells scraped from "old" flasks and seeded into a new one)

At 12–13 weeks, more or less, cell lines usually become "senescent." The cells become rounded and the cultures die out.

Figure 4.1 How cell lines and continuous cell lines are derived. Continuous cell lines arise from normal cells by some kind of spontaneous change or "transformation." Except for their immortality, continuous cell lines behave like normal cells in culture. We refer to them throughout this book *as if they were normal.* Wherever we use the term *transformed cell,* we mean cell lines *derived from* continuous cell lines (by exposing them to radiation, chemical carcinogens, or oncogenic viruses) and that *behave like* cancer cells.

cell systems is that they provide "pure" untransformed cells and "pure" transformed counterparts that can then be compared. Particularly useful have been the "temperature-sensitive mutants" discovered along the way. **Temperature-sensitive mutants** are cell lines that express transformedness only at certain temperatures. At other temperatures, they revert to the *un-*transformed phenotype. By providing a means by which to turn transformation on or off quickly, these mutants make it possible to evaluate the *tightness* of connections between chemical changes and other features of transformedness.

We will move on now to describe how *actual* cancer cells look under the microscope.

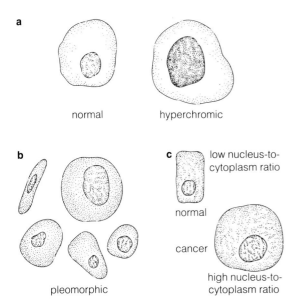

a

normal   hyperchromic

b

c low nucleus-to-cytoplasm ratio

normal

cancer

high nucleus-to-cytoplasm ratio

pleomorphic

Figure 4.2 (**a**) Hyperchromatism; (**b**) pleomorphism; and (**c**) the difference in nuclear-to-cytoplasm ratio in a normal cell, versus in a cancer cell

Cancer Cells Look Different

When a **pathologist** (a medical specialist who evaluates structural and chemical changes associated with disease) looks at cancer under the microscope, he or she sees tissue that lacks the high level of structural organization seen in normal tissue. The degree of deviation from normal varies from one type of tumor to another.

"Fixed," static sections of tumor tissue stained with hematoxylin and eosin (H&E)* often give the impression of motion, disarray, and even "anger" to observers with a little imagination. Some of the disarray is caused by the presence of variable amounts of dead cells, connective tissue, and infiltrating white cells. Actual cancer cells are often clearly recognizable, mostly because of their **hyperchromatism**—

more strongly stained chromatin and larger nuclei (see Fig. 4.2**a**). When a pathologist is evaluating a tumor, blue is bad!

There are other important features of cancer cells. Cancer cells tend to be **pleomorphic**—they have variable sizes and shapes (Fig. 4.2**b**). Cancer cells have a high nucleus-to-cytoplasm ratio; their nuclei are disproportionately large (Fig. 4.2**c**). In a group of cancer cells, there will tend to be more cells undergoing mitosis than in normal tissue—and often there is a large number of *abnormal* mitotic figures (Fig. 4.3). Cancer cells have unusually prominent nucleoli. Lastly, cancer cells tend to be anaplastic—they tend to be less well differentiated than the cells of surrounding normal tissue. Liver tumor cells don't look quite like any normal liver cells. Some cancer cells are so poorly differentiated that it can be difficult to identify the tissue of origin.

Cancer Cells and Differentiation

As a fertilized human egg divides and divides again, the individual cells in the expanding mass become different from one another. Ultimately, some results of this process look like "fully differentiated" liver, kidney, skin, and muscle cells.

For a long time it was thought that all cancer cells emerged from fully differentiated normal cells that had "*de*differentiated" as a consequence of transformation. It was thought that cells that had reached their mature appearance reverted—in the direction of embryologic forms—when "hit" by a carcinogen. Later it was more generally believed that cancer cells all come from the small numbers of undifferentiated cells already present in normal tissue (see Fig. 4.4).

Today, we know that genes (oncogenes—see Chapter 7) previously turned off during differentiation can be reactivated by carcinogenic agents. We also know that it is possible to cause the cells at one level of differentiation to become transformed into less well-differentiated cells by exposing them to carcinogenic agents. There are

---

*A mixture of dyes that colors the cytoplasm red and the nucleus blue.

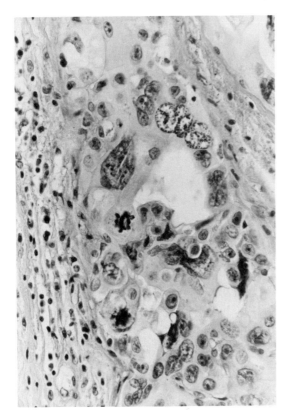

Figure 4.3 Two mitotic figures in a breast carcinoma (special type: medullary carcinoma) × 150. (Photo courtesy Professor Per H. B. Carstens, Department of Pathology, University of Louisville School of Medicine)

Cancer Cells Behave Differently

The spread of cancer from a primary tumor to regional lymph nodes and to other organs was noted by early physicians, and they must have deduced that cancer cells *behaved* abnormally. After it became possible to grow cancer cells and transformed cells in culture, a number of characteristic behavioral features of these cells were documented:

1. Altered contact inhibition of movement

2. Altered contact inhibition of cell division

3. Altered ability to recognize other cells

4. Altered intercellular adhesion

As we consider each feature in turn, note that they all have *something to do with the cell surface.*

Diminished Contact Inhibition of Movement

If a small clump of normal cells is placed in fresh medium in a tissue culture flask, the cells will slowly migrate along the glass or plastic surface outward. Ambercrombie (1975) showed that this migration resulted from cell-contact regulation of movement. Through time-lapse photography, he showed that, as a migrating cell made contact with another cell, forward motion stopped; after a short time, the cell began moving off in another direction. In experiments in which colonies of normal and then transformed cell lines were placed in a flask and allowed to migrate toward one another, cells of normal colonies stopped when they encountered the advancing edge of the other colony. Under the same circumstances, colonies of transformed cells climbed over and past one another (Fig. 4.5). The normal phenomenon has come to be called **contact inhibition of movement**. This feature appears to be lost or at least diminished in malignant cells.

In culture, normal cells form nice, orderly monolayers, whereas transformed cells pile up.

also other indications that the differentiated state is quite plastic. Blau et al. (1985) showed, for example, that when muscle cells are fused with various *differentiated* nonmuscle cells from different species, muscle gene expression is activated in the nonmuscle cells.

Although it is still not entirely clear, it may be that human cancer can arise by the transformation of either partially differentiated cells or from at least some kinds of more fully differentiated cells. It may simply be easier (require fewer changes) to transform undifferentiated cells (see Chapter 7; see also the section *Growth,* below).

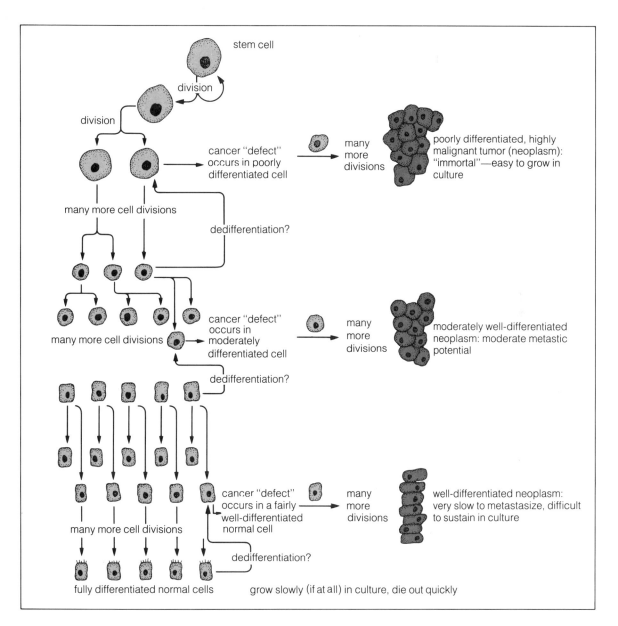

stem cell

division

division

cancer "defect" occurs in poorly differentiated cell

many more divisions

poorly differentiated, highly malignant tumor (neoplasm): "immortal"—easy to grow in culture

many more cell divisions

dedifferentiation?

many more cell divisions

cancer "defect" occurs in moderately differentiated cell

many more divisions

moderately well-differentiated neoplasm: moderate metastic potential

dedifferentiation?

many more cell divisions

cancer "defect" occurs in a fairly well-differentiated normal cell

many more divisions

well-differentiated neoplasm: very slow to metastasize, difficult to sustain in culture

dedifferentiation?

fully differentiated normal cells   grow slowly (if at all) in culture, die out quickly

Figure 4.4 The normal differentiation of cells (left) and the origin of poorly differentiated, moderately well-differentiated, and well-differentiated neoplasms. The relationship between differentiation and metastatic behavior is far from tight—poorly differentiated cancers *tend* to be highly metastatic, however.

This apparently results from the fact that the transformed cells are oblivious to contact inhibition of movement.

Diminished Contact Inhibition of Cell Division

If normal cells are placed in a tissue culture flask under the appropriate conditions, the cells begin to divide, moving outward, until the flask is covered with a single layer of cells that looks like a flagstone patio. At this point cell division ceases. If a few of the cells are scraped off, cells in that region begin dividing again until the blank space is filled in.

Such experiments indicate that normal cells quit dividing at "saturation density," not because they run out of nutrients, not because of accumulated waste, but because of "full contact" with other cells. When they are surrounded, they simply quit dividing. This kind of contact inhibition is sometimes called **contact inhibition of growth**.

Cancer cells generally lack or exhibit diminished contact inhibition of growth. Cancer cells continue to divide even after the bottom of a culture flask is covered. Apparently oblivious of other cells, cancer cells go right on dividing; they even pile up. They look less like a flagstone patio and more like a pile of flagstones dumped off the back of a truck.

The General Defect in Cell-to-Cell Recognition

It makes sense that normal cells *are* growth- and movement-inhibited by contact with other cells. This pattern helps explain how liver and skin cells stay where they belong and why livers and kidneys only get so big.

The fact that cancer cells are defective in these traits helps explain (1) the invasion of normal tissue by tumor cells, (2) the spreading of cancer, and (3) the fact that cancer manifests itself as lumps. The basis of these contact-

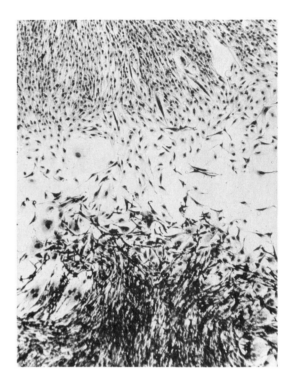

Figure 4.5 A normal (above) and a morphologically transformed colony (below) of Syrian hamster embryo cells. (Photo courtesy of Dr. J. Carl Barrett, National Institute of Environmental Health Sciences. *Science* Vol. 212, cover, June 19, 1981. © 1981 by the AAAS. Used by permission.)

mediated properties of normal cells and their alteration in the cancer cell must certainly involve both the cell surface and some kind of intercellular chemical interaction or recognition. Quite a number of studies have clearly indicated that normal cells can "recognize" and interact with one another chemically.

If a sponge is disassociated into individual cells and then mixed with cells of other strains of sponge, the cells from the same strain "find" one another and form multicellular clumps. Similarly, if rat cells and mouse cells are mixed, rat cells sort themselves out, forming aggregates with other rat cells, and mouse cells aggregate with other mouse cells. Moscona (1956) showed that if kidney and liver cells from the same species were mixed, pre-existing individual liver

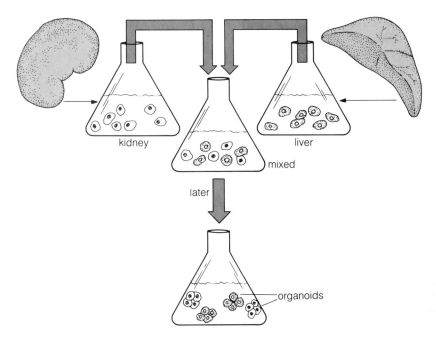

Figure 4.6 Moscona's experiment illustrating the adhesive specificity of cells of different organs in the same species

cells formed tiny liver "organoids," and kidney cells did likewise (Fig. 4.6). Liver cells did not bind to kidney. All such examples of selective adhesion suggest the presence of very highly specific cell surface recognition systems normally serving to segregate and then stabilize cells into differentiated tissues. Cancer cells tend not to adhere to other cancer cells very well, and so naturally there is a great deal of interest in the chemical basis of cell-cell recognition and adhesion.

So far, we know that among the chemicals involved in cell-cell recognition are certain divalent cations, notably calcium and magnesium, and sugar-containing macromolecules that can be stripped off the surface by trypsin (indicating that they are glycoproteins). Whatever macromolecules are interacting from cell to cell, it is most likely the *distribution* of arrays of the molecules—a kind of molecular Braille—that accounts for the specificity. One compelling reason for such an explanation is that if liver has a different code from kidney—even in the same

animal, as indicated by Moscona's experiments—there are too few different kinds of sugars on the surface to account for the number of different codes that would be required by the many kinds of tissue present in every animal. Just a few different kinds of glycoproteins could, however, be arranged in a large number of different patterns.

It has been suggested that enzymes may be involved in the initial stages of cell-cell adhesion. Glycosyl transferases, for example, are enzymes able to attach sugar residues to the carbohydrate portion of glycoprotein molecules. They put the finishing touches on protein-sugar complexes. It may be that such enzymes on *one* cell bind to the residues of their substrates on the *other*, accounting for the specific initial attachment of one cell to another. If not enzymes and substrates, then something very much like this process must account for the apparently very specific association of like cells.

We should be prepared to find out that many kinds of cell surface changes might all lead to the same end—the effective failure of the cell to know when it meets up with another cell. A recognition code could be disturbed by *additions* and *changes* as well as outright *deletions* of the molecules directly and indirectly involved.

It is not hard to imagine some kind of molecular hand-and-glove interaction between adjacent cells serving to appraise each cell of the existence of the other. If the glove does not fit very well because of some change in either the hand or the glove, the cells act as if they were alone. Molecular hands and gloves are probably made of glycolipids and glycoproteins.

Growth

Above all else, cancer cells are different in the way they divide. The very fact that neoplasms express themselves as lumps indicates that cancer cells increase in number faster than do the cells of surrounding normal tissue. Actual measurements of many different kinds of human tumors indicate that the average human neoplasm doubles every two months. Since the cell cycle time of cancer cells is generally not much different from that of normal cells, this rate means that only a fraction of the cells in a tumor are dividing at any one time. The fact that neoplasms become lumps indicates that, whatever the fraction is, it is enough to keep cell division ahead of cell death or loss. This imbalance contrasts with the case in mature normal tissues capable of growth, where cell division matches cell loss. What keeps too high a fraction of cancer cells in the so-called growth fraction? This is one of the burning questions in cancer research—and, indeed, in all of cell biology.

A Catalog of Changes in the Cancer Cell Surface

The preceding discussion suggests that one very plausible answer to the question "How do 'cancer genes' express themselves initially?" is "They are expressed as alterations in the cell sur-face." Many changes in the cancer cell surface have been well documented.

Often cited as the first clear demonstration that there are surface differences between normal and cancer cells was the work of D. R. Coman (1944) in the 1940s. He showed that tumor cells could be pulled apart more easily than their normal counterparts.

Driven by interest in basic cell biology, the basic biology of tumor cells, and in finding ways to control and cure cancer, there has since been, and continues to be, an enormous research effort directed at the cancer cell surface. The result to date has been the cataloging of a long list of things that are true about the cell surface. These along with some cytoplasmic and nuclear changes are summarized in Figure 4.7.

Nearly all the known changes in the cell surface are still under active investigation. We still need to know if, and just how, these changes influence overt behavior features of cancer cells and, indeed, just how *general* these changes are.

In the next few pages, we will describe what we know so far about the nature and possible significance of the most profound and important of these changes. We'll begin with glycoproteins and glycolipids.

Among the generalized changes in cell surface glycoproteins and glycolipids found in cancer cells are the following:

1. New glycoprotein molecules appear on the surface.

2. Some of the same glycolipid and glycoprotein molecules found on normal cell surfaces appear to be changed on transformed cell surfaces; some of these appear to be incompletely processed.

3. Certain high-molecular-weight glycolipids and glycoproteins are missing.

4. Another family of protein-carbohydrate complexes called *proteoglycans* are represented on the cell surface and in the intercellular matrix. These, too, appear to change in association with malignancy. Because these are large, negatively charged molecules in a position to inter-

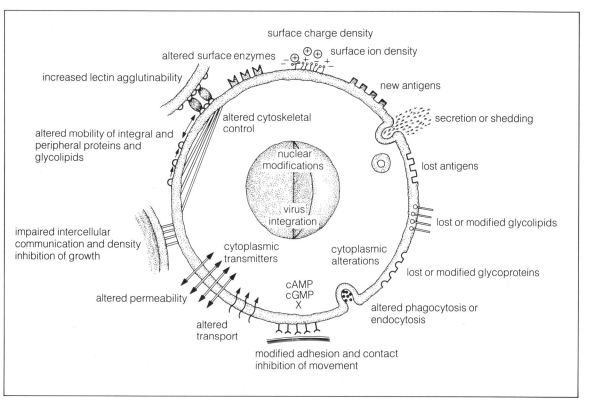

Figure 4.7 Summary of the cell surface and cell surface-related alterations generally seen in cancer cells. (Adapted from Nicholson by permission of the author and Elsevier Biomedical Press.)

fere with the chemistry of the cell surface, it is important that the synthesis of certain of them increases in cancer cells. (Few clear generalizations about the relationship between proteoglycans and cancer have emerged thus far; we mention them only in passing.)

All this could be summarized by saying that some new molecules appear, some of the regular molecules are lost, and some of the regular molecules are changed.

Let's consider some of the specifics.

Glycoprotein Changes

Transformation is almost invariably associated with alterations in cell-surface glycoproteins (Smets and Van Beek, 1984). Although in some

instances the complexity of malignant cell glycoproteins is increased, the trend, by far, is toward a lower protein content of the transformed cell surface. Many of the glycoproteins that *are* present are altered, mostly by being simpler. Much evidence shows that transformed cells have deranged mechanisms by which polysaccharides are made and attached to proteins.

LETS Consider Fibronectin Among the most profound or overt cell surface changes associated with transformation is the *loss* of a large glycoprotein, at first unimaginatively called Large External Transformation-Sensitive protein, or LETS. LETS was found by Yamada and others (see Willingham et al., 1977, and Hynes, 1986) to have something to do with adhesion. When investigators added LETS to red blood cells, it caused them to clump. LETS also caused the aggregation of previously disaggregated, transformed kidney cells and isolated cells derived from chicken embryos. It has also been observed that LETS levels are greatest in normal cells at rest, and that they decline to near zero during cell division—suggesting the possibility of a basic role in controlling cell division.

As interest in LETS gathered steam, it was discovered that LETS was really a glycoprotein known by another name, *fibronectin*. **Fibronectin** is a large-molecular-weight glycoprotein found in soluble form in the blood of vertebrates and on normal cell surfaces. It is a component of the matrix or stroma (Chapter 3) in which cells are imbedded. Fibronectin is an anchoring molecule. Together with various proteoglycans, collagen, and elastin, fibronectin forms a fibrillar network that holds cells in place in tissue. It is also believed to serve as an organizing grid for the integral proteins of the cell surface. It acts like an exoskeleton, in other words, holding receptor molecules in particular arrays. Fibronectin also influences organization inside the cell. Fibronectin molecules apparently interact specifically with actin filaments within the cytoplasm, probably via proteins that span the cell membrane (see Hynes, 1986). Perhaps it is through this interaction that fibronectin also has something to do with the shapes of cells. When fibronectin is removed from fibroblasts, they lose their spindle shape, round up, and develop numerous microvilli, making them look much like transformed cells. All of this suggests that fibronectin may lie close to a "primary defect" in cancer cells.

Hynes (1986) suggests that the simplest explanation for why cancer cells have low levels of fibronectin associated with their surfaces is that cancer cells stop making fibronectin. Although there is some evidence for this, there is also evidence that cancer cells may make a defective form of fibronectin—a form they cannot hold on to. Cancer cells may also make a defective transmembrane fibronectin-binding protein, and there is some evidence that cancer cells may break down fibronectin as soon as they make it

(see below). In any case, it seems to be more than coincidental that cancer cells are deficient in fibronectin and that this substance plays important roles in cellular organization, cell-to-cell adhesion, cellular migration, and normal cytoskeletal structure.

Protease Power Plasma fibronectin levels rise in the blood of cancer patients, and fibronectin is shed into the medium in which transformed cells are growing. It could be that all this is a direct consequence of a rise in **protease** (the general name for enzymes that break up protein molecules) secretion by cancer cells. The proteases may simply clip the fibronectin connections to the surface, allowing it to float away.

Transformed cells secrete "plasminogen-activating factor," which (as one might guess) activates plasminogen. It actually converts plasminogen, an inactive protease, into plasmin, the active form. The secretion of plasmin and other proteases may be part of a general mechanism by which cells lose fibronectin.

The possibility that protease secretion or activation may be a "first cause" in the expression of the malignant phenotype is suggested by experiments in which it has been shown that when normal cells are treated with exogenous proteases, they begin to behave like transformed cells. Additional support for this possibility comes from experiments in which it was shown that abnormal behavior of transformed cells can be reversed or at least modulated by protease inhibitors. Other contributing evidence comes from the observation that certain normally masked features of the *normal* cell surface appear to be uncovered or exposed in the transformed cell.

Glycolipid Changes

In vitro experiments with fibroblast cell lines and their virus-induced transformants indicate that glycolipid changes may be another general attribute of transformation. In general, the glycolipid content of transformed cell membranes is *reduced*; also, the complexity of membrane glycolipids is reduced—terminal sugar groups are often missing. Experimental evidence indicates that these changes are attributable to reduced synthesis and incomplete processing. Perhaps the fact that transformed cells are continually dividing simply doesn't leave the glycolipid synthesizing and processing machinery enough time to finish its work.

The Functional Significance of Cell Surface Changes in Cancer

The importance of changes in cancer cells goes beyond academic biochemistry. At the most fundamental level of tumor cell biology, glycoprotein changes apparently mean changes in receptor configurations on cell surfaces and a resultant disability to respond to other cells and to chemical signals from other parts of the organism. Glycoprotein changes are also important to immune defense against cancer because they are a means (as antigens) by which the cells that bear them might be recognized by the immune system.

Alterations in the Cell Membrane as a Control Panel   In Chapter 3, we introduced the concept of how the membrane of an individual cell is involved in converting signals from the "organism at large" into intracellular action. You may recall that the enzyme, adenyl cyclase, which is bound to the inside of the cell membrane is influenced by extracellular hormones that bind to receptors on the outside. Adenyl cyclase converts intracellular ATP to the "second messenger," cyclic AMP or cAMP, which is an important regulator of the things that go on inside the cell.

Work by Ira Pastan and others (1975) has shown that cAMP levels fluctuate with the state of cellular activity. Levels are generally high in resting normal cells and are low in dividing cells, including cancer cells. Another important regulatory molecule, cyclic guanosine monophos-

phate (cGMP), has been found to vary in a way opposite that of cAMP. Cell division is usually associated with *low* cAMP levels and *high* cGMP levels. Cyclic GMP has been found to stimulate RNA synthesis in some cells, and tumor promotors (see Chapter 8) have been found to influence cAMP levels.

Although these changes may simply be part of a long list of secondary characteristics generally true of "turned-on" cells, the key regulatory position of cAMP makes it especially interesting to cancer researchers. Conceivably, the decreased cAMP level seen in transformed cells is a major primary stimulus or key to autonomous growth. If membrane changes turn out to be among the key initial expressions of malignancy, the very next change in the cascade of events leading to the full expression of malignancy could well be suppression of adenyl cyclase and a drop in cAMP levels. Especially intriguing is the observation that transformation traits such as roundedness and diminished adhesiveness can be restored to normal when transformed cells are prevented from degrading cAMP, causing its levels to rise toward normal.

Tumor-Associated Antigens   In Chapter 3, the point was made that our immune systems are designed to deal with foreign proteins and other foreign "antigenic" substances. We could just as easily have used the word *new* in place of *foreign*. Human immune systems conduct a survey early in neonatal life and declare all proteins there at that time to be "self." Proteins that show up after that survey are dealt with by the immune system as if they were parts of hostile, foreign organisms. As might be expected from the fact that *new* proteins and protein complexes appear on the surfaces of cancer cells, cancer cells are often immunologically distinguishable from their assumed or actual normal counterparts (see Chapter 14).

Some such antigenic differences can be recognized only by *other* species, the so-called **heterologous antigens**. Some can be recognized by other members of the same species, the **alloantigens**. Alloantigens are the kinds of antigens—

such as histocompatibility antigens and blood-type antigens—that make it difficult to achieve successful organ and tissue transplants and that make it necessary to cross-match blood before giving transfusions.

Sometimes tumor cells bear **isoantigens**, tumor-associated antigens that the tumor-bearing animal recognizes as new or foreign. Some of these are antigens of tumor-inducing viruses; others are simply *neo*antigens associated with the transformed state. Some, if not all tumor-specific antigens may be altered histocompatibility antigens; that is, a "normal" histocompatibility antigen of the host, modified beyond recognition as far as the immune system is concerned. Some antigens found on cancer cells are immunologically identical to fetal antigens—antigens found in that tissue normally, but only in the fetal state. Such antigens are apparently expressed as a result of the reactivation of genes turned off at the end of fetal development. Unfortunately, while the existence of tumor-specific antigens has been demonstrated in many cell-culture and animal-tumor models, the evidence for tumor-*specific* antigens in human tumors is very weak. Most human tumors do, however, exhibit tumor-*associated* antigens, antigens that normally appear only during embryologic development or that appear in lesser amounts in normal cells. We will have much more to say about antigens later in Chapter 14.

The fact that cell surface protein changes are detectable immunologically has tremendous practical significance even though we may not have the slightest idea what the antigenic substance actually *does* on the cell surface. Examples of the uses of immunological properties of tumors in detection, diagnosis, and treatment of cancer are discussed at length in later chapters.

Altered Permeability and Membrane Transport
Materials are transported at generally higher rates across the membranes of transformed cells. Materials that show enhanced uptake include glucose, other sugars, and certain amino acids. Enhanced transport is consistent with the greater metabolic demand for certain raw materials characteristic of cancer cells and parallels a similar change seen in normal cells undergoing cell division. Increased transport of sugars and amino acids is probably not a *primary* change *responsible* for the malignant state; it is rather more likely that whatever triggers malignant behavior ultimately also increases transport. Still, the fact that cancer cells are different with respect to transport is important. Perhaps ways could be developed to selectively retard transport across cancer cell membranes and thereby help control the expression of malignancy.

Altered Secretion: Export   Another dimension of transport is of course *export*. Export is abnormal in cancer cells. While this fact may reflect changes or problems with many aspects of the cell, including the integrity of the membrane, it is most likely the result of both (1) the excess production of *normal* secretions and (2) the "inappropriate" secretion that result from the "inappropriate" activation of normally turned-off genes. In Chapter 12 we look at abnormal secretions from the viewpoint of their *general* effects on the host. Of direct relevance to the present discussion is the fact that "proteases" are among the things abnormally exported.

Altered Cell-to-Cell Junctions   Cells make connections with one another that are far more elaborate than simple contact. Among the discrete types of junctions (anatomically distinct kinds of points of contact) between cells are (1) **tight junctions**, junctions that appear to function as seals between cells and that appear to be derived from the fusing of parts of the plasma membranes belonging to adjacent epithelial cells; (2) **desmosomes**, (Fig. 4.8) junctions that appear to function as structural anchoring points possibly serving in tissue organization; and (3) **gap junctions**, which are actually channels between adjacent cells, through which cells may exchange chemical substances.

Junctions appear to be deranged in at least some cancer cells. Decreases in the number of desmosomes have been reported in cervical carcinoma as well as in tumors of breast, skin, and liver. If failure to form organizational and communicative junctions proves to be generally true of cancer cells, this may be part of the general reason why cancer cells characteristically don't communicate or otherwise relate to one another very well.

Changes in Surface Charge   If transformed cells are placed in an electric field, they tend to be drawn toward the positive pole. Although this is also true of normal cells, transformed cells move faster (Fig. 4.9), indicating that cancer cells are more negatively charged than their normal counterparts. This enhanced negative-charge density has been linked to phospholipid and nucleic acid changes but mostly to glycoprotein changes. Negative charges associated with transformation are nearly all reduced if the cell is treated with the enzyme neuraminidase, an enzyme that removes sialic acid residues from glycoprotein molecules.

Cell Membrane Summary   A number of changes in the cell membrane have been found to be associated with the transformed state. Changing cyclic nucleotide levels, membrane fluidity, surface receptors, protease activity, and the like are *all* good candidates as primary changes from which the rest of the malignant state may unfold. Yet it is not known how, or even *if*, all these changes are related to one another or to other features of the transformed cell in terms of cause and effect. In other words, we don't yet have a unifying concept that describes just how the cell membrane fits in the overall scheme of transformation and tumor cell behavior. The relationships among "oncogenes," cell membrane changes, and transformation (see Chapter 7) will continue to be a major focus of cancer research.

Cytoskeleton Alterations in Cancer Cells

In cancer cells, microfilaments and microtubules are not well organized. They exist in pieces

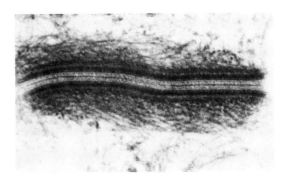

Figure 4.8 A desmosome (a type of cell-cell junction) joining two cells in a squamous cell carcinoma (× 70,000). Note the "tonofilaments" inserting into a plaque on the inner side of each plasma membrane with some filaments crossing over from cell to cell, forming a dense intercellular line. (Photo courtesy of Professor Per H. B. Carstens, Department of Pathology, University of Louisville School of Medicine)

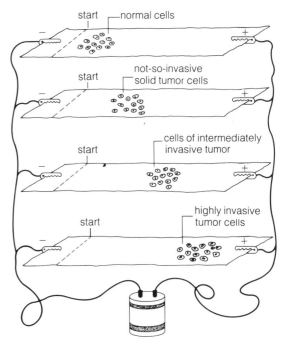

Figure 4.9 In one experiment, when normal cells and cancer cells were placed on an appropriate support strip in an electrical field, the more malignant cells moved most toward the positive pole, indicating greater electronegativity.

rather than in finished form. As indicated earlier, microfilaments and microtubules are important in maintaining the shapes of cells and in "setting" the character of the cell surface. Microfilaments and microtubules are also deranged in normal cells during division, and it is not known if this fact has any specific significance with respect to cancer.

Changes in the Nucleus and in the Regulation of Genetic Machinery

Among the changes often seen in cancer-cell machinery by which genetic plans are "translated and transcribed" into protein (Chapter 3) are the following:

1.   Transfer RNA is different; it may have too many or too few methyl groups (CH_3) attached.

2.   Some differences appear in proteins that regulate genes.

3.   Differences appear in the enzymes involved in nucleic acid synthesis.

4.   As previously pointed out, cancer cells often exhibit abnormal mitoses and they have large nuclei with prominent nucleoli.

5.   Almost all cancer cells seem to have unusual numbers of chromosomes but very few such abnormalities—such as the Philadelphia chromosome associated with leukemia (see Chapter 16)—appear to have any consistent relationship to cancer.

All these differences are potential influences of the expression of malignant state, but their actual significance is unknown.

It now appears that the most likely primary defects in malignant transformations involve normally quiescent, normal host-cell oncogenes activated in different ways by viruses and other carcinogenic agents. Some oncogenes prescribe products that activate certain enzymes—some of the same enzymes that are activated when cell-surface receptors bind to growth factors. Other oncogene products apparently mimic activated cell surface receptors and others mimic growth factors; the products of still other oncogenes regulate the expression of other genes in the nucleus. What we know of oncogenes thus far seems to suggest that they all have something to do with one or more parts of a complex chain of molecular interactions involved in the control of cell division and suggests that transformation is something that can be induced in more than one way. We will consider oncogenes and their products fully in Chapter 7. For now, let's consider some of the general things that have been discovered about regulator substances in cancer cells and some other possibilities that have been proposed.

Growth and Differentiation Inducers

Various gene-control factors have been described that induce transformation; other factors have been described that reverse or inhibit the expression of "transformedness." Perhaps such factors are balanced in normal cells, unbalanced in cancer (see Marx, 1986). Perhaps some cancer cells are unable to respond to growth-suppressor factors; perhaps others are chronically stimulated. It seems likely, in any case, that interrelated, on/off gene-regulating switches control both cell division and differentiation and that some correct sequence of switching brings the division of embryonic cells and other stem cells to a controlled endpoint. Anything that interferes with the normal cascade of gene/gene-product interaction leads to cancer—abnormal growth and differentiation.

Sachs (1986) and others, using normal and leukemic blood cells (all of which are derived from the same multipotent stem cell in the bone marrow), have isolated and characterized both growth inducers and differentiation inducers, and have found, among other things, that:

1.   Growth inducers and differentiation inducers are different proteins; growth inducers cannot cause stem cell derivatives to mature; if anything, differentiation inducers inhibit growth.

2. The actions of growth inducers and differentiation inducers are coupled. *Different* growth inducers stimulate cells at different stages of differentiation to produce *different* inducers of differentiation at different times. The result? Variable *numbers* of different *types* of differentiated cells derived from the same stem cell type. Since terminally differentiated cells usually no longer divide, differentiation must ultimately neutralize *growth* inducers.

If growth inducers induce the production of differentiation inducers that bring an end to growth, this would amount to an orderly way of reaching a final, quiet, configuration of differentiated cells. Sachs suggests that whereas normal cells depend on other cells for growth inducer, cancer cells either need little or no growth inducer, or they make their own. Cancer cells have also been found to have a defective coupling of growth and differentiation (see Sachs, 1986). Not only do the cancer cells not need growth inducer, even when it is supplied artificially, growth inducer fails to stimulate the production of differentiation inducer. The result? Steadily dividing cells that are not differentiated. Instead of a quiet configuration, cancer.

As stated earlier, all of this suggests that the normal processes of cell division and differentiation are driven and guided by a highly synchronized sequence of gene activation and gene suppression. Although the work of Sachs and others suggests that sequences involved may be complex and will thus take some time to unravel, the potential payoff in terms of possible breakthroughs in cancer therapy is enormous. Imagine, for example, how nice it would be to find differentiation inducers that cause cancer cells to differentiate and stop dividing.

Trigger Protein

In our discussion of the cell cycle in Chapter 2, it was pointed out that there is a "restriction point" in the G-1 phase of the cycle. Once the restriction point is passed, the cell is irreversibly committed to another division. The cell will either divide or literally die trying. Although it is not known what determines whether a cell will go beyond this point—what triggers cell division, in other words—cancer researchers would clearly like to know because in cancer cells, something keeps the trigger pulled. Pardee and others (see Rossow et al., 1979) have hypothesized that cells must accumulate a certain amount of an unstable "trigger" protein (also called "U," for unstable, protein) in order to reach and pass the restriction point. Any condition or thing that would tend to reduce the rate of protein synthesis by cells—say, crowding or starvation—would tend to lengthen G-1 because it would take longer for "U" protein to accumulate. Unless protein synthesis proceeds faster than "U" protein breaks down, a cell could *never* reach R. Such a model would explain many experimental observations about cell division and its control. It has been suggested that if indeed there is a "trigger protein" operative in normal cells, perhaps cancer cells make it faster or make a more stable variety. Since we don't yet know if there is such a protein, we obviously do not know yet just how it might trigger DNA synthesis, how it might be related to growth inducers, or how it otherwise sets the cell division cycle into motion.

Chalones

Skin, liver, kidney, and other tissues contain specific chemical substances able to arrest or retard the growth of cells in those specific tissues. These substances, called **chalones**, are believed to help account for the fact that organs such as the liver get just "so big" and then stop growing. Each normal liver cell theoretically produces some liver chalone. When the right number of liver cells are present, enough chalone is produced, collectively, to halt further growth of liver. If part of the liver is removed, the chalone level drops and liver cells start dividing and continue until the right number is present once again.

Could it be that cancer cells are deficient in their ability to make chalones or to respond to them? Maybe. Some cancer cells have in fact been found to contain greatly reduced chalone levels. It is not known how chalones might be related to the regulatory molecules described above.

Altered Metabolism

Biochemists and biologists have long been intrigued by the possibility that some key metabolic differences could account for all the overt differences between cancer cells and normal cells. Maybe some metabolic pathway is speeded up. Maybe some metabolic regulator fails to regulate. Such possibilities have been explored since about 1920, and many biochemical-metabolic differences have been catalogued.

In 1930 **Otto Warburg** published a book on the metabolism of tumors in which he suggested that neoplasms may originate from normal cells because of a defect in their respiratory pathways (Chapter 2) for which they compensate by increased glycolysis. Normally, glycolysis is greatly suppressed in the presence of oxygen. This phenomenon is called the **Pasteur effect**. Warburg found that cancer cells engage in anaerobic glycolysis and in a concomitant, rapid utilization of glucose even in the presence of oxygen. Although it does seem to be generally true that cancer cells burn up sugar faster than their supposed normal counterparts, the "Warburg theory" has little standing today. For one thing, any rapidly growing tissue needs more glucose; increased glycolysis is most likely a *secondary* consequence of increased rates of cell division. Also, many kinds of neoplasms have since been found to have normal glycolytic rates, and many normal tissues have been found to have glycolytic rates that *exceed* those of tumors. Cancer cells apparently do *not* have a universal defect in their ability to "respire."

Twenty-five years ago, **Jesse Greenstein** published *The Biochemistry of Cancer*, in which he proposed that all tumors seemed to share certain common enzymatic patterns—including some that had to do with respiration. This proposal also fell by the wayside as exceptions were catalogued.

Other attempts have been made to formulate similar "unifying" descriptions of cancer biochemistry, but none have stood up. When **Harold Morris** developed his series of transplantable liver tumor lines*—all derived from rat liver—it quickly became clear that tumor cells have widely different biochemical characteristics, even when the tumors come from the same organ of the same species.

Over the last few decades, **George Weber** (1972, 1977) and his coworkers took advantage of the fact that the Morris hepatomas spanned a wide range of growth rates and degrees of differentiation to see if there were any correlations between enzyme patterns and growth rate and/or differentiation. Although correlations have been found, certain pathways are enhanced and others diminished with increasing growth rate, and so forth, it is most likely that these are all *secondary* effects. They happen because cells *are* dividing and are not likely the *cause* of uncontrolled division.

The bottom line? Cancer cells do generally have certain metabolic features in common—features they share with other rapidly dividing cells such as those found in embryos and fetuses. There is no evidence for any key metabolic change that accounts for the difference between normal cells and cancer cells.

---

*Morris ultimately developed dozens of transplantable hepatoma lines that came to be known as the **Morris hepatomas**. All the lines were induced by feeding rats carcinogens and then transplanting the resulting tumors from rat to rat over many transplant generations. Morris made the lines available worldwide to investigators interested in them because they exhibited a spectrum of growth rates ranging from fast to slow and a spectrum of degrees of differentiation. They enabled scientists to study the ramifications of metabolic and other features of malignancy in cells that otherwise came from the same organ of the same species.

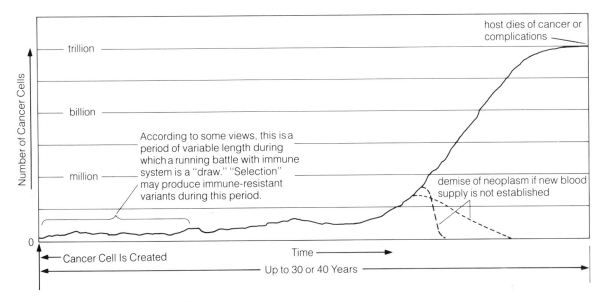

According to some views, this is a period of variable length during which a running battle with immune system is a "draw." "Selection" may produce immune-resistant variants during this period.

host dies of cancer or complications

demise of neoplasm if new blood supply is not established

Number of Cancer Cells

trillion

billion

million

0

Cancer Cell Is Created

Time

Up to 30 or 40 Years

Figure 4.10 The generalized natural history of a neoplasm

Tumorigenesis

The term *tumorigenesis* refers to the development of a neoplasm after the initial carcinogenic event—after a cancer cell first appears. It is far more than simple cell division that carries the initial cancer to the large mass stage, where it may contain billions or even trillions of cancer cells.

The natural history of a typical tumor is depicted in Figure 4.10. It would be impossible for a few cancer cells to graduate to a large mass without lots of help. Cancer cells need to be nourished and oxygenated just like any other living cells. If simply divided, they would quickly outgrow their blood supply and they would then wither and die. They flourish—temporarily, at least, because they are somehow able to induce the development of blood vessels and they somehow induce the development of supporting structures—connective tissue and intercellular cement.

As it grows, a neoplasm may wage a running war with the host's immune system, the survivors possibly becoming increasingly resistant to the immune system. A neoplasm evolves—its more slowly dividing cells fall by the wayside, and the fast-growing cells "take over." In a "malignant progression," the tumor becomes increasingly hostile. In some cases, selective progression is actually accelerated by therapy. The most susceptible cancer cells are killed by initial treatment, leaving the more resistant cells to survive. At some point in the process of tumorigenesis, cells begin to invade adjacent tissues and ultimately break away to metastasize. The next chapter is devoted to invasion and metastasis.

Summary

Many things happen to cells as they become cancer cells. Although a few of these changes may be the keys to all the others, no particular feature of malignant cells has yet been found to have such fundamental importance. Among the possible key expressions of "oncogenes" still under active consideration are protease secretion, decreased cAMP and increased cGMP, and altered cytoskeleton, altered glycoprotein and glycolipids on the cell surface.

The quest continues. It is driven both by the desire to fully understand the basic biology of tumors and to identify differences that can be exploited in detection, diagnosis, and treatment of cancer—even before the biology is fully understood.

References and Further Reading

Abercrombie, M. 1975. The Contact Behavior of Invading Cells. In *Cellular Membranes and Tumor-Cell Behavior*. Baltimore, Md.: Williams and Wilkins.

Bell, G. I. 1978. Models for the Specific Adhesion of Cells to Cells. *Science*. 200:618–27.

Blau, H. M., Pavlath, G. K., Hardeman, E. C., et al. 1985. Plasticity of the Differentiated State. *Science*. 230:758–66.

Bog-Hansen, T., ed. 1981. *Lectins-Biology, Biochemistry, Clinical Biochemistry*, Vols. 1–3. New York: DeGruyter.

Bretscher, M. 1984. Endocytosis: Relations to Capping and Cell Locomotion. *Science*. 224:681–86.

Burger, M. M. 1975. Surface Properties of Neoplastic Cells. In Weissmann, G., and Claiborne, R., eds. *Cell Membranes*. New York: Hospital Practice.

Chen, L. B., Gallimore, P. H., and McDougall, J. K. 1976. Correlation Between Tumor Induction and the Large External Transformation Sensitive Protein on the Cell Surface. *Proc. Natl. Acad. Sci.* 73:3570.

Coleman, P. L., Fisherman, P. H., Brady, R. O., and Todaro, G. J. 1975. Altered Ganglioside Biosynthesis in Mouse Cell Cultures Following Transformation with Chemical Carcinogens and X-irradiation. *J. Biol. Chem.* 250:55.

Coman, D. R. 1944. Decreased Mutual Adhesiveness, a Property of Cells from Squamous Cell Carcinomas. *Cancer Res.* 4:625–29.

Curtis, A., and Pitts, J., eds. 1980. *Cell Adhesion and Motility*. Cambridge Univ. Press.

Edelman, G. M. 1976. Surface Modulation in Cell Recognition and Cell Growth. *Science*. 192:218–26.

Fishman, P. H., and Brady, R. O. 1976. Biosynthesis and Function of Gangliosides. *Science*. 194:906–15.

Freshney, R. I. 1983. *Culture of Animal Cells: A Manual of Basic Technique*. New York: Liss.

Gottlieb, A. A., Plescia, O. J., and Bishop, K. H. L., eds. 1975. *Fundamental Aspects of Neoplasia*. New York: Springer-Verlag.

Hall, S. S. 1985. The Fate of the Egg. *Science 85*. November, pp. 40–49.

Hatanaka, M. 1974. Transport of Sugars in Tumor Cell Membrane. *Biochim. Biophys. Acta*. 355:77.

Hynes, R. O. 1979. *Surfaces of Normal and Malignant Cells*. New York: Wiley.

Hynes, R. O. 1986. Fibronectins. *Scientific American*. 254(6):42–51.

Inbar, M., Rabinowitz, A., and Sachs, L. 1969. The Formation of Variants with a Reversion of Properties of Transformed Cells. III. Reversion of the Structure of the Cell-Surface Membrane. *Int. J. Cancer*. 4:690.

Kolata, G. B. 1975. Microvilli: A Major Difference Between Normal and Cancer Cells? *Science*. 188:819–20.

Mannino, R. J., and Burger, M. M. 1975. Growth Control and the Mitotic Cell Surface. In Gottlieb, A. A., Plescia, O. J., and Bishop, K. H. L., *Fundamental Aspects of Neoplasia*. New York: Springer-Verlag.

Marx, J. L. 1976. Cell Biology: Cell Surfaces and the Regulation of Mitosis. *Science*. 192:455–57.

Marx, J. L. 1974. Biochemistry of Cancer Cells: Focus on the Cell Surface. *Science*. 183:1279–82.

Marx, J. L. 1986. The Yin and Yang of Cell Growth Control. *Science*. 232:1093–95.

Moscona, A. A. 1956. Development of Heterotypic Combinations of Dissociated Embryonic Chick Cells. *Proc. Soc. Expl. Biol. Med.* 92:410–16.

Nicolson, G. L. 1976. Transmembrane Control of the Receptors in Normal and Tumor Cells. II. Surface Changes Associated with Transformation and Malignancy. *Biochim. Biophys. Acta*. 450:1.

Nicolson, G. L., and Poste, G. 1976. The Cancer Cell: Dynamic Aspects and Modification in Cell Surface Organization. *New England J. Med.* 295(4):197–203.

Nicolson, G. L., and Poste, G. 1976. The Cancer Cell: Dynamic Aspects and Modification in Cell Surface Organization (Second of Two Parts). *New England J. Med.* 295(5):253–57.

Pastan, I. H., Johnson, G. S., and Anderson, W. B. 1975. Role of Cyclic Nucleotides in Growth Control. *Ann. Rev. Biochem.* 44:491–522.

Pitot, H. C. 1974. Neoplasia. A Somatic Mutation or a Heritable Change in Cytoplasmic Membranes? *Journal of the National Cancer Institute.* 53:905–11.

Pitot, H. C. 1978. *Fundamentals of Oncology.* New York: Dekker.

Pollack, R. E., and Hough, P. V. C. 1975. The Cell Surface and Malignant Transformation. *Ann. Rev. Med.* 25:431.

Rapin, A. M. C., and Burger, M. M. 1975. Tumor Cell Surfaces: General Alterations Detected by Agglutinins. *Advances in Cancer Res.* 20:1–91.

Robbins, S. L., and Cottran, R. 1984. Pathologic Basis of Disease. Philadelphia: Saunders.

Rossow, P. W., Riddle, V. G., and Pardee, A. B. 1979. Synthesis of Labile, Serum-Dependent Protein in Early G_1 Controls Animal Growth. *Proc. Natl. Acad. Sci., USA.* 76:4446–50.

Ruddon, R. W. 1981. *Cancer Biology.* New York: Oxford University Press.

Rüdiger, H. 1984. On the Physiological Role of Plant Lectins. *Bioscience.* 34(2):95–99.

Rush, B. F., and Blackwood, J. 1980. How Do Cancers Grow? *Contemporary Surgery.* 17:41–55.

Sachs, L. 1986. Growth, Differentiation and the Reversal of Malignancy. *Scientific American.* 254:40–47.

Sharon, N. 1974. Glycoproteins. *Scientific American.* 230(5):78–86.

Sharon, N. 1977. Lectins. *Scientific American.* 236(6):108–16, 118–9.

Smets, L. A., and Van Beek, W. P. 1984. Carbohydrates of the Tumor Cell Surface. *Biochim. Biophys. Acta.* 738:237–49.

Symington, T., and Carter, R. L. 1976. *Scientific Foundations of Oncology.* Chicago: Heinemann Medical Books/Yearbook Medical Publishers.

Thompkins, G. M. 1975. The Metabolic Code. *Science.* 189:760–63.

Weber, G. 1972. Molecular Correlation Concept: Ordered Pattern of Gene Expression in Neoplasia. GANN Monograph on Cancer Research 13:47–77.

Weber, G. 1977. Enzymology of Cancer Cells (First of Two Parts). *New England J. Med.* 296(9):486–92.

Weinhouse, S. 1973. Metabolism and Isozyme Alterations in Experimental Hepatomas. *Federation Proc.* 32:2162–67.

Willingham, M. C., Yamada, K. M., Yamada, S. S., et al. 1977. Micro-filament Bundles and Cell Shape Are Related to Adhesiveness to Substratum and Are Dissociable from Growth Control in Cultured Fibroblasts. *Cell.* 10:375–80.

Neoplasms?? This is supposed to be a book about cancer! Well, it is, but it is also a book about the abnormal growth of cells—neoplasms if you will, the most important of which is cancer—or malignant neoplasms or malignant tumors, or malignancies . . .

We need to define a few terms before we go on.

5

Classifying and Naming Neoplasms

A Dictionary of Oncology

Tumor   A swelling; a defined mass of tissue (such as a neoplasm) or accumulation of fluid that is not part of normal body architecture.

Neoplasm   Literally, a new growth; a defined mass of tissue that is not part of normal body architecture *and that results from cell division* outside the influence of normal growth regulation. "Tumor" is a more general term. When is a tumor not a neoplasm?—When it, the "lump," is a result of something *other* than cell division; a parasitic mass or a chronic abscess, for example.

Lesion   Any diseased tissue, including neoplasms.

Neoplasia   The process by which a neoplasm arises—the relatively autonomous growth of cells.

Hyperplasia   "Extra" cellular growth resulting in a larger than usual number of cells (Fig. 5.1). A "normal" example of hyperplasia is callus formation. A good pathological example is a toxic goiter of the thyroid, in which excess thyroid hormone is produced.

Hypertrophy   An increase in size of some organ or tissue resulting from an increase in size of the cells, but not in the number of cells. A good example is the increase in the size of the racket arm of a tennis player.

Metaplasia   Process by which one normal cell type is replaced by another normal cell type (Fig. 5.2). An example is the replacement of columnar epithelium by squamous epithelium (see Chapter 3). Squamous metaplasia occurs in the lung in response to irritation by cigarette smoke, for example. This metaplasia is apparently caused by the redirection of epithelial stem cells, usually as a response to the environment.

Dysplasia Disordered tissue; a condition in which cells are abnormally variable in size, shape, and organization (Fig. 5.3).

Although dysplasia and metaplasia do *not necessarily* give rise to cancer, some types of dysplasia—dysplasia of the uterus, for example—may indeed be a first stage of a progression of changes leading to frank malignancy (see the section on "precancerous conditions" below).

Anaplasia Tissue composed of very primitive-looking cells lacking the normally high degree of tissue organization and resembling early embryonal tissue (Fig. 5.3). The term *undifferentiated* is very nearly identical to *anaplastic*, the adjective derived from *anaplasia*.

Benign neoplasm A neoplasm that is incapable of metastasis (see entry for *metastasis*). Benign neoplasms are often encapsulated; their cells are usually similar to normal cells; they usually grow slowly and exhibit few mitotic figures (Fig. 5.4).

Malignant neoplasm Cancer; a neoplasm that *does* invade and metastasize. Malignant neoplasms are not usually encapsulated; the cells

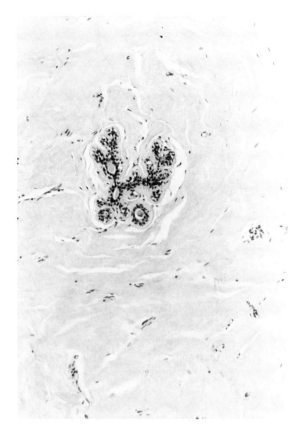

Figure 5.1 An example of benign hyperplasia. Sclerosing adenosis (with fibrosis) of the lobular epithelium of the breast. This condition is common in older women. (× 65). (Photo courtesy of Professor Per H. B. Carstens, Department of Pathology, University of Louisville School of Medicine)

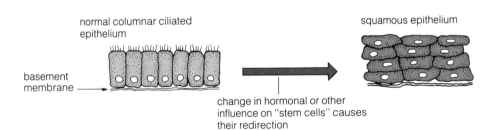

Figure 5.2 Squamous metaplasia. **Metaplasia** is the replacement of normal tissue structure with some other kind of *normal* structure. Shown here is squamous metaplasia, a condition in which normal *columnar* epithelium is replaced by normal *squamous* epithelium. Metaplasia is apparently the result of the "redirection" of stem cells by changes in environmental influences. Under normal local environmental influences, these stem cells give rise to columnar cells. When hormone stress levels or other influences change, the same stem cells give rise to squamous cells.

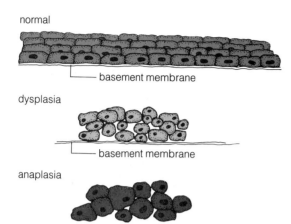

normal

basement membrane

dysplasia

basement membrane

anaplasia

Figure 5.3 Dysplasia is a condition in which the normal "ordered" and "regular" appearance of tissue gives way to tissue in which the cells are irregular in shape, size, and organization. **Anaplasia** is a condition in which the normal, "ordered," and "regular" appearance of cells in tissue gives way to tissue in which cells look primitive—like the cells in an early embryo.

of most malignant neoplasms are relatively undifferentiated (anaplastic); and malignant neoplasms sometimes grow much more rapidly than normal tissue (Fig. 5.4).

The most important difference between benign and malignant neoplasms is the potential for metastasis. Although there are (also) normal cells that abnormally spread to other locations (see Chapter 6), this migration is so rare and relatively inconsequential that metastasis is the closest thing to an absolute difference between normal cells and cancer cells that there is. All other differences are much more relative.

Malignant tumor In practice, this term has the same meaning as "malignant neoplasm." Technically, however, "malignant neoplasm" has the more precise meaning. See the distinction between tumor and neoplasm, made earlier.

Cancer In everyday use, this word is a synonym for "malignant neoplasm." The word *cancer* is derived from Greek and Latin words for "crab." Supposedly the invasive growth pattern of malignant neoplasms looked to some early physicians like a crab.

Malignancy This is another synonym for "malignant neoplasm."

Primary malignant neoplasm (or *primary malignant tumor*) A malignant neoplasm in its position of origin—as opposed to a secondary tumor, which is a metastatic mass.

Oncology Literally, the study of tumors, but in practice the study of malignant neoplasms or the study of cancer.

Metastasis Secondary neoplasm derived from a neoplasm that originated in another location.

Benign or Malignant?

When the pathologist looks at a biopsy of a tumor under the microscope, the most important decision to be made is whether to call the tumor benign or malignant. If the pathologist considers it benign, this means that he or she does not expect the tumor to metastasize and, unless it is in a "bad" location or happens to be producing harmful secretions, it is not likely to harm the patient. If the pathologist says "malignant," on the other hand, his or her belief is that the tumor *is* aggressive and may spread to other locations. While a doctor may suspect benign or malignant conditions just by seeing a neoplasm grossly, it is not until the pathologist looks at the tumor under a microscope that the definitive diagnosis can be made.

Since the pathologist cannot watch the cells of a tumor "behave," he or she has to rely on morphological features and other indirect information in assessing the fundamental character of a neoplasm. What do pathologists look for?

Benign neoplasms usually have a smooth, round contour; sometimes they even have a capsule of connective tissue surrounding them (Fig. 5.4a). Benign tumors tend to have orderly cellular arrangements and the cells tend to be well differentiated; that is, they resemble the normal cells of the tissue in which they arise. **Malignant neoplasms**, on the other hand have irregular borders projecting into (invading) adjacent tissue; the arrangement of cells is not orderly; individual cells vary greatly in shape and size; they have large nuclei with prominent nucleoli, and the nuclei are hyperchromic (are colored darkly with nuclear stains); some of the cells may be caught undergoing mitosis; and some of the mitotic figures may be abnormal. Unfortunately, these distinctions do not always hold up; the criteria for malignancy may be different even for different kinds of cancer arising in the same organ.

Over the years, pathologists have recorded the outcome regarding various types of malignant neoplasms arising in different organs in different kinds of patients. The long-term follow-up of patients with neoplasms of particular morphologic and histologic types has revealed that each type of cancer has a particular natural history with characteristic sequences of progression. To take advantage of the predictive value of this historical record, the pathologist needs information other than what can be extracted from the biopsy in order to make a **diagnosis** (name the condition). It may be helpful, for example, to know the tumor's exact location, its color, and other gross features. For some tumors, the age and sex of the patient may be all-important in arriving at an exact diagnosis and at a **prognosis** (prediction of what is likely to happen).

Benign Tumors That "Look" Malignant

Complicating the life of surgical pathologists considerably is the existence of lesions, some of them not even neoplastic, that *look like* invasive cancer. Certain benign adenomas of the breast look so much like cancer that they have resulted in unnecessary mastectomies. Mononucleosis, rheumatoid arthritis, and *Herpes zoster* infections sometimes produce hyperplasias of lymph nodes that resemble lymphomas (Rosai and Ackerman, 1979). Will it be drastic surgery, conservative surgery, or no surgery? The surgeon waits for the pathologist to tell him or her "how

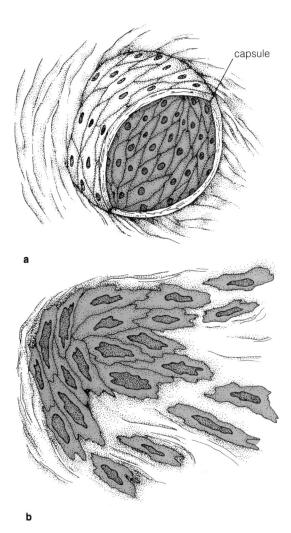

Figure 5.4 "The Good, the Bad, and the Malignant" . . . (**a**) The cells of **benign neoplasms** look almost normal, they grow slowly, and the benign neoplasm tends to remain encapsulated. The cells of benign neoplasms do not invade, and they do not metastasize. (**b**) The cells of **malignant neoplasms** range from looking *somewhat* different to looking *much* different from normal cells; they grow invasively, and they tend to metastasize. Malignant neoplasms tend not to be encapsulated.

badly the tumor is likely to behave" from the appearance of the cells under the microscope.

The work of a surgical pathologist can be compared in some respects to deciding from a photograph of a crowd of people which of the crowd are apt to misbehave. With most tumors this is not much of a problem; it's almost as if the "good guys" wore white hats and the "bad guys" all wore black hats. Masses of most kinds of cancer cells are practically unmistakable. In some cases, it is not so easy, however. The morphology and biological behavior of tumors do not always match up.

The Further Classification of Neoplasms

The most basic and most useful division of neoplasms is that based on behavior, the two divisions being "benign" and "malignant." The next most basic division is that based on the kind of tissue that gives rise to the tumor. One such logical grouping is the following (Ritchie, 1962):

Neoplasms of epithelial tissue

Neoplasms of connective tissue

Neoplasms of blood cell-generating and immune system tissue (this is a special division of connective tissue neoplasms; there are many important kinds of cancer in this category and so it gets a "division" of its own)

Neoplasms of nervous tissue

Neoplasms that contain cells of more than one kind of stem cell origin

Miscellaneous neoplasms

Benign neoplasms of epithelial tissue include warts (**epidermal papillomas**) and gastric polyps. The corresponding malignant neoplasms of epithelial tissue include epidermoid squamous cell carcinomas (skin cancer) and gastric carcinoma (stomach cancer).

Benign neoplasms of connective tissue include fibromas and osteomas. Fibrosarcomas

and osteogenic sarcomas are examples of malignant neoplasms of connective tissue.

There are both benign and malignant neoplasms that arise from blood cell-generating (**hematopoietic**) and immune system tissues; Hodgkin's disease and leukemia are two relatively common malignant examples. There are also benign and malignant counterparts arising from nerve tissue. A neuroma is benign; a neuroblastoma is malignant.

Tumors of mixed or multiple origins consist of more than one type of tissue. An adenofibroma, for example, consists of both epithelial cells and a fibrous stroma. Such neoplasms are commonly found in the breasts of younger women.

Immunohistochemical Classification

The National Cancer Institute recently set out to systematically evaluate solid tumors to see if the *antigens* present in tumors can be used to classify the neoplasms. If it turns out that certain antigens *can* be correlated with tumor behavior, then perhaps a more fine-tuned system of classification can be established—along the lines of tests used to identify bacteria. Such a system would take some of the guesswork out of selecting anticancer drugs and would improve the accuracy of prognoses. *Immunohistochemical* refers to methods by which cellular antigens—including particular enzymes or other characteristic components of particular types of cells—can be identified by reaction with antibodies the evidence for which can be seen under the light microscope or electron microscope. These tools enable the pathologist to refine the identification of particular types of cells. We will discuss this topic further in the chapter on detection and diagnosis.

An Imperfect System of Names and Naming

As strange as it might seem, there is no single system of naming malignant neoplasms in use throughout the world. The World Health Organization (WHO) recognized as early as 1952 that a universally accepted classification by histologic type was essential for all tumors if treatment results and mortality rates from different institutions and different countries were to be evaluable. Committees of pathologists from member nations have established standard nomenclature for at least 24 tumor sites (WHO, 1978), but much work is still to be done.

A generalization about naming tumors that *nearly* always holds true is that benign neoplasms have names containing a fragment of the name of the tissue from which the neoplasm arises plus the suffix "-oma." **Neuromas** are benign tumors of nerve tissue; **chondromas** are benign neoplasms of cartilage; and **fibromas** are benign tumors of fibrous connective tissue.

Unfortunately, more than a few exceptions exist to this general system of naming neoplasms. **Hepatomas** are not, as the name implies, benign; they are malignant neoplasms of liver cells. And a melanoma is really a malignant neoplasm, as is myeloma.

Malignant neoplasms are subdivided according to the type of tissue from which they arise. **Sarcomas** (*sarc-* "fleshy"; *oma-* "neoplasm") come from tissue that arises from mesoderm or mesenchymal tissues. **Carcinomas** are malignant neoplasms that arise in epithelial tissue.

Carcinoma in situ (in place) is a designation used for localized carcinomas that have all the characteristics of malignancy but that have not yet penetrated the basement membrane (Chapter 3). Left untreated, carcinoma *in situ* will almost invariably progress to invasive cancer.

So! The names of neoplasms *sometimes* indicate benign or malignant and the embryonic tissue of origin. They also indicate other important features. Some names of tumors indicate the organ from which the tumor arises; for example, a **gastric carcinoma** arises from the epithelial tissue of the stomach (the prefix *gastro-* means "stomach"). Other names of tumors are based on the name of the individual who gave the first complete description of that tumor, such as

Hodgkin's disease, Wilms' tumor, and Burkitt's lymphoma. "Papillary" (or parts of the word *papillary*) describes a particular growth form of a neoplasm. An **epidermal papilloma**, for example, is a benign neoplasm arising in the epidermis and that grows in a "papillary" form—as a fingerlike projection. **Epidermal papilloma** is another name for a wart.

Many traits revealed in a neoplasm's name have practical importance for cancer therapy. Just having a name—even one that may not be very descriptive—serves the purpose of linking a very particular form of cancer to all past medical experience with that *particular* cancer. Historical experience, in turn, gives the therapist and, indirectly, the patient a basis on which to develop expectations. Different kinds of cancer can behave *very* differently even when they arise from the same tissue of the same organ. Consider skin cancer, for example.

There are three very distinct behavioral types of skin cancer. **Basal cell carcinomas** of the skin only rarely metastasize, and even then the appearance of secondary neoplasms usually takes many, many years. Basal cell carcinomas are almost always curable, even when therapy is initiated very late. **Squamous cell carcinoma** is more likely to spread, and usually does so via the lymphatics. In sharp contrast to these two types, malignant melanoma—a neoplasm that arises from the pigment cells of the skin—metastasizes so fast that the metastases are sometimes discovered *before* the *primary* tumor has been identified.

Also, neoplasms of the *same* basic tissue type can behave quite differently in different organs. It is not enough to know that one is dealing with a squamous cell carcinoma. Squamous cell carcinomas of the lung bronchi tend to cross the basement membrane very early and to metastasize via the myriad blood vessels of the lung. Probably because the uterine cervix is poorly vascularized in comparison to the lung, squamous cell carcinomas of the cervix metastasize late, usually only after they have become fairly large.

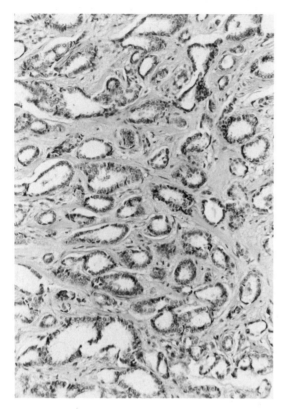

Figure 5.5 A well-differentiated neoplasm—tubular carcinoma of the breast. Note the tubules lined with uniform epithelial cells and surrounded by abundant fibrous tissue. This neoplasm is malignant and—although it rarely does so—it can invade blood vessels and lymphatics and metastasize (× 60). (Photo courtesy of Professor Per H. B. Carstens, Department of Pathology, University of Louisville School of Medicine)

Grading and Staging

Before treatment can be started or even planned, the physician must know as much about the tumor as possible. Basically, the physician must know (1) what the tumor has in fact done so far (extent), and (2) what it is likely to do from the point of detection on. Determining the extent is called **staging**; stating what the neoplasm is *likely* to do is called **grading**. Grading is based on the morphological appearance of the tumor cells; specifically, the degree of their departure

from normal states of differentiation (degree of anaplasia). This analysis is made with a microscope, by a pathologist.

For most cancers, three grades are used. **Grade I neoplasms** closely resemble normal tissue and are said to be well differentiated (Fig. 5.5). **Grade II neoplasms** are moderately differentiated, and **Grade III neoplasms** are those that are poorly differentiated (Fig. 5.6). While grading has little prognostic value with certain kinds of cancer—melanoma, for example—it is *highly* correlated with prognosis with other kinds of cancer. For chondrosarcomas of bone for example, the five-year survival rate is 78 percent for well-differentiated variants but only 22 percent for poorly differentiated types (Rosai and Ackerman, 1979). In general, grading is a useful way of linking specific subtypes of neoplasms to the prospects of patient survival (**prognosis**) and to the likely effectiveness of different therapeutic approaches.

The International Union Against Cancer and the American Joint Committee on Cancer have attempted to standardize the clinical staging of cancer by means of the so-called **TNM system**. The "T" here represents the tumor itself and refers to the degree of *local* extension of the primary tumor or its size. The "N" stands for "nodes" and refers to the extension of the tumor to regional and distant lymph nodes. The "M" represents "metastasis" and refers to whether or not the tumor has spread to distant sites. The TNM system considers each of these factors in order in arriving at the degree of advancement or at the developmental stage of a neoplasm.

The overall staging of a neoplasm is accomplished by some combination of several approaches. **Clinical staging** is the estimation of the extent of disease, arrived at by direct physical examination, blood tests, and by looking at the tumor indirectly via X-rays or directly by **endoscopic examination** (looking inside the body with a light tube). **Radiographic staging** is done via CAT scans, arteriography, or radioisotopic scanning (see Chapter 16). **Surgical staging** is done by exploring the extent of the tumor surgically.

Staging serves several purposes. The stage of a neoplasm in a particular patient is an indicator of the chances of that patient surviving. Staging also helps therapists plan treatment. If, for example, it is known that a particular breast neoplasm has already spread to the brain and to bone, there is no need to do radical, mutilating surgery designed to "get all" of the tumor. The rigorous use of staging information also makes possible the comparison of the results of experimental treatments at different institutions—it makes it more likely that "apples are being, and will be, compared with apples." This comparability is important, because a drug that might be very effective at one stage may have little or no effect at a more advanced stage.

The degree or correlation between prospect for survival and stage varies from one kind of cancer to another. In general, however, tumors are often completely curable in their early stages. A general example is epithelial cell cancers in which the tumor has not yet penetrated the basement membrane (Chapter 3). A more specific example: colon cancer of "Dukes" System Stage A (meaning that the tumor is restricted to the bowel wall) gives the patient a 90 percent probability of living beyond five years. At Stage C, wherein the tumor has spread to regional lymph nodes, five-year survival is reduced to 20 percent (Rosai and Ackerman, 1979).*

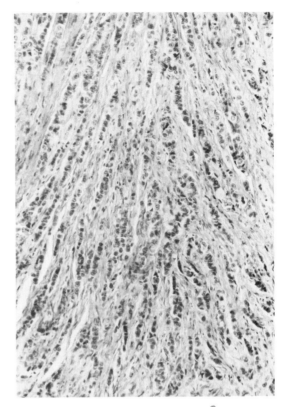

Figure 5.6 A poorly differentiated neoplasm. Infiltrating ductal carcinoma of the breast. Note the malignant cells growing in trabeculae (rows) without any lumina surrounded by fibrous tissue ($\times$ 60). (Photo courtesy of Professor Per H. B. Carstens, University of Louisville School of Medicine)

Precancerous Lesions and Conditions

A number of growth irregularities of tissue are called "precancerous." This term has been applied so indiscriminately, however, that it has little meaning in denoting the actual potential for giving rise to cancer. For some precancerous conditions, the development of cancer is inevi-

table. For others, the "extra" risk of cancer can be disregarded.

Human beings with a genetic condition called **familial polyposis** in which the inside surface of the colon is covered with fleshy projections called **polyps** (Fig. 5.7) have a definite high risk of developing colon cancer—usually in their early thirties. So great is the risk that patients with familial polyposis are regularly advised to consider having their colons removed even before any cancer is detectable. On the other hand, **adenomatous polyps** of the colon are relatively unlikely to give rise to cancer. Still other kinds of polyps of the colon are apparently free of *any* malignant potential.

---

*Duke's classification** is used by pathologists in reporting the results of their examination of resected colorectal cancer surgical specimens. Duke's A = to, but not through the muscle layer of the bowel; Duke's B = through muscle layer to outer casing of bowel; Duke's C = to regional mesenteric lymph nodes.

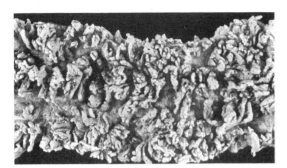

Figure 5.7 Multiple polyposis of the colon. (Photo courtesy of Professor Per H. B. Carstens, University of Louisville School of Medicine)

A heritable precancerous condition in which the development of cancer is inevitable is **xeroderma pigmentosum**. Xeroderma pigmentosum is a skin disease caused by defective repair mechanisms for the DNA damage induced by ultraviolet light. This condition, which is marked by an ultrasensitivity to sunlight, gives rise to basal cell carcinomas, squamous cell carcinomas, and malignant melanomas. The victims often die of cancer before age 20 (Rosai and Ackerman, 1979).

Another precancerous lesion truly associated with malignancy is **Hutchinson's freckle**, a flat, pigmented growth irregularity most often found in the cheeks of elderly patients. It is generally thought that if a patient with Hutchinson's freckle lives long enough, a malignant melanoma will arise from the freckle.

Other "precancerous conditions" with a relatively *low* risk of cancer include **leucoplakia** of the mouth and other mucous membranes (marked by atypical epithelial tissue structure), uterine epithelial dysplasias and hyperplasias, and Paget's disease of bone (gives rise to osteosarcoma and other bone cancers).

Summary

The most important determination to be made about a neoplasm is whether it is benign or malignant, and this is not always a straightforward, simple matter. Some benign tumors look malignant, and there is uncertainty about the malignant potential of certain "precancerous" conditions. After the exact location and tissue of origin of a neoplasm are pinpointed, some additional prognostic information may be derived by determining the "grade" of the malignancy—how well differentiated the cells are. Staging is the determination of how far advanced a cancer happens to be.

The advance of cancer is the subject of the next chapter.

References and Further Reading

Elias, J. 1982. *Principles and Techniques in Diagnostic Histopathology.* Park Ridge, N.J.: Noyes.

Ritchie, A. C. 1962. The Classification, Morphology and Behavior of Tumors. In H. Florey, ed., *General Pathology.* Philadelphia: Saunders.

Robbins, S. L., and Cotran, R. 1984. *Pathologic Basis of Disease.* Philadelphia: Saunders.

Rosai, J., and Ackerman, L. V. 1979. *The Pathology of Tumors.* American Cancer Society Professional Education Publication. New York: American Cancer Society.

World Health Organization. 1978. *A Coded Compendium of the International Histological Classification of Tumors.* Geneva: World Health Organization.

In his book *Recherches du Cancer,* published in 1820, the French physician Joseph Claude Anselme Recamier (1774–1852) introduced the term *metastasis* to describe the *secondary* growth of cancer in the brain of a patient with breast cancer. This description carried the understanding of cancer a step beyond the earlier recognition of local invasion and the spread of cancer to regional lymph nodes. Medicine quickly came to recognize metastasis as the crux of the cancer problem.

Were it not for metastasis, curing cancer would be a simple matter because surgery would almost always achieve cure. But metastasis spreads destruction to critical organs throughout the body, which makes cancer impossible to simply excise. Metastasis is clearly the worst feature of a disease that is sometimes simplistically described as "the uncontrolled division of cells." Thus one key to finding a cure is a better understanding of those factors that influence the detachment of cells from the primary tumor, their movement into the circulation, and their implantation in other locations (Fig. 6.1). We have some idea what these factors are, but we are a long way from a complete understanding.

6

The Spread of Cancer

Invasion and Metastasis

Cancer Cells and Cells That Are Similar

Some normal cells of the human body can move about. In their role as scavengers and defenders, white blood cells (leucocytes) can leave blood vessels and "invade" tissue in response to infection, trauma, and other stimuli. Leucocytes thus share some key behavioral features with cancer cells, but there are some important differences. An especially important difference is that blood cells normally lose their ability to divide when they enter the general circulation. Cancer cells do *not* surrender this option.

Invasion and metastasis also resemble the behavior of the cells of normal embryos. Embryonic cells migrate, they invade, and they establish new growth where they come to rest. We saw in the preceding chapter that embryonic cells differ from cancer cells in that *embryonic cells follow a genetic program that has a nonchaotic end point*—namely, the limited development of tissue having a functional interrelationship with all other tissues.

Still other examples of noncancer cells express metastatic behavior. Cells from the chorion (one of the membranes of the placenta) can be found surviving in lungs of pregnant women (Tarin, 1976). Such cells nearly always die shortly after the birth of the fetus when the hormone environment changes—but then, certain types of cancer respond to hormonal changes in a similar fashion. Pitot (1978) points out that viable bone-marrow fat cells sometimes spread to distant sites after fractures. Another example is the spread of endometrial cells (cells from the lining of the uterus) to various locations in the abdomen (**endometriosis**).

All of the foregoing examples suggest that there may be something to learn about metastasis by studying normal cells. Perhaps all cells capable of exhibiting invasive and/or metastatic properties share some key chemical or surface structural features.

Metastasis as an Entity and a Process

The metastatic sequence is illustrated in Figure 6.2. Metastasis begins with local invasion and ends with secondary tumors at remote sites. Between these points are a number of discrete steps that include (1) continuous extension of the tumor along paths of least resistance; (2) detachment of cells, or clumps of cells, that are disseminated via lymphatics and blood vessels; (3) arrest of tumor cells at distant sites; and (4) reinvasion by the tumor cells, this time out of the circulation into tissues where (5) the tumor cells secrete various factors that help create an environment conducive to the growth of the secondary tumor.

The Stages of Metastasis

Invasion

Except for the amoeboid movement that enables lymphocytes and other cells of the immune system to move in and out of tissue spaces, the tissues of the human body are normally *not* freely permeable to the migration of cells. This leads to the question, what is it about the cancer cell and its cell surface that enables it to invade?

Willis (1973) and Nicolson et al. (1977) list at least five factors that are possibly important in enabling invasiveness: (1) pressure buildup resulting from the expanding mass (producing mechanical forces that figuratively "inject" cancer cells into tissue), (2) cell motility (cancer cell motility is relatively uninhibited by contact), (3) loss of cellular adhesiveness (changes in cell properties such as adhesiveness could make cancer cells "slippery"), (4) phagocytic properties (cancer cells may eat their way out), and (5) production of toxins or enzymes that, respectively, damage and digest adjacent tissues, allowing cancer to extend. It may be that all of these factors are important in invasion by cancer cells.

Pressure and Fracture Lines Perhaps the first thing that the crablike extension of cancer into normal tissue suggests, is that the extension is a result of the buildup of pressure. Uncontrolled division would certainly produce rather densely packed, expanding masses of cells that must certainly exert pressure on adjacent tissues. Indeed, tumors do seem to extend into normal tissue along "natural fracture lines"—into spaces that could be expected by an architect to "part" in response to pressure (see Easty and Easty, 1976).

Further support for this concept is that expanding tumors often seem to be stopped by "capsules"; that is, by architectural barriers to fracture. Kidney capsules, for example, seem to be able to contain tumors and to limit—or at least redirect their extension.

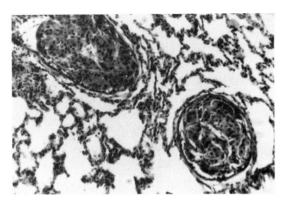

Figure 6.1 Two clusters of metastatic hepatoma cells in the lung of a rat (× 30). (Photo by the author. Originally published in C. E. Kupchella et al., 1981. Used by permission.)

Pressure spreading is an attractive hypothesis. However, apparently it does not tell the whole story. Cancers in experimental systems in which pressure is *known* to be *non*existent still exhibit invasiveness, clearly indicating that pressure is not the *only* factor involved.

Enzymes / Spreading Factors Do cancer cells digest their way through normal tissues by secreting enzymes? At one time it was a popular notion that certain kinds of bacteria had the ability to secrete hyaluronidase, an enzyme that digests intercellular "cement." Hyaluronidase came to be called "spreading factor" and was

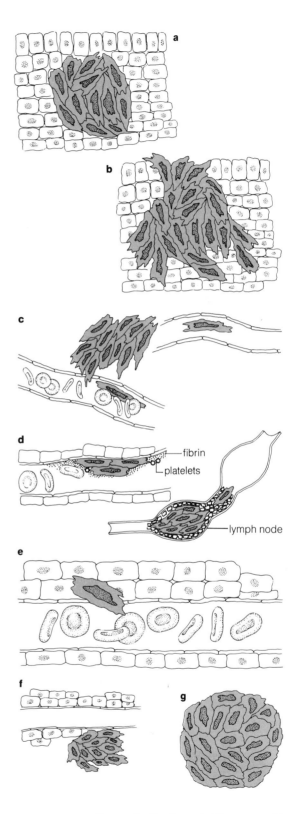

Figure 6.2 The stages of metastasis. The metastatic cascade occurs in a series of stages. The entire sequence is shown here, including (**a**) the establishment and growth of the primary tumor, (**b**) the invasion of adjacent tissue and body cavities, (**c**) the invasion of vascular and lymphatic channels and discontinuous extension via the bloodstream and/or the lymph "stream," (**d**) the arrest of tumor cells and clumps of cells in lymph nodes and/or on the vascular epithelium, (**e**) the penetration of vascular walls (extravasation) by the tumor cells, (**f**) early proliferation of metastatic cells and the establishment of a blood supply, and (**g**) the growth of the secondary tumor into a discernible mass. Cells can also escape from the *secondary* mass, and the entire process can be repeated, giving rise to *tertiary* neoplasms.

believed to play a role in the invasion of normal tissues by bacterial cells. As time went on, this concept fell out of favor. Very little positive correlation was found between invasiveness and whether or not a particular bacterial species could synthesize and secrete hyaluronidase. All this research nevertheless suggested the possibility that tumor invasion may be aided by enzyme secretion.

Many types of malignant neoplasms have been found to shed enzymes capable of altering ground substance. Nakajima and colleagues (1983) recently reported that the more highly invasive and metastatic sublines of a spectrum of B16 melanoma lines had more of the enzymes that are able to digest the glycosaminoglycans of the extracellular matrix—suggesting that cancer cells may slip into and out of the circulation by digesting the cement between cells.

The picture is still not crystal clear. Some highly invasive tumors have negligible degradative enzyme capacities while some relatively noninvasive tumors have been found to have *high* degradative enzyme activities. Recent evidence does show, however, that there is a fairly good correlation between invasiveness and the secretion of plasminogen activator—a protease activator (see p. 60). The strongest statement that can be made in summary is that enzymes "probably" facilitate invasion to a "limited" degree in "some" neoplasms.

Do Cancer Cells Kill Their Way Out? Another possible mechanism of invasion is that cancer cells kill their way through adjacent normal tissue. Cancer cells *do* have the ability to kill normal cells; however, this effect is thought to be a result of competition for nutrients and/or to disruption of blood supplies. There has been no definitive demonstration that cancer cells produce poisons that serve as a principal mechanism of invasion.

Migration as a Factor As described in Chapter 4, the experiments of Abercrombie and others have shown that cancer cells do *not* exhibit the same degree of contact inhibition of migration

seen in normal cells. This suggests, of course, that cancer cells may actually move under their own power into adjacent tissues. The migration of transformed animal cells grown in tissue cultures *into* and over other cells further suggests that such a mechanism would be operative even in the absence of "pressure buildup."

A number of investigators have suggested that there may actually be chemical stimulants to invasive migration. It has been proposed for example, that tumor cells tend to move according to acid-base gradients; that is, they move from high or low acidity to zones of relative neutrality. Easty and Easty (1976) describe a possible "chemotactic" influence (based on data presented by Koono, Ushijima, and Hayashi (1974) suggesting that cancer cells may secrete a substance that causes cells and tissues in remote locations to secrete a *second* chemical that serves as a "beacon" for the migrating cancer cell.

Slippery Cells Many of the changes that take place in cancer cell surfaces could well contribute to invasion. Cancer cells do not adhere to one another or to various substrates as well as normal cells, suggesting that their surface properties make them "slipperier" than normal cells. Perhaps this trait helps them "slip" between normal cells in the process of invasion.

Invasion Summary Obviously, a number of factors contribute to invasiveness in cancer. Research to date, rather than having provided definitive answers, seems simply to have identified a number of possibilities, all of which still seem viable to some degree.

Local Extension

The first consequence of invasion could be called "local extension." Willis (1973) lists the primary and anatomical *routes* of local extension of cancer as (1) tissue spaces, (2) lymph vessels, (3) blood vessels, (4) coelomic cavities, (5) cerebrospinal spaces, and (6) epithelial cavities.

Neoplasms may, according to Willis, extend into any one of these cavities, channels, and spaces, without loss of overall continuity; that is, without breaking away from the parent mass. Willis stresses the importance of invasion along *venous channels*, claiming that this route is seen in at least *half of all fatal cancers*.

Breaking Away: Discontinuous Extension

Once the extension of a tumor carries it into a body cavity or into a blood or lymphatic vessel, cells break away from the main mass rather regularly. Although single cells can break away from tumor masses, cancer cells are much more likely to break away as emboli or *clusters* of cells. Experimental observation has indicated that for every gram of adenocarcinoma in a rat, as many as a million cells or cell clumps were released into the blood in a twenty-four-hour period (see Glaves and Weiss, 1976). As we will see in the next section, most of these cells perish—but it doesn't take many survivors to cause problems.

Metastasis by Contact? It has been suggested that skin cancer might be transplanted by contact between a neoplasm and an "opposite" area of skin; for example, from one lip to another (see Willis, 1973). Metastasis by contact implantation appears that it might occur in tumors of the urinary tract and perhaps the lung. Willis, however, also says that what *appears* to be spread by contact may actually be the simultaneous development of independent tumors spread through blood or lymph channels.

Regional Extension: Metastasis to Lymph Nodes For many types of cancer, the very first evidence of disseminated disease presents itself as a mass in the lymph nodes (Fig. 6.3) that drain the area or region of the body carrying the primary tumor (see Chapter 3). Usually these secondary tumors come from emboli carried to the lymph nodes by the *down*stream flow of lymph. Occasionally, upstream lymph nodes become infiltrated by metastatic cancer. This exception is thought to be a result of blockage or the reversal of lymphatic flow, allowing cancer cells to migrate upstream.

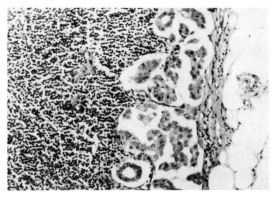

Figure 6.3 Metastasis of tubular carcinoma of the breast in a lymph node. Note the recognizable tubular pattern at the bottom of the photo (× 250). (Photo courtesy of Professor Per H. B. Carstens, University of Louisville School of Medicine. Used by Permission of the American Journal of Clinical Pathology, Volume 58, pp. 231–238, 1972.

Involvement of lymph nodes can be very rapid or very slow, depending on the neoplasm. In some animal tumor models, regional lymph node metastasis can be demonstrated a few days after implantation of a transplantable tumor. *In humans, lymph node involvement is found in about half of all fatal cancers.* The readiness with which cancer spreads to lymph nodes varies considerably from one human cancer to another (see Willis, 1973).

The variability of lymph node involvement in clinical cancer is at least partly a result of the fact that many things can happen to the cancer cells that become lodged in lymph nodes. They may die as a result of a local inflammatory reaction; they may wither and die because of lack of the proper environment; they can grow into a discernible lump; or they can remain dormant for reasons unknown (see Fig. 6.4).

It was once thought that the filtering action of the lymph nodes was responsible for nodal metastasis, but experimental investigation has revealed that filtration is a relatively minor factor and perhaps some sort of physiochemical cell surface and lymph node interaction is also important in whether or not cancer cells become lodged in lymph nodes.

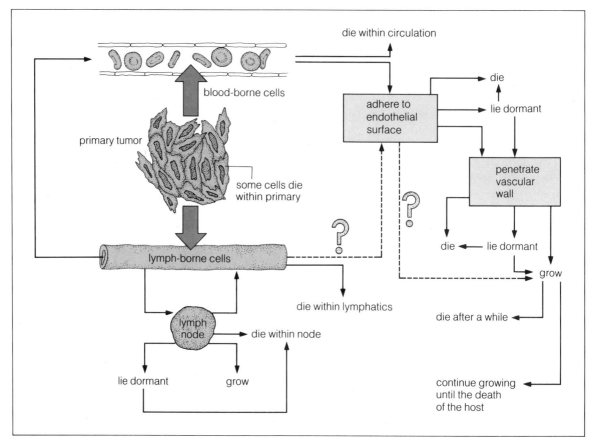

Figure 6.4 Very few of the viable cells shed from a tumor mass survive to become established as a metastasis. Illustrated here are some of the many possible fates of shed tumor cells.

The Transport of Cancer Cells to Distant Sites

Gravitational Dissemination within Body Cavities

Neoplasms frequently extend into, and invade body cavities such as nasal and pharyngeal cavities, the uterus, bladder, and bronchi of the lung, until the cavities are literally filled up with cancer. During the spread of cancer over the serous membranes of larger body cavities such as the pleural and peritoneal cavities, cancer cells sometimes break away and gravitate to the lower reaches of such cavities. Gravity, therefore, can be a casual factor in metastasis.

The Spread of Cancer through Lymphatic Vessels The lymphatic vasculature of the human body is illustrated in Chapter 3. An important feature of this system is that the main lymphatic trunk enters the venous system just before the veins enter the heart. Thus, the lymphatic and blood vessel systems of the body are interconnected, and cancer cells that reach the lymphatics are able to get into the bloodstream as well. Lymphatic drainage channels appear to be a common route by which tumors spread locally and regionally, perhaps reflecting a favorable environment for the survival of cancer cells in the lymphatic vessels.

Transport via the Bloodstream While some cancer cells that get into blood are believed to get there via the lymphatics, it is generally believed that the more aggressive cancer cells that reach the bloodstream get there through direct invasion of capillaries and veins. Willis claims that while the local spread of cancer may well occur predominantly through the lymphatic vessels, metastatic spread to remote organs and tissues is almost invariably the result of cells being transmitted through the bloodstream.

The mechanism by which cancer cells enter the bloodstream is not known. Apparently, arteries are only rarely invaded by cancer cells. It has been suggested that this resistance to invasion may be a result of high pressures, enzyme inhibitors (such as collagenase inhibitors) found in arterial walls, and/or the relative impermeability of the artery vessel wall. Cancer cells do enter capillaries, however, and they do enter veins.

What happens to cancer cells once they get into the bloodstream? In the blood, aggregates of cancer cells interact with one another, with platelets, with various soluble substances in the bloodstream, and with elements of the immune system. This interaction gives metastatic cells additional complex characteristics, some of which are possibly important in the eventual arrest and establishment of metastatic tumor masses.

Only a very small fraction of the cancer cells that "leave home" via the bloodstream—or in any other way—become successful colonists of distant places. Most of them perish. The circulatory system is really a very hostile environment. We tend to think of it as being otherwise because of the system's role in nurturing the cells of our tissues. But while it is good to have the circulation pass nearby, to be inside the circulatory system is a different matter. It would be roughly equivalent to a roller-coaster ride during a violent hurricane or tornado or maybe to going over Niagara Falls without a barrel.

The Clinical Significance of the Presence of Cancer Cells in the Blood

Dozens of less than perfect methods are described in the literature for recovering and identifying the cells shed from solid tumors in peripheral blood. The results of such work have been equivocal. Cancer cells do appear in large numbers in the blood but usually very late in the growth of the primary tumor. Most importantly, the presence of cancer cells in the blood offers very little prognostic significance. Perhaps, this fact is a consequence of the facts that cancer cell survival in the bloodstream is very low and that it is difficult to detect and identify cancer cells in the blood. At any rate, although the demonstration of cancer cells in the blood is of little prognostic value, histological evidence that cancer has invaded blood vessels near the primary tumor is generally accepted as a *bad* sign.

Arrest

If a metastatic cancer cell or a cluster of cells adrift in the circulatory system is to become established as a metastatic tumor, it must first come to rest. This fact raises some important questions: Why would a cell having invaded its way out of tissue, and having become detached from the parent tumor, stop somewhere and "crawl back into" normal tissue? What could possibly stop a cell that obviously has a tendency to "slip away"? Such a cell might be expected to spend the remainder of its life as an aimless drifter in the bloodstream.

A number of factors have been found in identifying those qualities of cells and hosts that determine when and how cancer cells adhere to

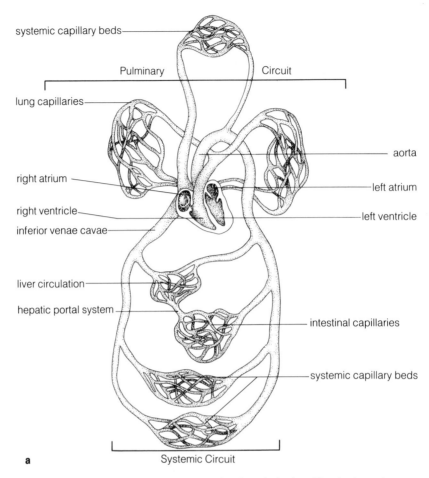

systemic capillary beds

Pulminary   Circuit

lung capillaries

aorta

right atrium

left atrium

right ventricle

left ventricle

inferior venae cavae

liver circulation

hepatic portal system

intestinal capillaries

systemic capillary beds

a   Systemic Circuit

Figure 6.5 (**a**) The general plan of the circulatory system, showing the principal capillary beds, and the general structure of (**b**) an artery, (**c**) a capillary, and (**d**) a vein.

epithelial surfaces of blood vessels. The four main factors involved are (1) *blood flow mechanics* (plumbing is important in establishing where cancer cells in the blood might become slowed down enough to even begin to become attached to the walls of blood vessels), (2) *blood coagulation factors*, (3) *immune system factors*, and (4) unknown features of the cancer cells themselves. In this section, we will spend most of our time with hemodynamic-mechanical and blood coagulation factors, discussing the role of the immune system and the cancer cell later.

Hemodynamic and Mechanical Factors

One popular notion about tumor cells is that they become lodged in places where large total cross-sectional area capillary beds (lung, brain, etc.) cause them to stall or slow down and/or where they become lodged because they are too large to pass through (see Fig. 6.5). A number of papers dealing with *morphological* aspects of the arrest and attachment of tumor cells leading to the establishment of metastasis are reviewed by Chew, Josephson, and Wallace (1976). While the

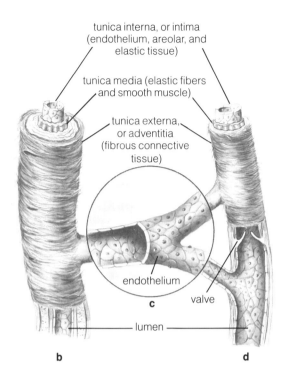

tunica interna, or intima (endothelium, areolar, and elastic tissue)

tunica media (elastic fibers and smooth muscle)

tunica externa, or adventitia (fibrous connective tissue)

endothelium

c

valve

lumen

b

d

mechanical trapping of tumor cells is both a simple and appealing idea, it does not seem to tell the whole story. Tarin (1976) cites a number of studies indicating that tumor fragments *do not necessarily* come to rest in the *first* capillary bed they enter. It has also been shown that cancer cells can ''squeeze'' through capillaries that ''look'' too small.

The major evidence against a simple trapping concept is that metastatic cancers simply do *not* faithfully exhibit distributions that support it. We'll discuss this fact further in the section on the preferential nature of metastasis, coming up.

Blood-Clotting Factors

A number of investigators (see Chew et al., 1976) present a picture of cancer cells, having once entered the bloodstream, becoming associated with both cellular and humoral constituents of blood. Platelets and fibrin may be the most important of these constituents. In studies with the Walker 256 rat tumor model, Chew et al. found the following: (1) *platelets* (see Chapter 3) were seen in almost every case in association with tumor cells attached to the vascular epithelium, (2) fibrin was present in the complex of platelets and tumor cells at the site of arrest, (3) as the fibrin-platelet complex disintegrated, the tumor cells remained attached to the blood vessel wall and then passed through the vascular wall by *destroying* cells of the vascular epithelium (rather than passing between cells) (see Chew et al., 1976).

Another observation in support of a role for platelets and fibrin in tumor cell arrest is that anticoagulants have been shown to *reduce* the frequency of metastasis (see Carter, 1976). Heparin, a well-known anticoagulant, has also been implicated as an antimetastatic agent (Tsubura et al., 1977). Tsubura, Yamashita, and Higuchi have also presented data illustrating that xylan sulfate, a sulfated polysaccharide, was also able to inhibit metastasis. They postulated that this compound worked by inhibiting some step in the coagulation cascade. Unfortunately, some conflicting results have been found (Carter, 1976; Gasic et al., 1973), and the overall effects of anticoagulants on tumor cell arrest are really quite unclear. The consensus in the literature seems to be that too little is known at the moment to even begin considering manipulating anticoagulation-coagulation forces for the purpose of treating and/or controlling metastatic cancer.

Again, to put metastasis into perspective, remember that *arrest* of tumor cells—as with all other aspects of metastatic dissemination—is a result of interaction between (1) the properties inherent in the cancer cells themselves and (2) factors and modifiers present in each host. Now let's focus on the properties of the tumor cells themselves, particularly in regard to the intriguing question ''Why do certain cancers give rise to metastatic secondary neoplasms in certain locations?''

Table 6.1 Patterns of Metastases. Sites of metastasis in 1,000 consecutive autopsied cases and in more than 100 cases each of breast, lung, and colon cancer.

Site of Metastatic Involvement	In 1,000 Consecutive Autopsies (%)	In 167 Cases of Primary Breast Cancer (%)	In 160 Cases of Primary Lung Cancer (%)	In 118 Cases of Primary Colon Cancer (%)
Abdominal nodes	50	44	29	59
Liver	49	61	40	65
Lungs	47	77	47	37
Mediastinal nodes	42	67	83	14
Pleura	28	65	28	14
Bone	27	73	33	9
Adrenal	27	54	36	14
GI tract	27	15	11	27
Diaphragm	20	25	16	11
Brain (cerebral)	18	9	43	—

Source: Bodansky, 1977. Used with permission of Raven Press.

Why Do Metastatic Deposits Occur Where They Occur?

Experience with human tumors clearly indicates that particular kinds of tumors tend to metastasize to particular places. Breast tumors tend to metastasize to the brain and to the lungs, lung tumors tend to metastasize to the brain, and prostatic cancer tends to spread to bone. The tendency for certain types of cancers to metastasize to certain sites, particularly the liver, lymph nodes, bones, lung, and liver is illustrated in Table 6.1. These data and others suggest that metastatic dissemination of cancer is far from random, raising the question "Why do these patterns arise?"

There are related intriguing questions. Why is it, for instance, that metastasis rarely occurs in the spleen? Or in the thymus? Why is it rather common for carcinomas (epithelial cell cancers) to metastasize to lymph nodes, while sarcomas (endothelial cell cancers) rarely do? Why are metastases only rarely seen in skeletal muscle or skin? Are vascular pressures and blood flow rates too high in muscle and skin to allow cancer cell to come to rest there? Or are other factors at work? And why do individual patients sometimes show completely nontypical distributions of metastatic disease (Tarin, 1976)?

Answers offered for these kinds of questions over the years have all revolved around mechanical factors: (1) tumors cannot become established in certain places because flow rates are too high and tumor cells cannot stop long enough to become attached and (2) cancer cells become lodged in capillary beds because blood flow rates are slow in capillaries and the passageways are small enough to trap cancer cells. But there are apparently some other possibilities. First, a "seed and soil" hypothesis suggests that certain tissues and organs have special characteristics that enable cancer cells to flourish. A corollary is that cells that travel to other sites and become lodged there never appear as metastases. A second hypothesis involves the receptors or recognition signals on the surface of cancer cells, causing them to associate with cells of particular organs and tissues (Fig. 6.6). A more recent hypothesis is that only in certain locations can metastatic cancer cells elicit the production (by surrounding cells) of growth factor(s) needed to support cancer cell-division.

Nicolson (1978) and others have shown that metastatic patterns do not really correlate all that well with patterns of blood flow and the locations of capillary beds. Fidler and Nicolson (1976) found that even after injecting B16 melanoma cells into the *left* ventricle of the mouse heart, in effect requiring that the cells pass through capillary beds *other than those in the lung first* (see Chapter 3), there was *still* preferential metastasis to lung. Similarly, Sugarbaker (1952) showed (using another model system) that cells injected into the left side of the heart did not develop metastasis in all peripheral organs. Clearly, capillaries do not *necessarily* stop all cancer cells.

Kinsey (1960) showed that if portions of normal lung were transplanted to various nonlung locations in an animal body, lung-seeking melanoma cells established metastasis in association with lung *and* the transplanted piece of lung but not anywhere else in the body. Control grafts using other organs ruled out the possibility that surgical disturbance itself had anything to do with metastatic deposits. And, since a transplanted piece of lung would be physiologically quite different in many ways from the normal lung, this experiment suggests that something about particular cancer cells causes them to bind to certain types of tissue. In other words, this finding seems to favor the "adhesive-specificity" explanation as opposed to simple plumbing differences or the "congeniality of soil."

Many experiments by Fidler and others have demonstrated that neoplasms are not homogeneous with respect to metastatic potential. By isolating single cells from a B16 mouse melanoma line, allowing these to grow, and then characterizing them as to their metastatic potential, Fidler found that the isolates had different tendencies to metastasize and that the tenden-

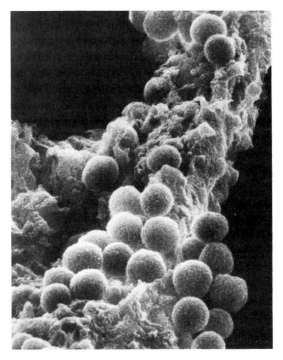

Figure 6.6 Scanning electron micrograph of mouse B16–F10 melanoma cells binding to mouse lung tissue (× 8,800). Even outside of mice, these metastatic tumor cells adhere preferentially to the tissue they colonize in a living mouse (see Netland and Zetter, 1984). (Photo by Netland and Zetter, 1984, cover. Copyright 1984 by the AAAS. Reprinted by permission of the authors and the publisher.)

cies were genetically faithful (see Fidler, 1978; see also Spremulli and Dexter, 1983).

Nicolson and Fidler were able to select sublines of B16 melanoma that preferred lung almost exclusively, and thus concluded that metastatic localization is *genetically* determined. A primary tumor is an aggregation of genetically *dis*similar cells having phenotypic shades of variation, including different metastatic preference.* The metastatic potential of individual cells

---

*Fidler and Hart (1982) say that this diversity may arise either by virtue of the multicellular origin of the primary tumor *or* by the "evolution" of diversity as a neoplasm develops from a single cell.

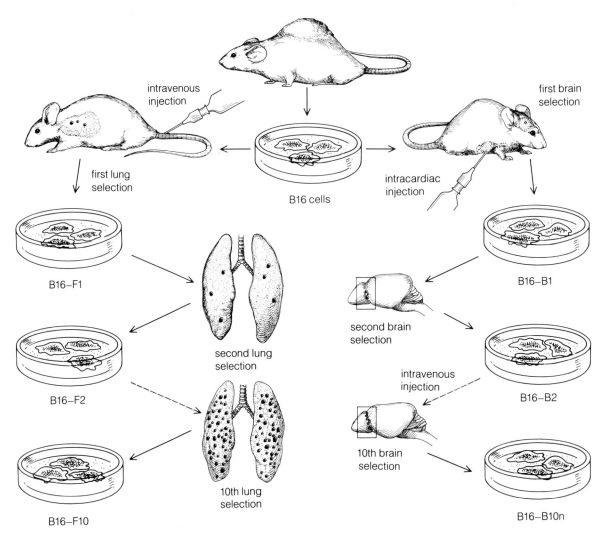

Figure 6.7 Selection of melanoma cell lines with enhanced ability to metastasize to lung (left) and to a particular part of the brain (right). The selections were accomplished by repeated isolation of tumor cells from the target organ, culturing them, and then injecting them into the tail veins of other mice. Highly lung-selective B16–F10 cells were produced by ten such cycles. Similarly, ten "selections" resulted in a B16–B10n cell line highly selective of rhinal fissure of the brain. (Adapted from Nicolson, 1979, p. 71. Used by permission of W. H. Freeman and Company.)

in a primary tumor is apparently quite variable, and genetic selection can establish lines from an individual tumor with high degrees of selectivity and efficiency of metastasis to particular organs (see Fig. 6.7).

Lung-seeking lines do not become lung-seeking lines because they become adapted to lung by spending a lot of time there. If a line is grown in lung (or brain), excised, and then reimplanted in the same organ ten times, the tendency to colonize that organ (when injected into the circulation) does not change. Apparently cells with particular metastatic preferences are present from the first.

The experiments just described notwithstanding, it seems likely that the "congeniality of soil" is also an important factor in metastatic distribution. In one experiment, Fidler and Nicolson radioactively labeled lung-preferring B16 melanoma cells and then injected these in different sites in mice. After a few hours, the B16 melanoma cells were found in *many* types of organs and tissues but mostly in the lung (Table 6.2). After two weeks, however, viable labeled cells were found only in the lung (see Fidler, 1976).

The implication of all of these findings is that the distribution of metastatic cancers is governed to some degree by factors other than circulatory "plumbing." The data also clearly suggest that the "congeniality of soil" hypothesis has some validity and that the adhesive-specificity hypothesis also has something to it. The data in Table 6.2 suggest that these factors may even somehow be related—that cancer cells may preferentially stop where they are more likely to survive.

Reinvasion

We find ourselves in the somewhat embarrassing position of, having been unable to give a definitive answer as to how cancer cells invade their way *out* of primary tumors and into blood vessels, now having to explain how they get back into tissue. Be that as it may, the next critical step in the metastatic cascade is the period between the point at which the cancer cell becomes attached to the wall of the vessel and the point at which it becomes established as a secondary tumor on the other side of the blood vessel wall.

While it may be that some metastatic deposits originate from cells that block a capillary, shut off blood flow, and begin to proliferate in place (and after a while, changes induced in and around the growing deposit may erase all evidence that the deposit originated in a capillary), the weight of experimental observation indicates that tumor cells most commonly must migrate out (Fig. 6.8) of the vasculature before they can establish a thriving "colony."

We have already indicated that of the cancer

cells that merely come to rest and attach to blood vessel surfaces, *most never become clinically manifest metastatic deposits.* Perhaps some are unable to get through the blood vessels and perhaps many of those that do are unable to establish a blood supply fast enough—and die because of the lack of oxygen or the buildup of toxic byproducts of metabolism. The trick, then, is to get through the blood vessel and establish supply lines quickly. The mechanism by which cancer cells move off the vascular highway back into the tissues is unknown. It seems likely that some form of **diapedesis**—the mode of invasion of white blood cells—is involved (Carter, 1976; Nicolson, 1979). The ability to slip through capillary vessel linings into tissue would require that cancer cells be highly deformable, and we have already mentioned they are sufficiently deformable to pass through capillaries smaller than they are.

Sato and Suzuki (1976) have studied various strains of transplantable ascites* tumors in the rat and have developed a way to measure deformability of tumor cells by recording the pressure required to "suck" a hemispheric bulge in cells (using a micropipette). They have compared metastatic potential and deformability, and concluded that deformability of tumor cells is a "potentially important" factor in metastasis.

Another possibility is that cancer cells destroy the cells that form capillary walls (see Fig. 6.5). Chew et al. (1976) observed that in the Walker 256 rat tumor line, tumor cells passed through the vascular wall after attachment, by destroying cells of the vascular epithelium.

Establishing a Beachhead: Angiogenesis

A cancer cell leaving the bloodstream and invading local tissue is not unlike an advancing army outdistancing its supply lines. Such a military

---

Ascites tumor cells do not adhere to one another to form *solid* tumors; rather, they exist as cell suspensions.

Table 6.2   Distribution of 200,000 Viable Radioactively Labeled B16 Melanoma Cells Injected I.V. into Normal C57B1/6 Mice. These data suggest that metastatic deposition may have a considerably dynamic nature in the early stages. The data also illustrate the "harshness" of the various environments into which metastatic cells travel.

Time of Death Post Injection	Number of Viable Tumor Cells			
	Lung	Liver	Blood[1]	Urine[2]
1 minute	136,000	2,200	3,750	—
5 minutes	105,700	7,600	2,200	—
10 minutes	130,500	9,350	2,600	100
1 hour	108,000	3,500	3,800	10,000
12 hours	5,500	700	1,050	10,500
1 day	1,700	600	580	1,700
3 days	450	200	40	0
14 days	400	0	0	0

[1]Per 1.0 ml blood.
[2]Urinary bladder and contained urine.

Source: Fidler et al., 1976. Used with permission of American Elsevier Publishing Co., Inc. and Dr. I. J. Fidler.

maneuver can be accomplished only by developing ways to live off the territory being invaded. Apparently, metastatic cancer cells come equipped to do just that. Or perhaps it would be more accurate to say that cells that come so equipped are the ones able to develop full-blown metastatic tumors.

Once cancer cells reinvade remote tissue, a number of things can happen. They may die, they may lie dormant for many years and then grow to a large size even well after the primary tumor has been removed, or they might immediately begin to grow to a large size.

According to Folkman and Tyler (1977), metastatic tumors cannot grow more than a few millimeters in diameter or achieve population densities of more than a million cells or so without having new blood vessels established to sustain them.

A number of studies have revealed that malignant tumors do not form their own blood vessels; they cause the host to make blood vessels for them (Folkman and Tyler, 1977; Knighton et al., 1983; Fett et al., 1985) via a chemical sub-

stance called *angiogenesis factor* or *tumor angiogenesis factor* (TAF).

Folkman and Tyler (1977) have presented some dramatic and interesting evidence that tumors are able to induce the formation of blood vessels and that this ability is more highly developed in cancer cells than in embryologic cells. Their experiments were based on inducing blood vessel growth into the cornea of rabbit eyes (Fig. 6.9).

The cornea does not normally have blood vessels. By placing fragments of embryologic tissue and tumor tissue in the cornea at variable distances from its edge, Folkman and Tyler and others have studied the ability of such implants to induce vessels to grow out from the edge of the cornea *to* the implant. Using this model, they have shown that normal tissues do *not* induce vascularization and that embryonic tissue will cause blood vessels to grow out only if implanted relatively close to the edge of the cornea. As illustrated in Figure 6.9, tumor implants induced the outgrowth of vasculature over a greater distance.

Another difference between embryologic and tumor tissue illuminated in this experimental model is that the intact blood vessels of *embryonic tissue* grafts lined up and became spliced to the vessels growing out from the edge of the cornea. In contrast, the original vessels within the *tumor* implant disintegrate, and new host vessels induced by the tumor and originating in the surrounding stroma take their place.

Recently, TAF has been isolated from human cancer cells by Burt Vallee and his associates at Harvard in collaboration with scientists at the University of Washington; they characterized the protein and named it *angiogenin* (see Fett et al., 1985). This achievement was a major breakthrough, not only because it should now be easier to find ways to block angiogenin and thus keep blood vessels from developing in tumors, but also because angiogenin may be useful in other areas of medicine. For example, it may be used to speed up the development of blood vessels in burns and other wounds, and/or to encourage the growth of new blood vessels in the heart after a heart attack.

According to Johnson (1976) and others, the sequence and process by which vasculature is established varies with tumor type and with the nature of the tissue invaded. At first, the metastatic tumor may grow for a while within an existing vascular network, eventually distorting it. After a while, new vasculature is developed, made up mostly of vessels with large sinusoidal spaces.

Overall, vascular perfusion of tumors is imperfect by normal tissue standards; that is, as the tumor grows, perfusion becomes less and less complete (Johnson, 1976).

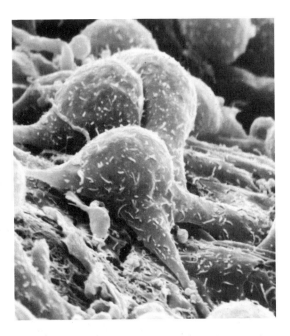

Figure 6.8 Scanning electron micrograph of metastatic melanoma cells invading the wall of a blood vessel (× 2,200). (Photo courtesy of Dr. Garth L. Nicolson, University of Texas, M. D. Anderson Hospital and Tumor Institute at Houston. Nicolson, 1979, p. 67. Used by permission.)

type of control is relatively absent in tumor tissue has been exploited as part of the basis for "therapeutic hyperthermia." Heat treatment is effective against tumor cells because the tumors cannot dissipate heat as fast as normal tissue. In addition, heat seems to reduce microvascular control still further, suggesting that multiple, sequential heat treatments might be advantageous. Such treatments are now being used experimentally in cancer patients.

Host and Treatment Factors in Metastasis

In some model systems, metastatic efficiency is related to hormone levels. Hormones may also, as we will see later, influence delay in the development of metastases. Hormones have also

Microvascular Control in Tumors

Apparently the vasculature of primary tumors and metastatic tumors is not able to respond to oxygen tension and heat as normal blood vessels do. Under conditions of low oxygen tension and temperature elevation, the capillaries and small vessels in normal tissue dilate. The fact that this

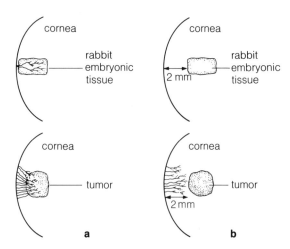

Figure 6.9 Angiogenesis. Illustrated here are the experiments of Folkman and Tyler (1977). Tumors are apparently able to release a diffusable chemical substance that stimulates nearby normal blood vessels to send out new capillaries that grow toward and eventually "nourish" the tumor. This substance is also apparently released by embryonic tissue but to a lesser degree. (**a**) Vascularization of embryonic tissue implanted in the rabbit cornea compared to tumor implanted in the cornea when both grafts are placed adjacent to the vessels at the edge of the cornea. (**b**) Comparison of corneal implants of embryonic tissue and tumor tissue when the grafts are placed at a distance from the vessels at the edge of the cornea. In this situation, the embryonic tissue is unable to attract new vessels, whereas the tumor graft does attract new vessels and becomes vascularized. (Adapted from Folkman and Tyler 1977, p. 96. Used with permission of Raven Press.)

been implicated in the arrest of tumor cells (Willis, 1973).

Age may be another factor. Willis (1973) cites studies carried out in the 1930s concluding that older rats were less susceptible to metastases than young rats.

The host may influence metastatic development in other ways, as suggested by the observation that metastatic efficiency is influenced by the site of experimental implantation of tumor cells. Certain strongly metastatic animal tumors (e.g., the Lewis lung carcinoma) become nonmetastatic when implanted in certain body cavities (Garattini, 1977).

And some of what looks like capricious metastatic behavior may well be due to vagaries of the host immune-defense system.

Metastasis and the Immune System

According to Nicolson (1978), protection against metastatic disease through immunization has been achieved in a number of experimental animal systems. Another important experimental observation suggesting that the immune system can defend against metastasis is that certain normally nonmetastasizing cells *will* metastasize in animals whose immune systems have been suppressed. It has long been known that human tumors found upon histological examination to be surrounded and/or infiltrated by cellular elements of the immune system have a more favorable prognosis.

More Harm Than Good? One key research question in tumor immunology has been "Why doesn't the host mount an immunologic response against neoplastic cells if they do indeed have antigens not found in normal tissues?" Research has made it clear that the immune system may even be guilty of treason. Tumor cells that are mildly immunogenic apparently can cause certain immunoglobulins to attach to their surfaces, making them "invisible" to the macrophages and other elements of the cell-mediated immune system. This interaction may also help cancer cells invade adjacent normal tissue and even increase the likelihood that cancer cells will metastasize.

Nicolson has suggested (1979) that lymphocytes may actually promote metastasis by clumping cancer cells—making them more likely to become trapped in capillary beds. It has been shown that in animals without mature T-cells the metastatic efficiency of B16 melonoma cells was *lower* than in normal animals (Nicolson, 1978). Apparently tumor immunity can markedly modify tumor metastasis in both positive and negative ways. This fact led Fidler and colleagues (1977) to suggest that immunologically sensitized experimental animals are really more appropriate animal models for studying the mechanisms of metastasis than "normal" animals. Obviously, metastasis and the immune system do not have a straightforward relationship.

Iatrogenic Factors

Ironically, certain aspects of cancer treatment have been found to adversely affect metastatic potential in both animals and human tumors. These include surgical manipulation, certain kinds of chemicals, drugs, and radiation.

Surgical Manipulation It has long been the practice for surgeons to exercise great care in handling and manipulating tumors as they are being resected. This care is based on the belief that cancer cells jarred loose during manipulation and surgical excision can become metastases. We refer here to the possibilities that tumor cells that can be transplanted directly by the surgeon's knife and that those jarred loose during surgery may be disseminated via vascular and lymphatic channels. Experiments have shown that *massaging* subcutaneous tumors in animals increases the likelihood of metastasis.

Drugs and Chemicals Pollard, Burleson, and Luckert (1977) have reported that both chloroform and halothane increased the rate and extent of metastasis to lungs in a mouse prostatic cancer model. These chemicals have their major effect on the liver, suggesting that perhaps their effect on metastasis is indirect, having to do with some role the liver may have in controlling metastasis.

Pollard et al. also report that the immune stimulant *Corynebacterium parvum* interrupted metastasis to the lungs. They also found that aspirin, an anti-inflammatory drug, interfered with metastasis. That the picture may be supercomplicated is suggested by conflicting reports that aspirin may enhance metastasis in some tumor systems (Brown, 1977). Such apparent conflicts may reflect differential effects of an agent on different stages of the metastatic process—

with different stages being limiting for different tumors. A promoter of plasmin, for example, may promote invasion by activating tumor cell proteases, but might retard tumor cell arrest by causing the dissolution of fibrin involved in arrest.

Radiation Enhancement of Metastasis Carter (1976) cites a number of studies indicating that prior irradiation of lung, liver, and kidney may make these organs more susceptible to the development of certain types of metastatic cancer. Controversy continues to rage over the notion that radiation enhances metastatic tumor development, however. Stjernswärd and Douglas (1977) have presented data showing that increased dissemination of cancer follows irradiation after primary surgical treatment of breast cancer. These workers discount the notion that this increase involves some suppressive effect of radiation on the immune system. Willis (1973) concluded his discussion of the matter of radiation-induced metastasis by saying that no solid evidence exists of radiation provoking metastatic spread. He suggests that the incriminating data may simply be a result of the positive effect of radiation on prolonging life—it allows people to live long enough for latent metastases to become apparent.

Metastasis as a Clinical Problem

The Recognition of Metastatic Potential

The patient diagnosed as having cancer but who shows no metastases presents a special problem to the clinician. Because treatment plans are based on whether or not disease has been disseminated, the diagnostician must try to determine through X-rays, scans, and other means if disease has spread. The clinician is often faced with tentative evidence of metastatic disease. In absence of histopathological confirmation of metastases, this problem is especially acute because of significant rates of false-positive and false-negative results using other methods.

It would obviously be very nice if a primary tumor could somehow be evaluated and the probability dissemination at a certain point in its tumorigenesis could be established. Unfortunately, we cannot yet make accurate estimates. As pointed out by Glaves and Weiss (1976), it is nearly impossible to assess the efficiency of metastatic spread of cancer in human beings, or to determine exactly when metastatic spread begins in the natural history of a tumor. The problems are multiple. One notable difficulty is that simple measurements of a neoplasm cannot distinguish between cells lost because of cell death and those lost through metastatic dissemination.

We do know that certain general types of tumors grow faster and are more likely to metastasize than other types of tumors. So far no morphological or histochemical attribute of cancer cells has been identified that correlates strongly with metastatic behavior.

Among the types of tumors that will rarely metastasize, regardless of degree of differentiation, are basal cell carcinomas of the skin. Some thyroid tumors (Carter, 1976) metastasize frequently even though they are well differentiated, so that overall, while morphologic characterization and the grade (Chapter 5) of a tumor is a good indicator of likely metastasis, other factors must also be operating that are not expressed morphologically or that we cannot yet identify.

The Latent Primary Tumor

It is not uncommon for metastatic disease to reveal itself even before the primary tumor has given any indication of its presence. In some situations, patients come in with broken bones and are later found to have a primary carcinoma of the thyroid with a metastasis to bone. It is not unusual in head and neck cancer to find a secondary mass in the neck that results from an unsuspected primary in some area of the head, neck, or even lung. Skin metastases may be the very first symptom of latent gastric cancer (Willis, 1973).

The Dormant Secondary Tumor

It is also not unheard of for malignant growth to appear in cancer patients many years after they were thought to be cured. In breast cancer, for example, metastases can appear in the vertebrae 30 years later. There has been enough documentation of this phenomenon to lead to the notion that metastatic tumor cells can actually remain *dormant*. It is not known, however, what causes metastatic tumor cells to go into and remain in a dormant stage or what causes them to eventually reemerge.

Wheelock et al. (1977) suggest that a number of clinically important questions are related to the dormancy of metastatic cancer. Some such questions are "How do tumor cells establish this state of dormancy and avoid destruction by immune defense mechanisms during this state? Are dormant metastases more likely with some types of tumors than others? Does the dormant condition result from a first slow, and then later accelerated, rate of tumor cell division—a turning on of cell division after a long period of being turned off, or is it a reflection of a gradual emergence from a long period during which the body is successfully combatting a metastatic tumor and for a while is able to stay even? Could special types of therapy be developed to deal with dormant tumor cells?" (see Wheelock et al., 1977).

Apparently, a number of factors can influence the rate of division of metastatic cancer; that is, can increase the division of metastatic cancer cells abruptly and possibly stimulate dormant metastatic cells to emerge from dormancy. Simpson-Herren et al. (1977) cite evidence that surgical removal of primary tumors and/or even sham surgical operations in experimental models stimulate the growth rate of metastatic lung tumors. This concept has received support in a number of studies and suggests that a primary tumor is able to repress or hold in some intermediate state of dormancy the metastatic cells present in the same body. Experiments in which sham surgery produced a similar effect suggest that the reason may be a little more complicated, possibly involving surgical suppression of the immune system.

The observation that taking out the primary tumor results in a spurt of growth in metastatic tumors suggests that drugs toxic to rapidly dividing cells might be used to special advantage immediately following surgery. And indeed, such strategies are employed, with success.

The Detection of Metastasis

We end our consideration of metastasis with a brief discussion of methods used to assess the presence of metastases.

Chemical Methods Earlier, we reviewed a number of differences between normal cells and cancer cells. Among the differences discussed were abnormal hormone secretions, abnormal secretions of certain enzymes, and the release of cell surface components into extracellular fluid, blood, urine, and cerebrospinal fluid. A number of strategies have been devised based on the persistence of abnormal secretions after the primary tumor has been resected. Alkaline phosphatase was one of the very first biochemical markers used to monitor the presence of metastases and human chorionic gonadotropin (HCG) has been one of the most useful of the peptide hormones (Bodansky, 1977). Of more recent vintage is the use of carcinoembryonic antigen assays in blood to find indications of tumors persisting after surgical excision. A number of other biochemical parameters have also proven useful in following the growth and/or progression of metastatic disease. These will all be considered in more detail in Chapter 16.

Radiographic and Radiologic Methods Radiographic techniques are also useful in the detection of metastatic deposits. In the lungs, the differential contrast between normal lung tissue and densely packed metastatic masses can be seen by X-ray (see Chapter 16). X-rays are also able to detect defects in bone produced by calcium resorption and other abnormalities of calcium deposition caused by the presence of met-

astatic disease. These methods are far from perfect. In recent years, routine radiographic analysis of the long bones has been found to be rather insensitive in the detection of disseminated disease, and the use of scans and imaging agents has become more popular (see Chapter 16). Radio-opaque materials put into the circulation reveal areas of the liver where the contrast medium is retained an extra length of time; that is, leaves a lingering "blush." This method takes advantage of the hemorrhagic character or abnormal vasculature within metastatic tumor masses. Other approaches to imaging metastatic lesions include use of radiolabeled antibody to tumor-associated-antigens as we discussed earlier. The radioactive antibody label reveals the presence of tumor through the interaction between the tumor antigens and the tagged antibody. Again, all these methods are discussed in more detail in Chapter 16.

Unfortunately, a number of things can cause false-negative findings in searches for metastases. Preoperative and postoperative workups miss metastatic disease later confirmed at autopsy. Gilbert and Kagan (1976) point out that defects must be at least 3 centimeters in diameter in order to be accurately detected as a metastatic lesion and that defects larger than 6 centimeters in diameter can be missed.

False-*positive* findings are obviously also a considerable clinical problem. Gilbert and Kagan cite a number of conditions responsible for false-positives, including gall bladder artifacts, cirrhosis of the liver, abcesses, and other types of benign diseases. All these errors show that we need *much* additional research aimed at improving the methods of detecting and evaluating metastatic cancer.

Summary

Metastasis is clearly the most significant feature of cancer. Contrary to what was once thought to be the case, the development of metastases involves much more than random survival of a very small proportion of the clumps of cells that break away from primary masses to become trapped in capillary beds. Rather, metastasis appears to result from a complicated interplay between host factors and a small subpopulation of cancer cells (in the primary mass) with the ability to invade adjacent tissue, enter the circulation, leave the bloodstream by passing through capillary walls, induce the development of a blood supply, and continue to proliferate. Difficulty in accurately assessing metastatic spread remains one of the biggest problems in clinical cancer treatment.

Cancer cells are different in many respects from normal cells. While many of these differences are subtle, they offer a considerable array of potentially exploitable differences and suggest numerous points of attack on cancer. The metastatic sequence—from invasion through the establishment of a vascular blood supply for a secondary tumor—offers some especially strategic points of attack on cancer (see Spreafico et al., 1977). Some very significant work has gone on in recent years, but we obviously have quite a way to go. The stimulus for additional work remains; improved understanding of metastasis is fundamental to any prospect for significant improvements in how we deal with cancer.

References and Further Reading

Ambrose, E. J., and Roe, F. S. C., eds. 1975. *Biology of Cancer.* 2nd ed. New York: Wiley.

Bodansky, O. 1977. Biochemical Criteria of Metastatic Growth in Human Cancer. In S. B. Day et al., eds., *Cancer Invasion and Metastasis: Biological Mechanisms and Therapy.* New York: Raven Press.

Braun, A. C. 1974. *The Biology of Cancer.* Reading, Mass: Addison-Wesley.

Brown, J. M. 1977. Effect of Cyclophosphamide and Other Drugs on Artificial Pulmonary Metastasis in Mice. In S. B. Day et al., eds., *Cancer Invasion and Metastasis: Biological Mechanisms and Therapy.* New York: Raven Press.

Cairns, J. 1975. The Cancer Problem. *Scientific American.* 233:64–78.

Carter, R. L. 1976. Metastasis. In T. Symington and R. L. Carter, eds., *Scientific Foundations of Oncology.* Chicago: Heinemann Medical Books/Yearbook Medical Publishers.

Chew, E. C., Josephson, R. L., and Wallace, A. C. 1976. Morphological Aspects of Arrest of Circulating Cancer Cells. In L. Weiss, ed., *Fundamental Aspects of Metastasis.* New York: American Elsevier.

Crum, R., Szabo, S., and Folkman, J. 1985. A New Class of Steroids Inhibits Angiogenesis in the Presence of Heparin or a Heparin Fragment. *Science.* 230:1375–78.

Day, S. B., et al., eds. 1977. *Cancer Invasion and Metastasis: Biological Mechanisms and Therapy.* New York: Raven Press.

Donati, M. B., et al. 1977. Hemostasis: An Experimental Cancer Dissemination. In S. B. Day et al., eds., *Cancer Invasion and Metastasis: Biological Mechanisms and Therapy.* New York: Raven Press.

Easty, G. C. 1975. Invasion by Cancer Cells. In E. J. Ambrose and F. S. C. Roe, eds., *Biology of Cancer.* 2nd ed. New York: Wiley.

Easty, G. C., and Easty, D. M. 1976. Mechanisms of Tumor Invasion. In T. Symington and R. L. Carter, eds., *Scientific Foundations of Oncology.* Chicago: Heinemann Medical Books/Yearbook Medical Publishers.

Fett, J. W., et al. 1985. Isolation and Characterization of Angiogenin, an Angiogenic Protein from Human Carcinoma Cells. *Biochemistry.* 24:5480–86.

Fidler, I. J. 1976. Patterns of Tumor Cell Arrest and Development. In L. Weiss, ed., *Fundamental Aspects of Metastasis.* New York: American Elsevier.

Fidler, I. J. 1978. Tumor Heterogeneity and the Biology of Cancer Invasion and Metastasis. *Cancer Research.* 38:2651–60.

Fidler, I. J., and Nicolson, G. L. 1976. Organ Selectivity for Implantation, Survival, and Growth of B16 Melanoma Variant Tumor Lines. *JNCI.* 57:1199–1202.

Fidler, I. J., Gersten, D. M., and Riggs, C. W. 1977. Quantitative Analysis of Tumor: Host Interaction and the Outcome of Experimental Metastasis. In S. B. Day et al., eds., *Cancer Invasion and Metastasis: Biological Mechanisms and Therapy.* New York: Raven Press.

Fidler, I. J., and Hart, I. R. 1982. Biological Diversity

in Metastatic Neoplasms: Origins and Implications. *Science*. 217:998–1003.

Fisher, B., and Fisher, E. R. 1976. Metastasis Revisited. In L. Weiss, ed., *Fundamental Aspects of Metastasis*. New York: American Elsevier.

Folkman, J. 1976. The Vascularization of Tumors. *Scientific American*. 234(5):58–73.

Folkman, J., and Taylor, S. 1982. Protamine Is an Inhibitor of Angiogenesis. *Nature*. 297:307–12.

Folkman, J., and Tyler, K. 1977. Tumor Angiogenesis: Its Possible Role in Metastasis and Invasion. In S. B. Day et al., eds., *Cancer Invasion and Metastasis: Biological Mechanisms and Therapy*. New York: Raven Press.

Garattini, S. 1977. Concluding Remarks on Cancer Dissemination and Metastases. In S. B. Day et al., eds., *Cancer Invasion and Metastasis: Biological Mechanisms and Therapy*. New York: Raven Press.

Gasic, G. J., et al. 1973. Platelet-Tumor-Cell Interactions in Mice: The Role of Platelets in the Spread of Malignant Disease. *Int. J. Cancer*, 11:704–18.

Gilbert, H. A., and Kagan, A. R. 1976. Metastasis: Incidence Detection and Evaluation Without Histological Confirmation. In L. Weiss, ed., *Fundamental Aspects of Metastasis*. New York: American Elsevier.

Glaves, D., and Weiss, L. 1976. Initial Arrest Patterns of Circulating Cancer Cells: Effect of Host Sensitization and Anticoagulation. In L. Weiss, ed., *Fundamental Aspects of Metastasis*. New York: American Elsevier.

Goldsmith, H. L. 1976. Collisions of Circulating Cells with the Vascular Endothelium. In L. Weiss, ed., *Fundamental Aspects of Metastasis*. New York: American Elsevier.

Harris, E. O., and Krane, S. M. 1974. Collagenases. Parts 1, 2, and 3. *New England J. Med*. 291:557–63, 605–09, 652–61.

Hewitt, H. B. 1976. Projecting from Animal Experiments to Clinical Cancer. In L. Weiss, ed., *Fundamental Aspects of Metastasis*. New York: American Elsevier.

Johnson, R. 1976. "Notes on the Vascular Physiology of Primary Tumors and Micro Metastases." In L. Weiss, ed., *Fundamental Aspects of Metastasis*. Amsterdam: North Holland.

Kinsey, D. L. 1960. An Experimental Study of Preferential Metastasis. *Cancer*. 12:674–76.

Knighton, D. R., et al. 1983. Oxygen Tension Regulates the Expression of Angiogenesis Factor by Macrophages. *Science*. 221:1283–85.

Koono, M., Ushijima, K., and Hayashi, H. 1974. Studies of the Mechanisms of Invasion in Cancer. III. Purification of a Neutral Protease of Rat Ascites Hepatoma Cells Associated with the Production of a Chemotactic Factor for Cancer Cells. *Int. J. Cancer*. 13:105–15.

Kupchella, C. E., et al. 1981. Tissue and Urinary Glycosaminoglycan Patterns Associated with a Fast, an Intermediate, and a Slow-Growing Morris Hepatoma. *Cancer Res*. 41:419–24.

Lash, J. W., and Burger, M. M., eds. 1977. *Cell and Tissue Interactions*. Society of General Physiologists Series, Vol. 32. New York: Raven Press.

Laurence, D. J., Munoro, J., and Meville, A. 1976. Biological Markers. In T. Symington and R. L. Carter, eds., *Scientific Foundations of Oncology*. Chicago: Heinemann Medical Books/Yearbook Medical Publishers.

Law, L. W., et al. 1976. Some Biological and Biochemical Properties of Soluble Tumor Antigens. *Ann. N.Y. Acad. Sci*. 276:11–25.

Mellgren, J. 1976. Quantitative Aspects of Metastasis in Experimental Animals. In L. Weiss, ed., *Fundamental Aspects of Metastasis*. New York: American Elsevier.

Moscona, A. A. 1956. Development of Heterotypic Combinations of Dissociated Embryonic Chick Cells. *Proc. Soc. Expl. Biol. Med*. 92:410–16.

McCutcheon, M., Coman, D. R., and Moore, F. B. 1948. Studies on Invasiveness of Cancer: Adhesiveness at Malignant Cells in Various Human Adenocarcinomas. *Cancer*. 1:460–67.

Nakajima, M., et al. 1983. Heparan Sulfate Degradation: Relation to Tumor Invasive and Metastatic Properties of Mouse B-16 Melanoma Sublines. *Science*. 220:611–13.

Netland, P. A., and Zetter, B. R. 1984. Organ-Specific Adhesion of Metastatic Cells in Vitro. *Science*. 224:1113–14.

Nicolson, G. L. 1978. Experimental Tumor Metastasis: Characteristics and Organ Specificity. *Bioscience*. 28(7):441–47.

Nicolson, G. L. 1979. Cancer Metastasis. *Scientific American*. 240(3):66–76.

Nicolson, G. L., and Milas, L. 1984. *Cancer Invasion and Metastasis: Biologic and Therapeutic Aspects*. New York: Raven Press.

Nicolson, G. L., et al. 1975. Tumor Cell Surfaces and Metastasis: Dynamic Changes in Neoplastic Membrane Structure and Their Relationship in Tumor Spread. In Symposium, 1975, *Cellular Membrane and Tumor Cell Behavior.* Baltimore, Md.: Williams & Wilkins.

Nicolson, G. L., et al. 1976. Cellular Interaction in the Metastatic Process. In Membranes and Neoplasia: New Approaches and Strategies. *Journal of Supramolecular Structure,* Supplement. 1:237–44.

Nicolson, G. L., et al. 1977. Cell Interactions in the Metastatic Process: Some Cell Surface Properties Associated with Successful Blood-Borne Tumor Spread. In J. W. Lash and M. M. Burger, eds., *Cell and Tissue Interactions.* Society of General Physiologists Series, Vol. 32. New York: Raven Press.

Nicolson, G. L., Winkelhake, J. L., and Nassey, A. C. 1976. An Approach to Studying the Cellular Properties Associated with Metastasis: Some *in vitro* Properties of Tumor Variants Selected *in vivo* for Enhanced Metastasis. In L. Weiss, ed., *Fundamental Aspects of Metastasis.* New York: American Elsevier.

Paget, S. 1889. The Distribution of Secondary Growths of Cancer of the Breast. *Lancet.* 1:571.

Pitot, H. C. 1978. *Fundamentals of Oncology.* New York: Dekker.

Pollard, M., Burleson, G. R., and Luckert, P. H. 1977. Factors that Modify the Rate and Extent of Spontaneous Metastases of Prostate Tumors in Rats. In S. B. Day, et al., eds., *Cancer Invasion and Metastasis: Biological Mechanisms and Therapy.* New York: Raven Press.

Raz, A., and Avri, B. 1983. Modulation of the Metastatic Capability in B16 Melanoma by Cell Shape. *Science.* 221:1307–10.

Robbins, S. L. and Cotran, R. 1984. *Pathologic Basis of Disease.* Philadelphia: Saunders.

Rodgers, J. E. 1983. Catching Cancer Strays. *Science 83.* June-August, pp. 42–48.

Sato, H., and Suzuki, M. 1976. Deformability and Viability of Tumor Cells by Transcapillary Passage, with References to Organ Affinity to Metastasis in Cancer. In L. Weiss, ed., *Fundamental Aspects of Metastasis.* New York: American Elsevier.

Schabel, F. M. 1975. Concepts of Systemic Treatment of Micrometastases. *Cancer.* 35:15–24.

Schirrmacher, V. 1985. Cancer Metastasis: Experimental Approaches, Theoretical Concepts, and Impacts for Treatment Strategies. *Advances in Cancer Research,* Vol. 43. New York: Academic Press.

Shimkin, M. B. 1977. *Contrary to Nature.* DHEW Publication No. (NIH) 76-720. Washington, D.C.: U.S. Public Health Service, Superintendent of Documents.

Simpson-Herren, L., et al. 1977. Kinetics of Metastasic Experimental Tumors. In S. B. Day et al., eds., *Cancer Invasion and Metastasis: Biological Mechanisms and Therapy.* New York: Raven Press.

Spreafico, F., et al. 1977. Current Status of Alternative, Selective, Antimetastatic Therapy. In S. B. Day et al., eds., *Cancer Invasion and Metastasis: Biological Mechanisms and Therapy.* New York: Raven Press.

Spremulli, E. N., and Dexter, D. L. 1983. Human Tumor Cell Heterogeneity and Metastasis. *J. Clin. Oncology.* 1(8):496–509.

Stjernswärd, J., and Douglas, P. 1977. Immunosuppression and Metastasis. In S. B. Day et al., eds., *Cancer Invasion and Metastasis: Biological Mechanisms and Therapy.* New York: Raven Press.

Sugarbaker, E. D. 1952. The Organ Selectivity of Experimentally Induced Metastases in Rats. *Cancer.* 5:606.

Sugarbaker, E. D., Thornthwaite, J., and Ketcham, A. S. 1977. Inhibitory Effect of a Primary Tumor on Metastasis. In S. B. Day et al., eds., *Cancer Invasion and Metastasis: Biological Mechanisms and Therapy.* New York: Raven Press.

Sylven, B., and Bois, I. 1960. Protein Content and Enzymatic Assays of Interstitial Fluid from Some Normal Tissues and Transplanted Mouse Tumors. *Cancer Research.* 20:831.

Symington, T., and Carter, R. L., eds. 1976. *Scientific Foundations of Oncology.* Chicago: Heinemann Medical Books/Yearbook Medical Publishers.

Symposium. 1975. *Cellular Membranes and Tumor Cell Behavior.* A collection of papers presented at the 28th annual symposium on Fundamental Cancer Research, M. D. Anderson Hospital and Tumor Institute, Houston, Texas. Baltimore, Md.: Williams & Wilkins.

Talmadge, J. E., Wolman, S. R., and Fidler, I. J. 1982. Evidence for the Clonal Origin of Spontaneous Metastases. *Science.* 217:361–62.

Tarin, D. 1976. Cellular Interactions in Neoplasia. In L. Weiss, ed., *Fundamental Aspects of Metastasis.* New York: American Elsevier.

Terranova, V. P., et al. 1984. Modulation of the Metastatic Activity of Melanoma Cells by Laminin and Fibronectin. *Science*. 226:982–84.

Tsubura, E., Yamashita, T., and Higuchi, Y. 1977. An Inhibitory Mechanism of Blood-Borne Metastasis by Sulfated Polysaccharides. In S. B. Day et al., eds., *Cancer Invasion and Metastasis: Biological Mechanisms and Therapy*. New York: Raven Press.

Van Putten, L. M., and Lelieveld, P. 1976. The Effects of Cytostatic Drugs and Radiotherapy on the Cell Cycle. In T. Symington and L. L. Carter, eds., *Scientific Foundations of Oncology*. Chicago: Heinemann Medical Books/Yearbook Medical Publishers.

Weiss, L., ed. 1976. *Fundamental Aspects of Metastasis*. New York: American Elsevier.

Weiss, P., and Scott, B. I. 1963. Polarization of Cell Locomotion in Vitro. *Proc. Natl. Acad. Sci.* (Wash). 50:330–36.

Welch, D. R., Bhuyan, B. K., and Liotta, L. A., eds. 1986. *Cancer Metastasis: Experimental and Clinical Strategies*. New York: Alan R. Liss.

Wheelock, E. F., et al. 1977. The Tumor Dormant State. In S. B. Day et al., eds., *Cancer Invasion and Metastasis: Biological Mechanisms and Therapy*. New York: Raven Press.

Willis, R. A. 1973. *The Spread of Tumors in the Human Body*. 3rd ed. London: Butterworth.

PART THREE
CARCINOGENESIS

Cancer doesn't just happen, something makes it happen. In this part of the book, we will consider the things that make cancer happen. We begin with a chapter devoted to the question "What *basically* goes wrong when a cell becomes a cancer cell?" Because cancer is a persistent trait once initiated and because the genes are the keepers of cellular "tradition," in Chapter 7 we will concentrate on genes and their role in cancer. In this initial chapter of Part III, we will explore the notion that key genes, called *oncogenes*, are responsible for the malignant condition.

In three of the chapters in Part III, we will consider the nature of the things that influence oncogenes or otherwise cause cells to express "cancerness." Nearly all of the specific causes of cancer fall into just three general categories: chemicals, radiation, and viruses. These will be considered separately in Chapters 8, 9, and 10, respectively.

But cancer is a response, a result. Cancer is what happens when cancer-causing agents interact with something. Cancer is a product of two things in an equation. "Cause" amounts to only one of them; the other is the nature of the gene-specified, gene-regulated life forms affected by these causes. There could be no carcinogens and no cancer if there were no living things. There are two reasons for driving this obvious point home. First of all, the fact that not all humans are created equal when it comes to susceptibility to carcinogens has considerable, immediate, practical importance. Secondly, no treatment of carcinogenesis could be complete without some consideration of the genetic and other host factors that enable "causes" to have such "effects"! Host factors in carcinogenesis are considered throughout Part III, and Chapter 11 is devoted to genetics and cancer.

An epilog to Part III focuses on the well-founded claim that cancer is largely an environmental disease. The epilog is a summary for all of Part III in that it looks at all the causes of cancer in terms of their sources. It also serves as part of the foundation from which we will later explore the next most obvious question, namely "What can we do to keep cancer-causing agents from causing cancer?"

In this chapter we are going to consider some generalizations about the genesis of cancer. It should be easier to appreciate carcinogenesis now that we have considered some of its results.

What causes cancer? Although it may seem at times that *everything* does, actually only some things do. Radiation causes cancer, and certain chemical substances cause cancer. Viruses cause cancer in many animals and have been implicated in at least a few human cancers. Radiation, chemical carcinogens, and viruses all share an ability to alter the genetic material directly and to alter the control of how genes are expressed.

Research to date indicates that carcinogenic agents work through a few *common* gene-affecting mechanisms, and this indication underlies our discussion of a unified concept of carcinogenesis in this chapter. Our focus will be on oncogenes. An **oncogene** is a piece of DNA found in an oncogenic virus or in a cancer cell, and able to bring about (at least partial) neoplastic transformation when it is introduced into another, otherwise normal cell. As we will see, more than one oncogene may be needed to bring about complete transformation in most model systems. The main point, for the time being, is that radiation, chemical carcinogens, and viruses all may create, activate, introduce, or otherwise bring cells under the influence of oncogenes (Fig. 7.1).

Philosophical Basis for a Unified Theory of Carcinogenesis

Although more than a hundred different kinds of cancer afflict human beings, all of the types and subtypes exhibit the same basic features of malignancy. Since all cancer cells behave in the same basic way, is it not reasonable to expect that the same *basic* thing goes wrong at the cellular level in all types of cancer?

True, we did catalog several dozen distinctive features of cancer cells in Chapter 4. Had we been even more exacting, we could have listed hundreds of things that are different about cancer cells. It is highly *un*likely that each of these

7
_____

Oncogenes and Carcinogenesis

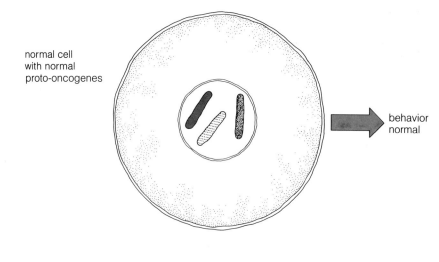

normal cell
with normal
proto-oncogenes

behavior
normal

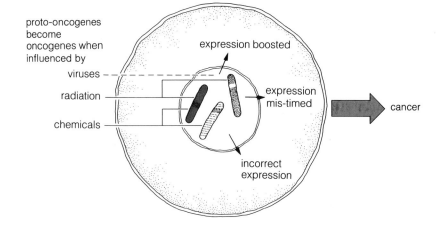

proto-oncogenes
become
oncogenes when
influenced by

viruses

radiation

chemicals

expression boosted

expression
mis-timed

incorrect
expression

cancer

Figure 7.1 A unifying explanation of carcinogenesis. All cells apparently have genes called *oncogenes* that when normally expressed specify normal growth. When these genes are expressed at the wrong time or to the wrong degree, when they are mutated by chemicals or radiation and thus misexpressed, when viruses inject bogus, uncontrollable copies, or when viruses inject genetic material into the genome in such a way as to cause the oncogene to be expressed at the wrong time or to the wrong degree—the result is cancer.

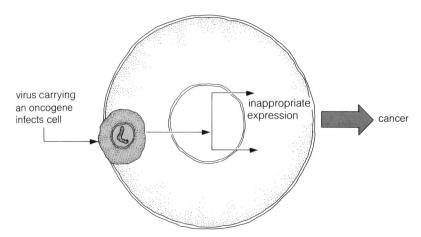

virus carrying
an oncogene
infects cell

inappropriate
expression

cancer

features is a result of a change in different, individual genes. It is more likely that the features of cancer cells are the result of a *cascade* of changes resulting from some smaller number of *primary* changes (see Chapter 4)—a few things gone wrong.

Before we get into the details of the nature of oncogenes, let's consider some historical background. Let's begin by looking at some of the evidence for the notion that cancer is a result of altered normal genes (mutations), and then by considering the possibility that cancer results from the activation of normal genes that should have been suppressed or shut off.

Cancer by Changes in Normal Genes?

When a cancer cell divides, the result is two identical cancer cells. Although, for reasons we will not go into here, this statement is not completely true, it is true enough to make the point that malignancy is a trait that is passed on during cell division like any other genetic trait. Evidence for the notion that this trait is the result of altered genes includes the following:

Cancer can be induced by radiation, and since the work of H. J. Muller in the 1930s radiation

has been known to cause genetic mutations. Cancer is induced by the very same wavelengths of radiation known to alter DNA.

Cancer can be induced by viruses, and viruses can insert both their own and extraneous genetic material into cells (Chapter 10).

Generally speaking, the ability of a particular chemical to induce cancer is related to its *ultimate* ability to change DNA.

Most often, when cancer has been found to be caused by a nonmutagenic chemical it has ultimately been found that the chemical is converted into a mutagen once it gets into the host.

Chromosome alterations are seen in many forms of cancer; for some cancers—many of the leukemias, for instance—there is a recognized, specific relationship between the cancer and a *certain* change in a *certain* chromosome (more on this later).

The potential for developing a rare few kinds of cancer—retinoblastoma, for example (see Chapter 14)—can be inherited directly from parents in the same way as other genetic features.

Transforming genes have now been isolated that differ from normal genes by just one nucleotide base, offering the first clear evidence that malignancy can in fact be induced by a single mutation (Weinberg, 1983).

In summary, there is both good circumstantial evidence and now some direct evidence that cancer can result from changes in genes. These changes include mutations of existing genes or the introduction of new genes, as in the case of virus-induced tumors.

Cancer by Gene Activation?

Earlier we reviewed the concept of cellular differentiation. The point was made that even though all body cells contain a full complement of some 30,000 to 50,000 genes, only relatively few genes are functional in any one cell. Differences between the cells of different tissues—between liver cells and nerve cells, for instance—are a result of the fact that a *different* few genes are operational in different kinds of cells. In Chapter 3, we considered hormones as one of the mechanisms by which a body is able to turn the genes of particular cells on and off. All this discussion is to remind the reader that genes can in fact be turned off, turned on, and even turned off and on again. Most genes are turned off.

The idea that cancer might be a result of the inappropriate activation of one or more genes arose mainly from the observation that cancer cells look and behave a lot like embryonic cells. Cancer cells often look like the embryologic forms of the cells from which they arise. In addition, cancer cells often bear embryonic antigens on their surfaces—that is, they express antigens usually only found on the surface of their embryologic counterparts. This finding suggests the possibility that one or more genes normally active only during the embryologic state become cancer genes if turned back on in an otherwise *partially* differentiated cell.

Often cited as circumstantial evidence for a gene-activation mechanism of carcinogenesis is the fact that under certain circumstances and under certain conditions malignancy can be reversed—converted back to normal—without any apparent mutagenic influence. Some examples: if a nucleus from a cancer cell in a frog is used to replace the nucleus of a newly fertilized frog egg, the egg goes on to become a normal frog free of cancer. Human neuroblastoma cells have been known to revert to what are apparently normal neurons. But these and other similar examples constitute only weak circumstantial evidence. Mutations can also spontaneously revert to normal and, just as with other genes, mutant genes may not always be expressed. In other words, reversibility in and of itself does not favor the gene activation theory over the gene mutation theory.

Until recently, one of the big problems with the gene activation theory is that there was no completely satisfactory way to explain how something other than a permanent gene mutation could be transmitted from cell to cell during division. Although it is plausible that a chemical substance could react with a repressor (Chapter 2) and thereby bring about *de*repression of a gene, such a substance should "wash out" with repeated cell division and allow the normal phenotype to reemerge.

In recent years, following the observation that oncogenes are often located physically next to the break in the chromosome breaks associated with cancer, it has been suggested that oncogenes can become activated by being separated from the genes that normally control them, or by ending up next to control sequences of DNA that activate them. But we are getting ahead of the story. Let's recap and then develop the whole oncogene story.

To summarize the gene activation concept: the possibility is real that some human cancers result from inappropriate activation of genes that were supposed to be permanently turned off. It is possible that some cancers are caused this way and that others are the result of mutation or the introduction of foreign genetic material. In the following section, we will take a look at how *both* of these mechanisms may be related through oncogenes.

Oncogenes

The reasoning and the sequence of discoveries that led to the identification of oncogenes went roughly as follows.

It has been known for a long time—since just after the turn of the century—that viruses can induce cancer in animals. In recent years so-called oncogenic viruses have been used routinely by cancer researchers to convert normal cells into transformed cells (Chapter 4). Not very long ago, using only very recently available techniques of genetic engineering, virologists began to isolate the viral genes or pieces of virus genetic material actually responsible for bringing about the transformation. In a short time they had isolated more than two-dozen such genes (Table 7.1).

When it was discovered that some *oncogenic* viruses apparently had *no* oncogenes, it was reasoned that perhaps in such cases viruses were somehow able to activate "oncogenes" already present in the target cells. When normal cells were examined for the presence of oncogenes, investigators were amazed to find that practically all normal cells had genes very similar to the "oncogenes" isolated from viruses. Naturally, this raised the question, "What are oncogenes doing in normal cells?" The answer apparently is "Very little, if anything." Normally, they are minimally active or even dormant. In some cases at least, transformation appears to be a result of the increased activity of a normal gene.

The normal counterparts of transforming oncogenes are now called **proto-oncogenes**. Research has revealed a number of ways in which such genes might become activated (see Land et al., 1983; Cline et al; Croce and Klein, 1985). The following list is partial: (1) viruses can bring uncontrollable oncogenes into a cell; (2) viruses (without oncogenes) can introduce genetic material that interferes with the control of proto-oncogenes such that they become more active (see Shen-Ong et al., 1984; Croce and Klein, 1985); (3) the number of oncogenes (proto-oncogenes) can increase, a process called *gene ampli-*

fication (see Brodeur et al., 1984); (4) oncogene mutations can result in a gene product that is more potent (see Guerrero et al., 1984); (5) genes that regulate oncogenes can undergo mutations that make them less able to regulate or restrain oncogenes; and (6) oncogenes can become "uncontrolled" (turned up or derepressed) when a chromosome breaks (see Hecht et al., 1984; Croce and Klein, 1985).

Now that we have the story in outline, let's consider more of the detail.

Viruses and Oncogenes

In the early 1970s, several different groups of investigators demonstrated that viruses able to cause sarcomas in chickens had a special gene that the investigators called the *src* gene (actually, *v-src*—oncogenes are now identified by three letter codes and a prefix. The prefix letter indicates whether the oncogene is viral, *v*, or cellular, *c*; the three-letter code indicates the animal from which the tumor arose and/or the tumor; *src* = sarcoma). The *v-src* gene was discovered by investigators working with a mutant virus unable to cause chicken sarcoma. When they compared the genetic machinery of mutant viruses with that of the normal virus—the one able to induce chicken sarcoma—they found that the mutant genome was shorter. A gene was missing.

The "missing" gene was isolated (from the normal or parent strain of the virus) and then characterized. With genetic engineering technology, the genetic material of the viruses was cut into pieces, copied many times by putting the pieces into bacteria, and then tested to see just which pieces could cause transformation when inserted into a test cell. (See Weinberg, 1983, for a description of the methodology by which oncogenes are isolated and identified.)

In the subsequent search for the src gene in other oncogenic viruses, several dozen different oncogenes have been found thus far (Table 7.1). But, as already indicated, the search also revealed that not all cancer-causing viruses *had* on-

Table 7.1 Some of the First-to-Be-Isolated Retroviral Oncogenes, Their Normal Hosts, Their Counterparts Found in Human Cancer Cells, and the Location and Activity of the Known Oncogene Products

Viral Oncogene	Retrovirus (Normal Host/Tumor)	Human Tumor(s) in Which c-Oncogene Is Found	Oncogene Products	
			Subcellular Location	Activity/Function*
abl	Abelson mouse leukemia	CML	Plasma membrane	Tyrosine protein kinase
erbA	Chicken leukemia		Cytosol	U
erbB	Chicken leukemia/ sarcoma		Plasma and intra-cellular membranes	Truncated epidermal growth factor receptor
ets	Chicken leukemia		U	U
fes/fps	Cat/chicken sarcoma	AML, CML, ALL; lung, breast, and kidney carcinoma	Cytoplasm (cytoskeleton(?)/ plasma membrane)	Tyrosine protein kinase
fgr	Gardner-Rasheed cat sarcoma		U	Hybrid of actin fragment plus tyrosine protein kinase
fms	McDonough cat sarcoma	Breast, kidney, lung, ovary, pancreas carcinoma; CML, Hodgkin's, AML (?)	Plasma and intra-cellular membranes	Truncated epidermal growth factor receptor
fos	Mouse osteogenic sarcoma	**	Nucleosol	U
B-lym		Human and chicken lymphoma	Nucleosol	U
mil	Mill Hill 2 chicken leukemia/carcinoma		Cytosol	Serine protein kinase
mos	Moloney mouse sarcoma/ plasmacytosis		Cytosol	Serine protein kinase
myb	Chicken myeloblastic leukemia	AML, ALL, CML, Hodgkin's and non-Hodgkin's lymphomas; breast and lung(?) carcinomas	Nucleosol	U
myc	Chicken myelocytomatosis, carcinoma	**	Nucleosol	DNA binding
raf	Rat (newborn) fibrosarcoma		Cytosol	Serine protein kinase
H-ras/K-ras	Rat sarcoma	**	Plasma membrane	GTP binding
N-ras		Leukemia(?) and carcinoma(?)	Plasma membrane	U
rel	Turkey reticuloendotheliosis		U	U

Table 7.1   (Continued)

Viral Oncogene	Retrovirus (Normal Host/Tumor)	Human Tumor(s) in Which c-Oncogene Is Found	Oncogene Products	
			Subcellular Location	Activity/Function*
ros	Chicken sarcoma		Plasma membrane	Tyrosine protein kinase
sis	Simian sarcoma		Cytosol/secreted	Chain of platelet-derived growth factor
ski	Chicken sarcoma		Nucleosol	U
src	Rous chicken sarcoma	Lymphosarcoma; CML	Plasma membrane	Tyrosine protein kinase
yes	Chicken sarcoma		Plasma membrane	Tyrosine protein kinase

Note: Human tumors studied include adenocarcinomas of the colon, small bowel, pancreas, ovary, uterus; carcinomas of kidney, lung, breast; Hodgkin's and non-Hodgkin's lymphomas; acute myelogenous leukemia (AML), chronic myelogenous leukemia (CML), acute lymphocytic leukemia (ALL).

*Oncogenes have recently been divided as follows:

Class 1	Tyrosine protein kinases found in cytoplasm
Class 1-related	Potential protein kinases
Class 2	Growth factors
Class 3	GTP-binding proteins in cytoplasm
Class 4	Nuclear proteins

**Carcinoma, sarcoma, leukemia, lymphoma. RNA of oncogenes *fos*, *myc*, H-*ras*, and K-*ras* is found in all types of tumors examined so far, whereas RNA expression of oncogenes *erbA*, *erbB*, *rel*, *sis*, and *yes* has not been found. Test results for RNA expression of *abl*, *fes*, *fms*, and *myb* indicate variation with cell type.

U: undefined

Source: Adapted from Peter and Tseng-Fung, 1984, p. 38. Reprinted with permission of Diagnostic Medicine, Medical Economics Co., Oradell, NJ.

cogenes. The possibility that transforming viruses without oncogenes activated proto-oncogenes already present in normal cells seemed reasonable especially in light of the fact that having or not having an oncogene was unrelated to the ability of a virus to reproduce. It was reasoned that the oncogenic viruses with oncogenes may have picked them up from animal cells infected by viral ancestors during the course of evolution (see Chapter 10 for a description of the way in which viruses reproduce via the cells of other organisms).

When it was first observed that normal animal cells often had stretches of DNA similar to those from viruses, it was thought that these common genes originated with viruses—that vi-

ruses had infected such cells way back in evolution and the virus genetic material became incorporated into the genome and just *stayed* there, being replicated any time a cell divided. Now it is believed that the common "oncogenes" actually originated in animal cells—that viruses picked up such genes from animal cells during "virus infections" and kept them. The most compelling evidence for this hypothesis is that all or at least *parts* of the oncogenes found thus far are divided into transcribed regions (called **exons**) separated by nontranscribed stretches of DNA called **introns**. This kind of fancy spacing is commonly found in animal cells, but not in retroviruses (RNA viruses—see Chapter 10). All this evidence stimulated the search for oncogenes in still more normal cells, leading to the discovery that proto-oncogenes are present in the normal cells of most, if not all, creatures, including mice, birds, humans, and even fruit flies (Bishop, 1982).

The virus-oncogene connection in summary—insofar as we can now determine (and speculate) from the few pieces of the puzzle in hand—is that during the course of evolution, viruses picked up a number of normal genes from various animal host cells, which became part of the viruses' genetic array, as oncogenes. When oncogenic viruses give these genes back to an animal cell during present-day infections, for some unknown reason the result often is malignant transformation. The oncogenes may have been changed (mutated) after the viruses got them so that they make too much product; the amount of viral oncogene product in chicken sarcoma cells is 100 times greater than the amount of normal "oncogene" product in normal cells (Cooper, 1982). Other possibilities are that oncogenes make product at the wrong time, or make product that is slightly different, more potent. Still another possibility is that the viruses transmit oncogenes in some kind of uncontrollable arrangement with pieces of viral genetic material.

Not all oncogenes have a (known) virus connection. In fact, oncogene research has generated two artificial groups of oncogenes, viral and cellular. The cellular category is made up of oncogenes isolated from cancer cells including human cancer cells and having the ability to transform, demonstrated in the so-called **NIH 3T3 transfection assay**. The abbreviation NIH stands for National Institutes of Health; *3T3* is the name of a mammalian cell line. In the transfection assay, 3T3 cells are given bits of DNA to see if the DNA can transform the cells.

It must be emphasized that while viruses are unquestionably linked to many kinds of neoplasms in animals other than humans, viruses have been implicated in only a few human cancers. Human cells may somehow be no longer generally responsive to viral oncogenes. In humans, oncogenes are apparently most often influenced by things other than viruses.

Oncogenes in Human Neoplasms

Oncogenes capable of transforming the NIH 3T3 line of mouse cells commonly used to test for transforming power have been isolated from many kinds of human neoplasms (see Cooper et al., 1984; Santos et al., 1984; Slamon et al., 1984; Bonner et al., 1984; Pelicci et al., 1984; Feig et al., 1984; Brodeur et al., 1984; and Yokota et al., 1986). Although similar genes can be isolated from *normal* cells, these cannot transform the NIH 3T3 cells. Apparently whatever converts proto-oncogenes to transforming oncogenes involves something more than just taking them out of context.

The Activation of Oncogenes

Earlier (page 109) we listed some of the ways in which oncogenes can become "activated". Let us now look at some of these mechanisms in detail, in light of experimental evidence.

Mutation and Oncogenes

Several groups of investigators collectively wondered about the difference between a quiescent oncogene or proto-oncogene of a normal cell and its counterpart in a cancer cell. They mass-produced a human bladder cancer oncogene and its counterpart from normal bladder cells, and began swapping pieces of the two kinds of genes to see just where the transforming gene locus was and how it differed from the analogous portion of the gene from normal cells. Using these techniques, at least three different groups of scientists found that the critical difference between the normal cell gene and the transforming oncogene was a single nucleotide base substitution—one base out of approximately

6,000. Thymine was replaced by guanine (see Marx, 1982c; the entire nucleotide sequence of the oncogene has been published by Reddy, 1983). This point mutation resulted in the substitution of valine for glycine as the twelfth amino acid in the gene's protein product. Also, the product of the transforming oncogene was 100 times more effective in bringing about malignant transformation than the proto-oncogene product. Until this discovery, it was generally thought that oncogenes brought about transformation simply—and only—by producing *more* of a normal product. Later Feinberg and colleagues (1983) found that this point mutation is apparently only *one* of the things that can cause this human oncogene to specify malignancy. They were unable to find the same mutation in the cells of ten other cases of human bladder cancer, nine cases of colon cancer, or in ten cases of lung cancer.

Chromosome Flaws and Oncogenes

It has been known for a decade that many neoplasms have characteristic breaks and other gross flaws, compared to the chromosomes of normal cells (Sandberg, 1980). **Chromosome-banding techniques** (the use of special stains to visualize the bands of differential chemical density in chromosomes—see Chapter 11) have revealed more subtle, but no less characteristic, chromosome defects associated with even more types of cancer. Some examples of the kinds of chromosome defects associated with cancer are the following.

Translocations involving Chromosomes 9 and 22 are seen in the cells of nearly all adult cases of chronic myelogenous leukemia (CML). Translocations involving Chromosomes 8 and 14 have been found in the cancer cells of virtually *all* cases of Burkitt's lymphoma evaluated. One study revealed a deletion of precisely the same chromosome locus in the neoplastic cells in 26 patients with small-cell lung carcinoma. There are many other examples (see Yunis, 1983; see also Chapter 11).

The fact that chromosomal aberrations such as these represent physical displacements of genes suggests the possibility that oncogene activation may consist of the movement of previously inactive or "sluggishly" active genes to locations adjacent to activator sequences of DNA—or movement of an oncogene *away from* genes that had been repressing it. This idea has received considerable impetus in the last few years with the discovery that oncogenes are, in fact, often physically located next to certain cancer-linked breaks in chromosomes.

Figure 7.2 illustrates the chromosome-oncogene connection associated with Burkitt's lymphoma. Chromosome 14 contains a region known to be the home of the "active" genes that code for the antibodies made by B-lymphocytes (see Chapter 14). B-lymphocytes happen to be the cells that are transformed in Burkitt's lymphoma. An oncogene designated *myc**, normally located on normally quiet (in B-lymphocytes) Chromosome 8, is characteristically translocated to Chromosome 14[†] next to an immunoglobulin gene (Gold, 1983). Apparently the *myc* oncogene of lymphocytes is activated by being translocated from a "sleepy" region of Chromosome 8 to one of several activated regions on other chromosomes (see Marx, 1982a). It has even been demonstrated that *myc* genes on Chromosome 14 are expressed at much higher levels than *myc* genes located on Chromosome 8—even in the same cell (see Rushdi et al., 1983).

---

*The cellular *myc* gene was implicated in cancer when it was discovered that a cancer-causing virus (which had no oncogene), in chickens inserted itself into the genetic material of chicken cells near, or next to, a normal gene, *myc*, that resembled oncogenes seen in other oncogenic viruses.

[†]In about 5 percent of the patients with Burkitt's lymphoma tested, there is instead an exchange between Chromosomes 8 and 22; in another 5 percent, there is an exchange between Chromosomes 8 and 2. It so happens that Chromosome 2 bears a gene that codes for one of the two light chains (see Chapter 14 for a description of immunoglobulin—antibody—structure) of the antibodies made by lymphocytes at about the point where the break occurs; Chromosome 22 carries the genes that code for the *other* light chain—again, where the break occurs.

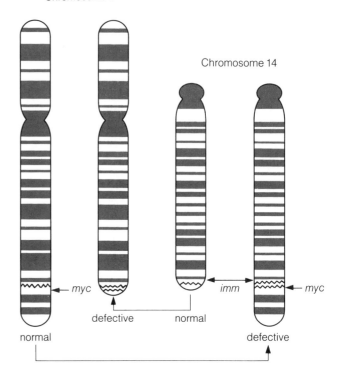

Chromosome 8

Chromosome 14

normal

myc

defective normal

normal

imm

myc

defective

Figure 7.2 The relationship between chromosome breaks and oncogenes in Burkitt's lymphoma. Burkitt's lymphoma affects B-lymphocyte cells, which normally make antibodies. An oncogene designated *myc* (see text) is normally located on Chromosome 8. In the most common break associated with Burkitt's lymphoma, the *myc* gene is translocated to Chromosome 14, where genes *(imm)* that specify immunoglobulins are located and which therefore is an "active" region of chromosome. The current view is that one of the general mechanisms of oncogene activation is the movement of oncogenes to activated regions of the genome. (Redrawn from Gold, 1983.)

Other Possibilities

Two more general mechanisms of activation of cellular oncogenes deserve some of the expanded consideration we have just given to viruses, direct mutations, and chromosomal rearrangements. They are (1) gene amplification and (2) enhancement of transcription. Gene amplification and enhanced transcription fall under what some investigators call the "dose hypothesis"; namely, that cancer can result if certain normal genes are overexpressed. Whatever the product of the gene is, according to this hypothesis, cancer is a result of there being too much of it.

Gene Amplification Gene amplification is the phenomenon in which many more than the normal number of copies of a particular gene appear in a cell. Although we do not know exactly how

gene amplification is controlled, it is a normal way by which cells increase gene products as needed—when large amounts of particular proteins are needed by **oocytes** (egg cells) in frog egg production, for example. Other things being equal, gene amplification results in more gene product because it results in more sites for synthesizing messenger RNA (see Chapter 2). Oncogene amplification may well be one of the general ways in which normal cells become cancer cells. The amplification of the *myc* gene and its near relative, for example, has been seen in several types of cancer. It has been reported to be amplified 30 to 50 times in human promyelocytic leukemia; the K-*ras* oncogene has been found to be amplified three to five times in cells derived from human colon cancer (see Land et al., 1983). Even greater amplifications have been reported in other human neoplasms (see Brodeur et al., 1984; Pelicci et al., 1984; and Kohl et al., 1984).

Enhanced Transcription The term *enhanced transcription* refers to a process that has also been implicated as one of the classes of oncogene activation mechanisms: the enhancement of the expression of a *normal* number of *normal* proto-oncogenes. Novel, more efficient, promotors (see Chapter 2) have been implicated in the activation of H-*ras* in rats (see Land et al., 1983); special pieces of DNA (enhancer sequences) may also be involved in some cases. Either by translocation or mutation, these may end up next to proto-oncogenes and enhance their expression (see Land et al., 1983).

There is no closure here. No sweeping generalization about the activation of cellular oncogenes is possible yet—save perhaps that control of oncogene expression can be lost in a number of ways. As will be seen in the next section, the loss of control of oncogene *expression* can likewise manifest itself in a variety of ways, depending on the nature of the products of the genes that are out of control.

What Do Oncogenes Do?
First the Good News

Perhaps the answer to the question "What do oncogenes do?" should begin with another question, "What do proto-oncogenes do?" Apparently proto-oncogenes play some basic role in the regulation of cell division. A number of them have been found to be maximally expressed at certain stages of embryonic development; the *myc* gene in particular has been found to be activated when the **hematopoietic** (blood-cell producing) **system** is being expanded in the fetal liver (Cline et al., 1984). In blood-vessel lining cells, *sis* (see Table 7.1) messenger RNA levels have been found to be low when the cells are in a differentiated mode and higher when the cells are proliferating (see Jaye et al., 1985). There is evidence that *myc*, *fos*, and other proto-oncogenes are activated by growth factors. All of this seems to suggest that proto-oncogenes may generally function whenever and wherever cells are called upon to divide—in embryonic development or later, during wound healing or liver regeneration (see Peter and Tseng-Fung, 1984). Whatever proto-oncogenes do, it is very likely that they serve some *basic* function, because they are so highly conserved in evolution.

Functional Classes of Oncogenes

It is unlikely that the 30 oncogenes found to be derived from cells and the 10 or so found in oncogenic DNA viruses thus far (see Table 7.1 for a partial listing) specify 40 different *kinds* of action. It is more likely that oncogenes fall into a few common, functional classes.

One classification divides oncogenes into those whose products (note that the reference here is to products, not the genes, themselves) are found in the nucleus and another whose products localize in the cytoplasm or the cell membrane. Nuclear oncogene products include those of *myb*, *myc*, *ski*, and *fos* oncogenes, among others; cytoplasmic products include those of *ras*, *src*, *erbB*, *neu*, *ros*, *fms*, *fes/fps*, *yes*, *mil*, *raf*, *mos*, and *abl* (see Table 7.1). These two "geographical" classes also seem to be functional subdivisions. Nuclear oncogene products generally confer immortality on cells and give them independence from exogenous growth factors. Cytoplasmic oncogene products generally promote **anchorage independence** (cells do not have to attach to something in order to grow) and seem to be associated in one way or another to the secretion of growth factors (see Weinberg, 1985). The two classes also appear to represent two different kinds of oncogene *activation*. Generally speaking, oncogenes of the cytoplasmic product class appear to be activated by mutations that lead to structural alterations in the proteins they encode. Examples include *ras*, *src*, *erbB*, *abl*, *fes/fps*, and *neu* oncogenes; exceptions include the cytoplasmic *abl* oncogene, which is altered by chromosomal translocation (as is the nuclear oncogene, *myc*) (Weinberg, 1985).

Again, generally speaking, nuclear oncogenes are activated by some form of deregulation in the nucleus.

The good news is that we have a good idea what at least some oncogenes do. Many of them code for protein kinases. A **protein kinase** is an enzyme that specializes in activating other enzymes and other kinds of molecules by attaching a phosphate group to them. The following oncogenes are among those that code for protein kinases, enzymes that attach phosphate specifically to the amino acid, tyrosine (and are thus called **tyrosine kinases**): *src, yes, fes, fgr, abl,* and *ros*; the products of *raf, mil,* and *mos* phosphorylate proteins at the amino acid, serine.

At least some oncogenes provide the specifications for the construction of protein kinases able to activate cell-surface proteins involved in cellular adhesion. Although it is not yet known exactly what these oncogene products do at the surface, they have been localized in **adhesion plaques**—structures involved in the adherence of cells to solid surfaces—structures known to be dismantled when cells are transformed (Bishop, 1982). This fact is certainly interesting in that (as indicated in Chapter 4) the cell surface is a likely place for a key malignant defect to be localized. Other oncogene-specified protein kinases—*ros* and *src* products, for example—may act by mimicking cytoplasmic signals normally generated when cell surface receptors combine with normal signal molecules, that is, by activating the molecules involved in the generation of second messenger molecules (Chapter 4). It appears that enzymes activated by certain oncogene-specified kinases are some of the same enzymes activated by **platelet-derived growth factor (PDGF)**. PDGF is a substance brought to wounds by platelets and released when platelets stick to jagged edges of damaged tissue (Chapter 3). (The function of PDGF is to stimulate certain kinds of cells to divide, as part of the wound repair process.)

Ultimately, oncogene-specified protein kinases may also be linked to *lipid* kinases (normally activated by certain hormones) and the phosphorylation of phosphatidyl inositol (PI). As pointed out by Weinberg and others, the phosphorylation of PI would, in turn, lead to the activation of the "second messengers"—diacylglycerol and inositol trisphosphate. The trisphosphate increases calcium ions in the cell and these, in conjunction with diacylglycerol, activate protein kinase C, which activates various enzymes. Calcium itself is another kind of second messenger, able through its interaction with a calcium binding protein called **calmodulin** to activate various enzymes and help bring about some of the changes associated with transformation.

Still other oncogene products may mimic growth factors (such as PDGF) more directly. In 1983, it was discovered that a particular oncogene, *sis* (isolated from a simian sarcoma virus believed to have originated in a woolly monkey), was 87 percent identical (in terms of its nucleotide base sequences) to part of the gene that codes for PDGF (Doolittle et al., 1983; Deuel et al., 1983). The discovery of the relationship between PDGF and oncogenes was a result of the convergence of work in several different laboratories. One group purified PDGF in 1979. In 1983, the same group, in collaboration with another group, determined the amino acid sequence of PDGF. Still another group determined the amino acid sequence of the *sis* oncogene. Another scientist, armed with a computerized databank of known amino acid sequences, compared the amino acid sequences and found that the two had many similarities—the *sis* oncogene product is nearly identical to one of the protein subunits of PDGF (see Graves et al., 1984). There is some evidence that the *sis* oncogene product may be able to activate the PDGF receptor by phosphorylating it (Leal et al., 1985).

Less than half of the known oncogenes act as protein kinases. Only one is known to possibly act as a growth factor. What about the others? There are other kinds of growth factors, and perhaps other oncogenes will be found to specify some of these. Some oncogene products may activate second messengers in ways other than phosphorylation.

Products of the *ras* oncogene family (H-ras,

K-ras, and N-ras) may function by activating ad-enyl cyclase; *ras* proteins appear to function as G proteins or **GTP-binding proteins**. GTP bind-ing proteins are found in a variety of tissues, where they are involved in the transduction of signals across the cell membrane when primary messenger molecules bind to receptors on the cell surface (see Downward et al., 1984; see also Fig. 7.3).

The *erbB* oncogene product serves as a sub-strate for protein kinase and is similar in struc-ture to the receptor protein for epidermal growth factor (EGF) (Marx, 1984a; Coussens et al., 1985). The receptor specified by *erbB* may behave as if it were activated and gives the signal to divide even in the absence of EGF—or per-haps, once normally activated it cannot be turned off (Marx, 1984a). The *fms* and *neu* onco-gene products are apparently also protein kinase substrates that appear to be variations of growth factor receptors (Rettenmier et al., 1985).

The oncogene *myc* encodes a protein that binds to nuclear material—probably DNA. The product of *myc* and other "nuclear" oncogenes apparently regulates or deregulates other genes, possibly other oncogenes (see Fig. 7.3) in ways yet to be discovered. Typically, the introduction of an oncogene into a normal cell causes many changes. A gene product that influences the expression of still other genes directly could be the basis of such **plieotropy**.

The picture that seems to be emerging thus far is that oncogene products impact various parts of a normal signaling cascade that begins with growth factors and other signals and ends with the activation of genes. The common effect of these products is independent growth—in-dependence generated by different oncogene products in different ways. Some oncogenes ap-parently specify the production of growth fac-tors. Some such oncogenes (e.g., *sis*) code for proteins able to act directly as growth factors; others (e.g., *ras*, *src*, *mos*, *fes*, *abl*, *fps*, *yes*, and *mil/raf*) code for proteins able to stimulate other genes to make growth factors (see Weinberg, 1985). Other oncogenes make products that ob-viate the need for growth factors. Among these

are oncogenes that code for growth factor recep-tors that may behave as if they have combined with growth factor even when they have not. The *erbB*, *neu*, and *fms* oncogenes code for pos-sibly defective growth factor receptors. Still other oncogenes code for messenger-generating proteins in the cytoplasm that would normally only be made when signals activate cell surface receptors. There is some evidence that the *ras* family of oncogene products may send false sig-nals to the nucleus, signals normally sent only in the presence of growth factors. Nuclear on-cogene products may free the cell from depen-dence on growth factors by simply doing what-ever their proto-oncogene counterparts do under the influence of exogenous growth fac-tors, even when there is no growth factor pres-ent. It is already known that growth factors normally stimulate *myc*, *fos*, and other proto-oncogenes. The *myc* and *fos* oncogenes may sim-ply be chronically turned on *myc* and *fos* proto-oncogenes.

The *bad* news is that oncogene products may fail to make cancer cells different enough from normal cells. When the existence of onco-genes was first imagined, a reasonable expecta-tion was that oncogene products would all be novel proteins that could be used to immunize human beings against similar proteins. It was, in other words, a basis for the hope that there one day will be a vaccine against all or most forms of cancer. Although the discovery of on-cogenes has given us a much better understand-ing of cancer, part of that understanding makes it clear why cancer is and will be a difficult thing to cure.

Cancer in Two Steps

Different oncogenes may be involved in differ-ent stages of carcinogenesis. In 1983, three groups of scientists reported that at least two genes are involved in the transformation of nor-mal cells into cancer cells. One of the genes ap-parently confers the "immortalization" dis-cussed in Chapter 4. A second step apparently

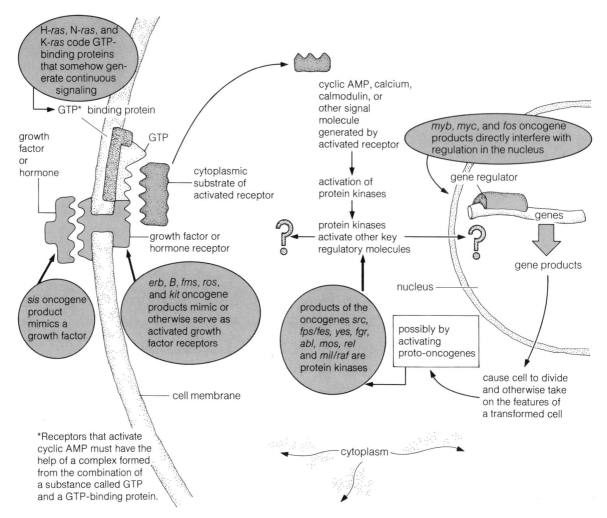

Figure 7.3 Normally, a "messenger" molecule such as a hormone or growth factor causes a cell to divide through a cause-and-effect cascade such as shown here. Also shown is what oncogenes might do to short-circuit this system.

makes the cell divide continually. The conclusion that at least two genetic changes must be involved in carcinogenesis was reached by Robert Weinberg and others at MIT, Earl Ruley and others at the Cold Spring Harbor Laboratory, and Robert Newbold and others at the Institute of Cancer Research in England. Each of these groups observed that the H-*ras* oncogene (Table 7.1) could not, by itself, cause normal cells to become cancer cells. The Weinberg group found

that the *myc* oncogene and the H-*ras* oncogene were *both* necessary for the conversion of rat embryo cells into cancer cells. The Ruley group found that baby rat kidney cells could be converted into cancer cells by the H-*ras* oncogene only if the cells had already been made "immortal" by another gene. And the Newbold group found that the H-*ras* oncogene could transform cultured cells only if they were made "immortal" by exposure to chemical carcinogens.

The Weinberg group suggested that the *myc* gene confers "immortality" and that the *ras* gene speeds up cell division. Apparently the order of the two steps is relatively unimportant.

There is also some evidence that there may be cooperation between oncogenes, or that there may be cascades in which the products of one kind of oncogene turn on oncogenes further down the chain. Philip Leder and his colleagues suggest that the *myc* oncogene can be activated by PDGF or the very similar product made by the *sis* oncogene. The *myc* oncogene, in turn, makes a product that may regulate still other genes in the nucleus of the cell (see Marx, 1983b).

Why did it take so long to discover that two or more genes may be involved? At least part of the reason is that much of the work involving only one gene was done with permanent cell lines—cells that *already* had gone through one of the required steps (see Chapter 4).

In any case, it now seems clear that two or even more oncogenes must be activated to bring about a complete transformation of a normal cell. Rarely has a single oncogene been found to be able to completely transform a normal cell (see Land et al., 1983). It may be that the cell's environmental circumstance determines if just one oncogene can transform it. If this is true however, it may mean that a second oncogene may simply be activated by certain cellular environments. Giving cells two, or otherwise artificially activating two oncogenes, may make them independent of whatever environmental circumstance allows a single oncogene to transform a cell (see Weinberg, 1985).

Summary and Prospects

In summary, genes able to induce cellular transformation were first recognized in work with oncogenic viruses. It was soon found that these genes were not unique to cancer-causing viruses; they are present and functional in normal cells of most if not all species. Oncogenes appear to be normal, functional, vital components of the genome. They specify cancer when their structure or their control systems are disturbed by carcinogenic agents in a number of different ways leading either to more *powerful* gene products or to *more* gene product. In many, if not all cases, more than one oncogene is apparently involved in the development of any one cancer, and the products of one oncogene may influence other oncogenes in a kind of chain reaction.

Now would be a good time to reflect on the connection between this chapter and Chapter 4, where we catalogued the features of cancer cells. "Features" are all determined by genes and by the way genes interact with each other and with one another's products.

We have made the case often that of all the genes and gene products involved in malignant transformation, most are probably secondary to changes or problems with a few primary genes. This likelihood suggests that "cancerness" is the net result of a cascade of action and reaction set in motion by one of a few key oncogenes or key groups of oncogenes.

Why do we keep using the word *few*? We know that it probably isn't many because cancer is not so rare as to be the result of accumulated, specific malfunctions in hundreds of genes. Cancer would be much less common if, let's say, a hundred different mutations were required for it to appear. Nor do we see the range of transformedness or cancerness we might expect if cancer involved lots of individual steps. Basically, a cancer cell is either a cancer cell or it isn't.

Yet, while it is conceivable that just one key gene may well be responsible for cancer through some kind of cascade effect, available evidence and logic suggest that it may take more—a few more—than one gene.

Consider Figure 7.4. Cellular behavior is a complex thing. In any system with an output—be it an impact, a product, or a behavioral feature—the output is a *net* result, a net expression of a number of individual, interconnected parts and processes, any one of which could go wrong. Heat pumps, automobiles, cities, human bodies, governments, and cells all have more than one way to go wrong.

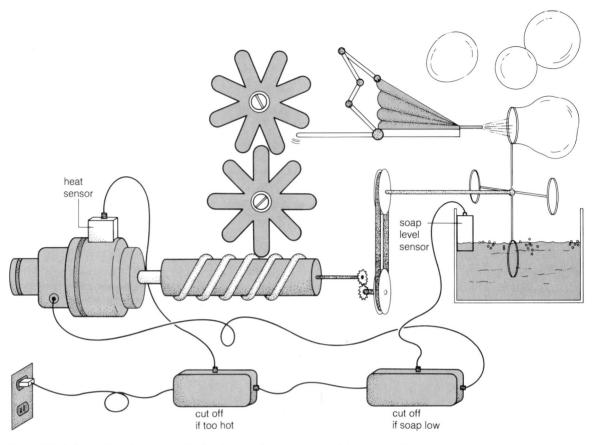

Figure 7.4 Cells are like other systems having "outputs" as a net result of the action of individual, interconnected parts.

heat
sensor

soap
level
sensor

cut off
if too hot

cut off
if soap low

Figure 7.3 suggests that there are many interconnections between genes and features of cells that determine how a cell will respond to its environment. The figure is simplistic and obviously incomplete; if we put even all of the little that we *know* about cells on the figure, it might have to be as big as a living room wall. Even as it is, the figure makes it clear that many things involving many genes can go wrong to cause a cell to misbehave. But just because many things *can* go wrong doesn't mean that they all *do* go wrong. There are probably weak spots, trouble spots. When a heat pump's coils overheat, the problem could be caused by a lot of things, but the cause is very often a faulty relay switch.

Maybe cancer cells have the equivalents of relay switches.

References and Further Reading

Becker, F., ed. 1975. *Cancer: A Comprehensive Treatise.* Vol. 1: *Etiology: Chemical and Physical Carcinogenesis.* Vol. 2: *Etiology: Viral Carcinogenesis.* New York: Plenum.

Bishop, J. M. 1982. Oncogenes. *Scientific American* 246(3):80–92.

Bishop, J. M., Rowley, J. D., and Greaves, M., eds 1984. *Genes and Cancer.* New York: Alan R. Liss.

Bonner, T., et al. 1984. The Human Homologs of the *raf (mil)* Oncogene Are Located on Human Chromosome-3 and Chromosome-4. *Science.* 223:71–74.

Borden, L. A., et al. 1984. Homologies Between Signal Transducing G Proteins and *ras* Gene Products. *Science.* 226:860–61.

Brodeur, G. M., et al., 1984. Amplification of N-*myc* in Untreated Human Neuroblastomas Correlates with Advanced Disease Stage. *Science.* 224:1121–24.

Cline, M. J., Slamon, D. J., and Lipsick, J. S. 1984. Oncogenes: Implications for the Diagnosis and Treatment of Cancer. *Annals of Internal Medicine.* 101(2): 223–33.

Cooper, G. M. 1982. Cellular Transforming Genes. *Science.* 218:801–06.

Cooper, G. S., et al., 1984. Characterization of Human Transforming Genes from Chemically Transformed, Teratocarcinoma, and Pancreatic Carcinoma Cell Lines. *Cancer Research.* 44(1):1–10.

Coussens, L., Yang-Feng, T. L., Liao, Y. C., et al. 1985. Tyrosine Kinase Receptor with Extensive Homology to EGF Receptor Shares Chromosomal Location with *neu* Oncogene. *Science.* 230:1132–39.

Croce, C. M., and Klein, G. 1985. Chromosome Translocations and Human Cancer. *Scientific American.* 252:54–60.

Decade of Discovery. 1981. NIH Publication No. 81–2323. Washington, D.C.: U.S. Department of Health and Human Services.

Deuel, T. F., et al. 1983. Expression of a Platelet-Derived Growth Factor-Like Protein in Simian Sarcoma Virus Transformed Cells. *Science.* 221:1348–50.

D'Eustachio, P. 1984. Gene Mapping and Oncogenes. *American Scientist.* 72:32–40.

DeVita, V. 1986. *Important Advances in Oncology* 1986. Philadelphia: Lippincott.

Doolittle, R. F., et al. 1983. Simian Sarcoma Virus *onc* Gene, *v-sis*, Is Derived from the Gene (or Genes) Encoding a Platelet-Derived Growth Factor. *Science.* 221:275–76.

Downward, J., et al. 1984. Close Similarity of Epidermal Growth Factor Receptors and *v-erb*-B Oncogene Protein Sequences. *Nature.* 307:521–27.

Favera, R. D., et al. 1982. Chromosomal Localization of the Human Homolog (*c-cis*) of the Simian Sarcoma Virus *onc* Gene. *Science.* 218:686–87.

Feig, L. A., Bast, R. C., and Cooper, G. M. 1984. Somatic Activation of *ras*^K Gene in a Human Ovarian Carcinoma. *Science.* 223:698–700.

Feinberg, A. P., et al. 1983. Mutation Affecting the 12th Amino Acid of the *c-Ha-ras* Oncogene Product Occurs Infrequently in Human Cancer. *Science.* 220:1175–77.

Gold, M. 1983. Cancer: When the Chromosome Breaks. *Science 83.* (4) September, pp. 16–17.

Graves, D. T., et al. 1984. Detection of *c-sis* Transcripts and Synthesis of PDGH-like Proteins by Human Osteosarcoma Cells. *Science.* 226:972–74.

Guerrero, I., Villasante, A., D'Eustachio, P., and Pellicer, A. 1984. Isolation, Characterization, and Chromosome Assignment of Mouse N-*ras* Gene from Carcinogen-Induced Thymic Lymphoma. *Science.* 225:1041–43.

Guerrero, I., Villasante, A., Croces, V., and Pellicer, A. 1984. Activation of c-K-*ras* Oncogene by Somatic Mutation in Mouse Lymphomas Induced by Gamma Radiation. *Science.* 225:1159–62.

Hecht, F., et al. 1984. Common Region on Chromosome 14 in T-Cell Leukemia and Lymphoma. *Science.* 226:1445–47.

Hunter, T. 1984. The Proteins of Oncogenes. *Scientific American.* 251(2) August, pp. 70–79.

Jaye, M., et al. 1985. Modulation of the *sis* Gene Transcript During Endothelial Cell Differentiation in Vitro. *Science.* 228:882–84.

Kohl, N. E., Gee, C. E., and Alt, F. W. 1984. Activated Expression of the N-*myc* Gene in Human Neuroblastomas and Related Tumors. *Science.* 226:1335–36.

Kuo, J. F., ed. 1985. Phospholipids and Cellular Regulation. Boca Raton, Fla.: CRC Press.

Land, H., Parada, L. F., and Weinberg, R. A. 1983. Cellular Oncogenes and Multistep Carcinogenesis. *Science.* 222:771–778.

Leal, F., Williams, L. T., Robbins, K. C., and Aaronson, S. A. 1985. Evidence That the *v-sis* Gene Product Transforms by Interaction with the Receptor for Platelet-Derived Growth Factor. *Science.* 230:327–30.

Leder, P., et al. 1983. Translocations Among Antibody Genes in Human Cancer. *Science.* 222:765–78.

Marx, J. L. 1982a. Cancer Cell Genes Linked to Viral *onc* Genes. *Science.* 216:724.

Marx, J. L. 1982b. The Case of the Misplaced Gene. *Science.* 218:983–85.

Marx, J. L. 1982c. Change in Cancer Gene Pinpointed. *Science.* 218:667.

Marx, J. L. 1983a. Cooperation Between Oncogenes. *Science*. 222:602–03.

Marx, J. L. 1983b. *Onc* Gene Related to Growth Factor Gene. *Science*. 221:248.

Marx, J. L. 1984a. Oncogene Linked to Growth Factor Receptor. *Science*. 223:806.

Marx, J. L. 1984b. Oncogenes Amplified in Cancer Cells. *Science*. 223:40–41.

Marx, J. L. 1984c. What Do Oncogenes Do? *Science*. 223:673–76.

Naharro, G., Robbins, K. C., and Reddy, E. P. 1984. Gene Product of *v-fgr onc*: Hybrid Protein Containing a Portion of Actin and a Tyrosine-Specific Protein Kinase. *Science*. 223:63–66.

Needleman, S. W., et al. 1983. Normal Cells of Patients with High Cancer Risk Syndromes Lack Transforming Activity in the NIH/3T3 Transfection Assay. *Science*. 222:173–75.

O'Connor, T. E., and Rauscher, F. J., eds. 1983. *Oncogenes and Retroviruses: Evaluation of Basic Findings and Clinical Potential*. New York: Alan R. Liss.

Oppenheimer, S. B. 1982. Causes of Cancer: Gene Alteration Vs. Gene Activation. *American Laboratory*. 14(11) November, pp. 40–46.

Pelicci, P., et al. 1984. Amplification of the *c-myb* Oncogene in a Case of Human Acute Myelogenous Leukemia. *Science*. 224:1117–21.

Peter, J. B., and Tseng-Fung, J. 1984. Oncogenes, Proto-Oncogenes and Cancer. *Diagnostic Medicine*. 7(9) October, pp. 36–49.

Pimentel, E. 1986. *Oncogenes*. Boca Raton, Fla: CRC Press.

Reddy, E. P. 1983. Nucleotide Sequence Analysis of the T24 Human Bladder Carcinoma Oncogene. *Science*. 220:1061–63.

Rettenmier, C. W., Chen, J. H., Roussel, M. F., and Sherr, C. J. 1985. The Product of the *c-fms* Proto-oncogene: A Glycoprotein with Associated Tyrosine Kinase Activity. *Science*. 228:320–22.

Roussel, A., et al. 1979. Three New Types of Viral Oncogene of Cellular Origin Specific for Haematopoietic Cell Transformation. *Nature*. 281:452–55.

Rushdi, A., et al. 1983. Differential Expression of the Translocated and the Untranslocated *c-myc* Oncogene in Burkitt Lymphoma. *Science*. 222:390–93.

Sandberg, A., ed. 1980. *The Chromosomes in Human Cancer and Leukemia*. Amsterdam: Elsevier/North Holland.

Santos, E., et al. 1984. Malignant Activation of a K-*ras* Oncogene in Lung Carcinoma but Not in Normal Tissue of the Same Patient. *Science*. 223:661–64.

Shen-Ong, G. L., et al. 1984. Activation of the *c-myb* Locus by Viral Insertional Mutagenesis in Plasmacytoid Lymphosarcomas. *Science*. 226:1077–80.

Slamon, D. J., et al. 1984. Expression of Cellular Oncogenes in Human Malignancies. *Science*. 224:256–62.

Weinberg, R. A. 1983. A Molecular Basis of Cancer. *Scientific American*. 249(5) October, pp. 126–43.

Weinberg, R. A. 1985. The Action of Oncogenes in the Cytoplasm and Nucleus. *Science*. 230:770–76.

Weinstein, B., and Vogel, H. J., eds. 1983. *Genes and Proteins in Oncogenesis*. New York: Academic Press.

Yoakum, G. H., et al. 1985. Transformation of Human Bronchial Epithelial Cells Transfected by Harvey *ras* Oncogene. *Science*. 227:1174–79.

Yokota, J., Tsunetsugu-Yokota, Y., Battifora, H., et al. 1986. Alterations of *myc*, *myb*, and *ras-Ha* Proto-oncogenes in Cancers Are Frequent and Show Clinical Correlation. *Science*. 231:261–65.

Yunis, J. J. 1983. The Chromosomal Basis of Human Neoplasia. *Science*, 221:227–36.

This chapter is about chemicals that cause cancer. The last chapter led us to expect that if chemicals play some kind of role in cancer, they must somehow be able to influence DNA. Chapter 7 should also have led us to expect that there may be more than one way by which chemicals influence DNA. Here are some of the things we will consider in Chapter 8:

The first connection between cancer and chemical substances was made 200 years ago.

Different kinds of chemicals "cause" cancer. Some are simple metallic elements; others are complex organic compounds.

The most important cancer-causing chemicals seem to be electron-seeking chemicals or chemicals that can be converted to such **electrophiles**. Certain electrophiles can react with electron-*rich* DNA, distorting DNA in the process.

Some chemicals, called **mutagens**, are able to react with DNA either directly or after metabolic activation, to cause mutations. Nearly all carcinogens are mutagens, and *most* mutagens are carcinogens.

Some chemicals, called **precarcinogens**, cannot react with DNA until they are converted by metabolism to other chemical forms, called **ultimate carcinogens**.

Other chemicals, called **promoters**, are neither mutagenic nor carcinogenic but are somehow able to speed up cell division. Promoters can "bring on" cancer if cancer has already been initiated.

Chemicals that can act as both initiators and promoters are called **complete carcinogens**. Carcinogens with little or no promotion power are sometimes called **initiators**.

It follows from the last two items that some chemicals *unable* to induce cancer on their own, may well be able to do so in *combination* with other chemicals.

Testing chemicals to see if they are carcinogenic presents a considerable problem. It is unethical

8
_____

Chemical Carcinogenesis

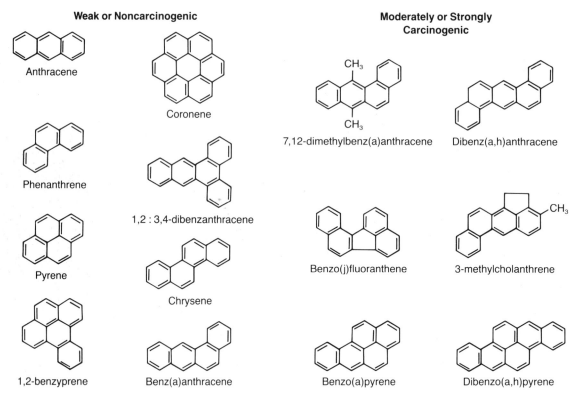

Figure 8.1 Some polycyclic aromatic hydrocarbons

to test chemicals on human beings, and animal tests are not 100 percent applicable to humans. Animal testing is very time consuming and expensive. Tests using bacteria or mammalian cells in culture can determine mutagenic potential very cheaply but they also present problems.

Historical Overview

There is no way to tell just when human beings first noticed a connection between chemicals and cancer. The first few people who saw a connection may well have been content to let others figure it out for themselves. They may have tried to tell others and failed to arouse much interest. Very early observers may even have written

down their observations, and the writings later were lost. We have only the preserved written record to go by.

According to the *written* record, an orderly sequence of steps linking chemicals and cancer began at about the time of the American Revolution. An English physician, Percival Pott, reported a high incidence of scrotum cancer among London chimney sweeps. Ten years earlier, another London physician, John Hill, had published *Cautions Against the Immoderate Use of Snuff*, describing a connection between cancer and snuff dipping. And an Italian, Bernardino Ramazzini, wrote in 1700 about breast cancer being somehow associated with being a nun. But the *thread* of the chemical carcinogenesis story actually begins with Pott.

Pott speculated that continuous exposure to soot among largely unwashed, preadolescent

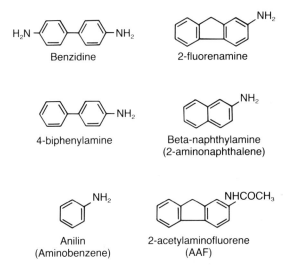

Figure 8.2 Some carcinogenic aromatic amines

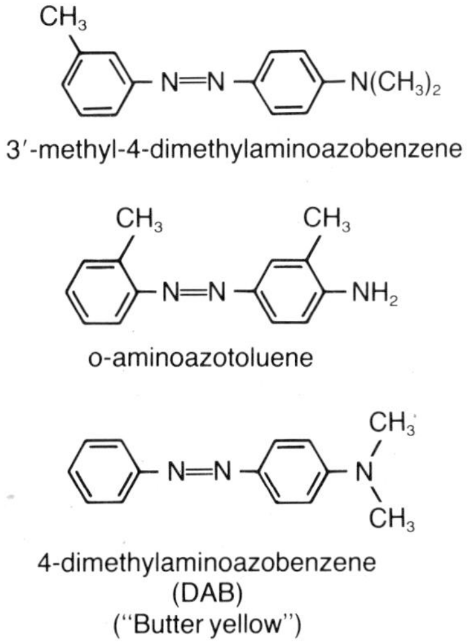

Benzidine

2-fluorenamine

4-biphenylamine

Beta-naphthylamine
(2-aminonaphthalene)

Anilin
(Aminobenzene)

2-acetylaminofluorene
(AAF)

3'-methyl-4-dimethylaminoazobenzene

o-aminoazotoluene

4-dimethylaminoazobenzene
(DAB)
("Butter yellow")

Figure 8.3 Some carcinogenic aminoazo dyes

chimney cleaners caused scrotal cancer in many of them as adults. This connection was probably widely assumed in Pott's day—the chimney sweeps themselves called scrotal cancer "soot wart." But Pott gets the credit because he wrote it down. One hundred years later, a German by the name of Volkman declared that the *tar* in soot caused cancer, because of his observation that tar workers were prone to cancer of the hands and forearms (see Shimkin, 1977). After another forty years, two Japanese workers, Katsusaburo Yamagiwa and Koichi Ichikawa showed that they could induce cancer on rabbit ears by repeatedly dabbing tar on them.

But tar is actually a complex mixture of chemicals, and it wasn't until 1930 that certain polycyclic hydrocarbons (Fig. 8.1) were identified as the carcinogenic ingredients in coal tar. A group of scientists headed by E. L. Kennaway at the Beatty Institute in London succeeded in isolating dibenz(a,h)anthracene and then benzo(a)pyrene from coal tar as the first pure chemical carcinogens. Many other polycyclic hydrocarbons have since been identified as strong carcinogens; others have been identified as moderate to weak carcinogens. Still other polycyclic hydrocarbons have been shown to have

absolutely no carcinogenic potential at all. This raises an obvious question: if being a polycyclic hydrocarbon doesn't assure carcinogenicity, what does? Let's finish bringing historical developments up to date before we explore this question.

Although we sometimes think of the age of chemistry as having been born with World War II, it started much earlier. In the years immediately after the American Civil War, dye factories sprang up throughout Europe and cancer sprang up with them. Already by 1895, German doctors had reported that aniline dye workers had unusually high incidences of bladder cancer. The problem-chemicals turned out to be a family of aromatic amines (Fig. 8.2), including aminoazo dyes (Fig. 8.3) found in the dye mixtures. In the early 1930s, Tomizu Yoshida reported from Tokyo that the aromatic amines o-aminazotoluene and 4-dimethylaminoazobenzene induced liver cancer in rats. Other aromatic amines have since been found to be carcinogenic but by no means are *all* aromatic amines or aminoazo dyes carcinogenic.

Long after the carcinogenic potential of aromatic amines was established, it was discovered that they did not act directly. An aromatic amine, beta-naphthylamine (see Fig. 8.2), able to cause bladder cancer when *fed* to many species of experimental animals, almost *never* causes bladder cancer if implanted *directly* in the bladder. The explanation for this was presumed to be that some necessary thing happened to beta-naphthylamine when it was eaten. Later work with this and other compounds confirmed that many chemicals able to cause cancer first had to be activated by metabolism—changed into the actual cancer-causing derivative.

In general use now are the terms *precarcinogen*, *proximate carcinogen*, and *ultimate carcinogen*. A **precarcinogen** is a chemical able to induce cancer only after metabolic remodeling. An **ultimate carcinogen** is the derivative that does the actual damage—by interfering with DNA. A **proximate carcinogen** is somewhere in between—it is a partly converted precarcinogen.

The search for carcinogens and for common denominators led to the cataloging of many different chemical classes of carcinogens. In addition to the polycyclic hydrocarbons and the aromatic amines already mentioned other "classes" of chemical carcinogens include (1) alkylating agents, (2) nitroso compounds, (3) various natural (as opposed to synthetic) chemical products, (4) metals, and (5) other inorganic compounds such as asbestos. Before we go on, let's summarize the nature and particular features of the chemical substances that make up each of these classes.

Categories of Chemical Carcinogens

What follows is a description of different classes of chemical carcinogens. Let's be clear about what it is that these classes of chemicals have in common before we jump in.

A **chemical carcinogen** is any chemical substance that when "given" to otherwise normal, previously untreated animals in some nonlethal dose, produces changes in DNA that lead to more malignant neoplasms than would appear in a similar group receiving none of the substance. Note that this definition does *not* distin-

guish between direct-acting carcinogens and those requiring metabolic activation. This definition does exclude chemicals that simply accelerate cell division (promoters) and chemicals that suppress the immune system, both of which would increase the number of neoplasms appearing in animals that had previously received very low or even subthreshold doses of carcinogens.

Polycyclic Aromatic Hydrocarbons

Members of the class of polycyclic hydrocarbons were the first chemical carcinogens identified but their significance as carcinogens extends well beyond the historical by virtue of their prevalence and their potency. The prevalence of polycyclic hydrocarbons is a result of the fact that these compounds are created in the incomplete combustion of coal, oil, leaves, tobacco, steak, and practically any other organic material that is burned. **Polycyclic** means "more than one ring in its structure." **Hydrocarbon** means "molecule consisting of hydrogen and carbon." **Aromatic** originally meant "having an aroma" and has now come to mean (in chemistry anyway) "having at least one benzene ring or related ring structure. Polycyclic aromatic hydrocarbons tend not to be direct-acting carcinogens; they have to be activated first. A review by Harvey (1982) gives a lucid account of the significance of this class of chemical compounds and the problem of chemical carcinogenesis, with a focus on their mechanisms of action. Some examples of polycyclic aromatic hydrocarbons are shown in Figure 8.1.

Aromatic Amines

Aromatic amines are aromatic compounds bearing amino groups (NH_2). Examples of carcinogenic aromatic amines are shown in Figure 8.2. Aminoazo compounds, including the aminoazo dyes discussed above, are characterized by having both an amine group and an azo group, $N=N$ (two nitrogen atoms sharing a double bond). Some representatives of this class of organic compounds are shown in Figure 8.3.

Nitroso Compounds

Nitroso compounds are characterized by the nitroso group, NO. Some carcinogenic nitroso compounds are illustrated in Figure 8.4.

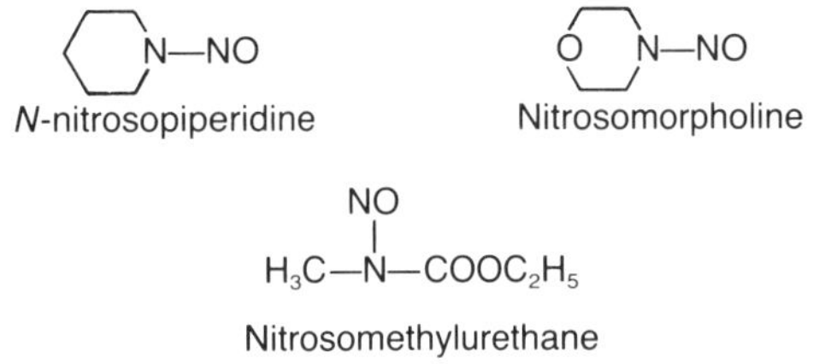

Alkylating Agents

Alkylating agents are chemicals that add alkyl groups* such as the methyl group, CH_3, to the compounds with which they react. This property apparently makes it possible for alkylating agents to act directly with nucleic acids. Some examples of alkylating agents are illustrated in Figure 8.5.

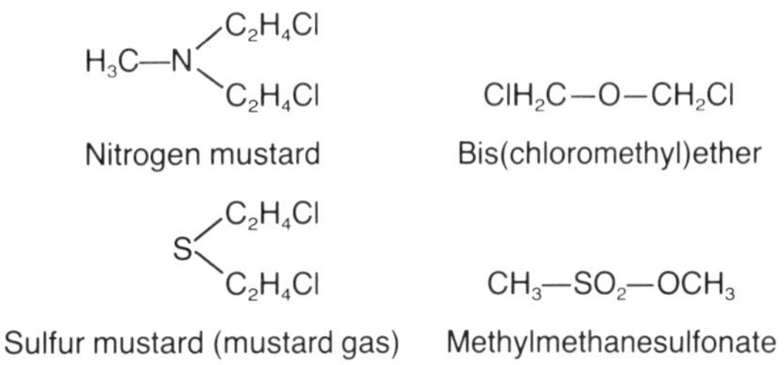

Metals and Other Inorganic Substances

The metals beryllium, chromium, cadmium, and nickel have been linked to neoplasms in both humans and other animals. Asbestos and arsenic have also been associated with *human* cancer. The radioactive isotopes (see Chapter 9) of a number of elements—including uranium, thorium, and radium—are carcinogenic, not because of their chemistry but because of the ionizing radiation they emit when they undergo radioactive decay. We will consider *this* kind of carcinogenesis in the next chapter.

Miscellaneous Natural Products

One of the most powerful carcinogens known is a "natural" product (we use quotation marks because even man-made chemicals are natural, really), aflatoxin (Fig. 8.6), made by the fungus

---

*An alkyl group is any univalent group or radical *typically* (though not always) derived from an aliphatic (straight-chain) hydrocarbon by removal of a hydrogen atom. Alkyl groups have the general formula $C_nH_{2n + 1}$. Examples include CH_3, C_2H_5, and C_3H_7.

Figure 8.4 Some nitroso compounds

Figure 8.5 Some alkylating agents

Aspergillus flavus. In 1960 thousands of young turkeys died mysteriously in England; it was later found that aflatoxin had contaminated the peanut meal fed to the animals. Other similar tragedies revealed that aflatoxin was not only toxic, it is also a powerful liver carcinogen in ducks, rats, trout, and monkeys.

Other "natural" carcinogens include safrole, an oil found in the roots of sassafras; cycasin, found in cycad nuts; a chemical found in the common bracken fern; and a number of alkaloids found in various plants. It turns out that many if not most plants contain toxins with carcinogenic potential. The structures of some carcinogenic natural products are illustrated in Figure 8.6.

Mechanisms of Chemical Carcinogenesis

What makes a carcinogen a carcinogen? What do the different classes of carcinogens just described have in common in terms of reactivity? We have talked about direct-acting carcinogens

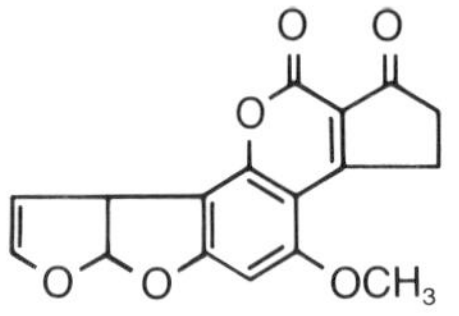

Aflatoxin B₁ (Fungi)

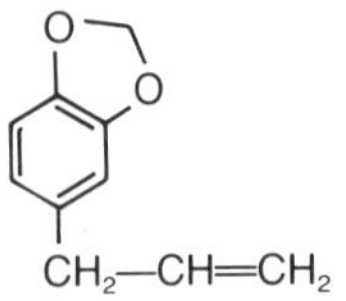

Safrole (Sassafras)

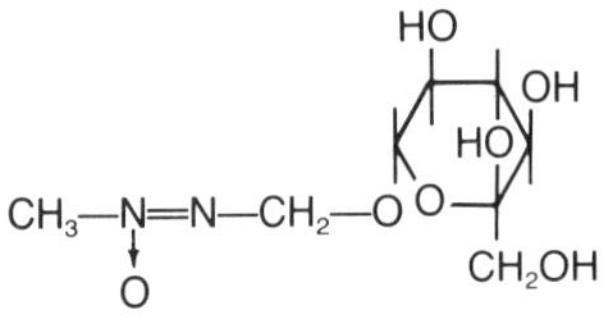

Cycasin
(Cycad plants)

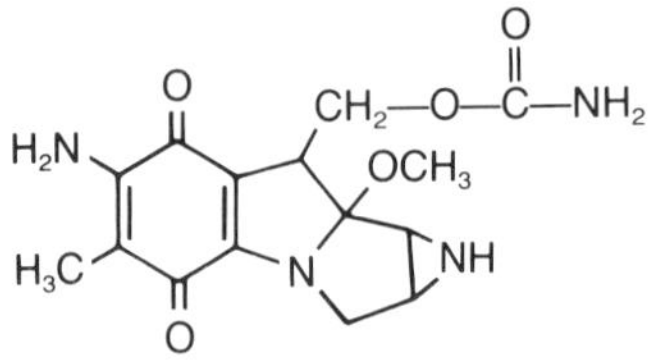

Mitomycin C (Fungi)

Figure 8.6 Some naturally occurring carcinogens

and "precarcinogens"—chemicals that must be converted into *ultimate* carcinogens before they cause cancer. What do direct-acting carcinogens and ultimate carcinogens share in terms of chemical reactivity?

It turns out that many, if not most, carcinogens are **electrophiles**—literally "electron-lovers," or electron-seeking chemicals. Electro-

philic chemicals are susceptible to entering mutually satisfying relationships with other chemicals that have electrons to *donate*. Proteins and nucleic acids (both RNA and DNA) all happen to be electron-rich, a fact that suggests that carcinogens could have RNA, DNA, and/or proteins as their ultimate molecular "targets."

We know that certain carcinogens bind to particular amino acids in the structure of proteins. Although it is conceivable that by forming covalent bonds with key proteins, carcinogens could alter the expression of DNA and thereby induce cancer, the actual significance of carcinogen-*protein* bonding to cancer is unknown. Most evidence indicates that carcinogens do their damage not through reaction with protein, and not through reaction with RNA, but through reaction with DNA.

Many carcinogens are known to react with particular nucleotide bases in DNA. Guanine is apparently the target of many alkalyating agents and aromatic amines, for example. Other nucleotide bases are preferentially "attacked" by other carcinogens. The details of the binding of carcinogens to DNA molecules are secondary in importance to the fact that the ultimate influence of carcinogens at the molecular level appears to be *in distorting DNA molecules* (see Fig. 8.7). If not repaired in time, the distortion may cause the DNA to be replicated incorrectly; this, of course, means "mutation." Figure 8.8 summarizes the kinds of carcinogen-induced chemical changes that alter the structure of DNA.

Much work over many years has revealed that most carcinogens (initiators, ultimate carcinogens, and complete carcinogens) are able to cause mutations in bacteria. Chemicals first found to be mutagenic to bacteria have always ultimately proven carcinogenic when tested in animals. Thus, nearly all, if not all, carcinogens appear to be mutagenic; most mutagens appear to be carcinogenic.

It should be emphasized again that carcinogens can, and no doubt do, also react with proteins and with RNA. The possibility that some carcinogens can cause cancer by reacting with these molecules is still open to question.

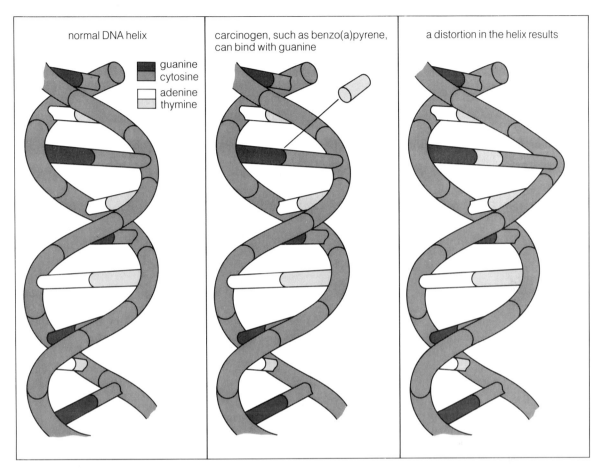

Figure 8.7 Most carcinogens either directly or indirectly combine with DNA and distort the helix. Shown here is benzo(a)pyrene combining with the nucleotide base, guanine. (Redrawn from *Decade of Discovery*, 1981, p. 47)

In the figure, the top panels are labeled:

normal DNA helix

carcinogen, such as benzo(a)pyrene, can bind with guanine

a distortion in the helix results

Legend:
- guanine
- cytosine
- adenine
- thymine

Chemical Carcinogens Vary Greatly in Potency

Electrophiles can be strongly or weakly electrophilic. They have different solubility properties, they come in different sizes, and they differ in other properties that influence their abilities to *get at* key parts of DNA molecules. No wonder, then, that studies with rodents have shown that *the potency of chemical carcinogens can vary by six orders of magnitude*—a millionfold (Ames et al., 1982); see Figure 8.9.

Chemical Carcinogenesis Is Dose-Dependent

There is a direct relationship between the amount of a carcinogen that a group of organisms gets and the number of neoplasms that appear in that group. At least, this statement is true within limits particular to each carcinogen (see Fig. 8.10). Exposure to carcinogens in single small doses produces additive effects—the number of tumors that result is proportional to that total cumulative dose.

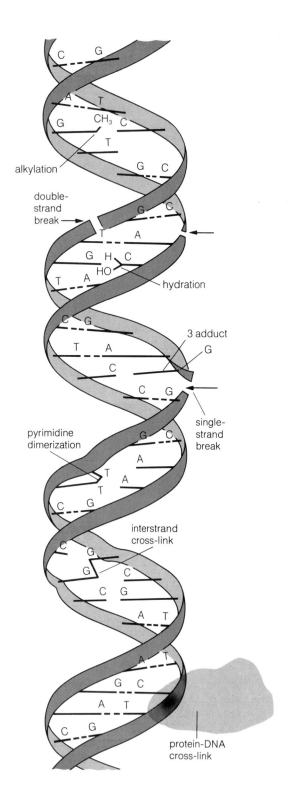

alkylation

double-strand break

pyrimidine dimerization

hydration

3 adduct

single-strand break

interstrand cross-link

protein-DNA cross-link

The Concept of "Threshold" May or May Not Generally Apply in Chemical Carcinogenesis

If a chemical causes cancer, will a very little bit of it cause cancer? This question has some practical importance in light of the fact that even if a dose causes cancer in just one in a million people, and if everybody in America gets that dose, there will be more than 200 cancers.

The question of threshold is still a question because it doesn't lend itself to experimental investigation. To determine if a dose will produce cancer in one in a million animals, the dose would have to be given to several million animals, and none given to several million more. The problem (see Fig. 8.10), then, is that even though there *is* some reason to believe that there is such a thing as threshold for some if not all carcinogens, based on a limited ability of cells to dispose of carcinogens and/or to repair the damage done to DNA (see Cornfield, 1977, and Hoel et al., 1983), we can't be sure.

Chemical Carcinogenesis Is Not Instantaneous

It takes time for cancer to appear after exposure to a carcinogen. Even super-powerful carcinogens require months to produce neoplasms in experimental animals. Weak carcinogens may have latency periods that exceed the life span of an animal. For a particular carcinogen, the larger the dose, the *shorter* the latency period. Cancers in human beings can appear 5 to 50 years after exposure to a cancer-causing agent. Occupational-cancer studies have shown, for example, that cancer of the liver, lung, or bladder can appear 30 years after peak exposures to vinyl chloride, asbestos, or benzidine, respectively.

Figure 8.8 Some of the different kinds of effects carcinogens have on DNA. (From Devoret, 1979, p. 4. Used by permission of W. H. Freeman and Company. © 1979 by Scientific American, Inc. All rights reserved.)

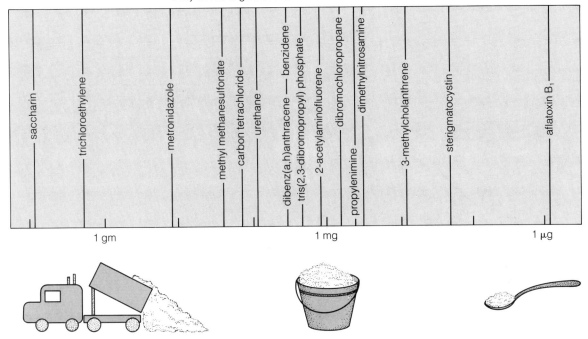

Daily doses to give 50% of animals cancer in "lifetime"

saccharin
trichloroethylene
metronidazole
methyl methanesulfonate
carbon tetrachloride
urethane
dibenz(a,h)anthracene — benzidene
tris(2,3-dibromopropyl) phosphate
2-acetylaminofluorene
dibromochloropropane
propylenimine
dimethylnitrosamine
3-methylcholanthrene
sterigmatocystin
aflatoxin B_1

1 gm   1 mg   1 µg

Figure 8.9 There are carcinogens and there are *carcinogens*! Gram for gram, some carcinogens are a million times more powerful than others. (From Maugh, 1978). The differences between a gram, a milligram, and a microgram are roughly proportional to the differences between a truckload, a bucketful, and a spoonful.

Chemical Carcinogenesis in Stages

Under some conditions, with certain experimental models, carcinogenesis is clearly divisible into an irreversible first phase called *initiation* and a reversible second phase called *promotion*. Isaac Berenblum first found that certain chemicals could not themselves cause cancer but could greatly increase the effects of chemicals that could. Berenblum's experiments are illustrated in Figure 8.11. In essence, he gave mice a carcinogen in doses so low that they would not be expected to produce tumors in the lifetime of any of the mice. He showed that other substances, which he called *promoters*, could not produce tumors in mice in *any* amount. If these promoters were applied *after* the subthreshold dose of the carcinogen, however, many tumors developed. These experiments showed that carcinogenesis occurs in stages—in some systems, at least—and made it necessary to speak of *initiators* and *promoters* rather than just *carcinogens*.

Initiators

What do initiators do? How do they initiate? The answer appears to be that most of them ultimately change and distort DNA by forming covalent bonds with DNA molecules. They induce mutations, in other words. Among the mutations they are able to induce, are some that specify malignant behavior. Permanent alterations of DNA would explain why initiation is irreversible and why the "initiated condition" is passed along to daughter cells in cell division.

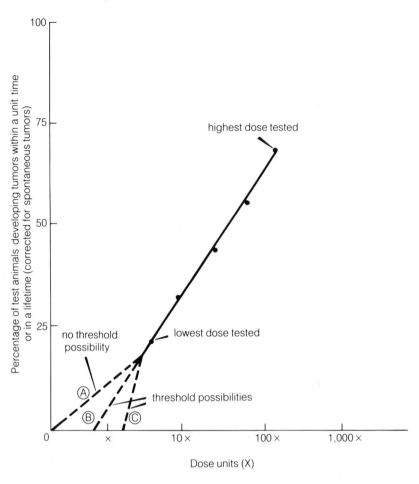

Figure 8.10 Assays of carcinogenicity are usually done at high doses because logistics and statistical constraints make it impossible to test doses low enough to generate cancers in small fractions of the animals exposed. A result of this dilemma is that we don't often know what happens between (1) the lowest dose that can be tested and (2) zero. (*Source:* Kupchella and Hyland, 1986, p. 444. Used by permission of Allyn and Bacon, Inc.)

Promoters

Promoters, as we've already noted, are chemicals that are not carcinogenic but that can increase tumor yields by shortening the latency of cancer development in cells in which cancer has already been initiated. It is important to recognize that *if* a body has cells in it in which cancer has already been initiated, the effect of promoters would be indistinguishable from that of a powerful, complete carcinogen. A class of chemicals called *phorbol esters* are the best-known chemical promoters; they are found in the oil of croton plants and in other plants.

It has long been suspected that there is a relationship between cancer and things that stimulate cell division. In the late 1940s, Rous showed that more tumors arose around holes punched in carcinogen-treated rabbit ears than in nonhealing areas of the same ears. It is well known that certain neoplasms of hormone-target tissue can be brought on faster by hormone doses known to stimulate cell division. It has also been known for some time that weak liver

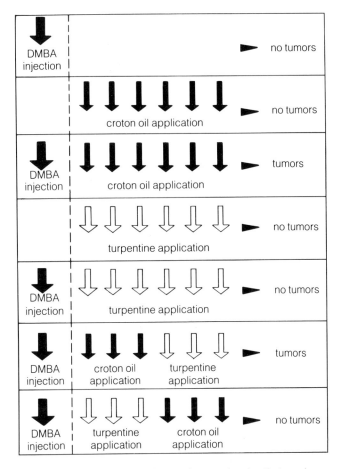

Figure 8.11 Isaac Berenblum's experiments showing that carcinogenesis may take place in stages. (*Source:* Kupchella and Hyland, 1986, p. 448. Used by permission of Allyn and Bacon, Inc.)

carcinogens unable to cause cancer in normal livers, *can* induce cancer in livers undergoing rapid cell division during regeneration.

During the early parts of this century, a theory perhaps best articulated by Virchow gave irritation and the cell division it induced a central role in carcinogenesis. Virchow believed that cancer arose because tissue was made to divide rapidly by some external stimulus: rubbing, chafing, bumping, or the like. But Virchow apparently had promotion and initiation mixed up. Irritation by itself cannot cause cancer, but it

may very well act as a promoter by stimulating cell division (see Konstantinidis et al., 1982).

What do promoters do? How do they promote? The exact mechanism is unknown but because they bind to the cell surface, they are believed to function through some kind of surface-mediated control of cell division, by activating a membrane-associated kinase (Kolata, 1983). They are believed to function after the fashion of certain growth-stimulating, membrane receptor-binding growth factors. Some promoters are apparently able to activate protein kinase C via

Table 8.1   "Promoters" That Play a Role in Human Cancer

Agent	Resultant Neoplasm
Dietary fat (calories)	Mammary adenocarcinoma (increased cancer incidence in general with excess caloric intake)
Cigarette smoke	Bronchogenic carcinoma Esophageal and bladder cancer
Asbestos	Bronchogenic carcinoma and mesothelioma
Halogenated hydrocarbons (TCDD [tetrachlorodibenzo-p-dioxin], PCBs [polychlorinated biphenyl compounds])	Liver*
Saccharin	Bladder*
Phenobarbital	Liver*
Hepatitis B virus	Hepatoma
Prolactin	Mammary adenocarcinoma*
Synthetic estrogens	Liver adenomas
Alcoholic beverages	Oral cancer
	Liver and esophageal cancer

*Promotion demonstrated in experimental animals but not in humans as yet.

Source: Pitot, 1981, Table 2, p. 267. Used by permission of the author and the publisher.

the polyphosphate system of hormone signal transduction discussed in Chapter 7.

Promoters may *also* indirectly damage DNA (see Marx, 1983). Certain promoters are known to generate highly reactive oxygen derivatives that lead to chromosome damage and other changes in DNA, which may in turn have the effect of amplifying or activating cellular oncogenes—without causing mutation.

Some researchers believe that bile acids stimulated by a high-fat diet act as promoters of human colon cancer (see Marx, 1978). Saccharin is apparently a promoter in rats if not in humans, and asbestos is probably also a promoter. In Chapter 1 we pointed out how asbestos enhances the cancer impact of cigarette smoke.

Cigarette smoke probably contains both initiators and promoters; this would explain why the cancer risk of smokers who quit drops significantly (see Chapter 13). Some promoters of hu-

man cancer are listed in Table 8.1. In conclusion, note that most known chemical carcinogens are complete carcinogens; they both initiate *and* promote.

Metabolic Activation

We have already discussed that many chemical carcinogens must be activated (undergo molecular remodeling by metabolism) before they are able to "initiate" a cancer. This realization simplifies the concept of carcinogenesis greatly by supporting the possibility that all carcinogens may ultimately have the same effect even though they themselves may be very different. Metabolic activation provides an explanation for why a carcinogen taken by mouth can produce a bladder cancer but is unable to do so when

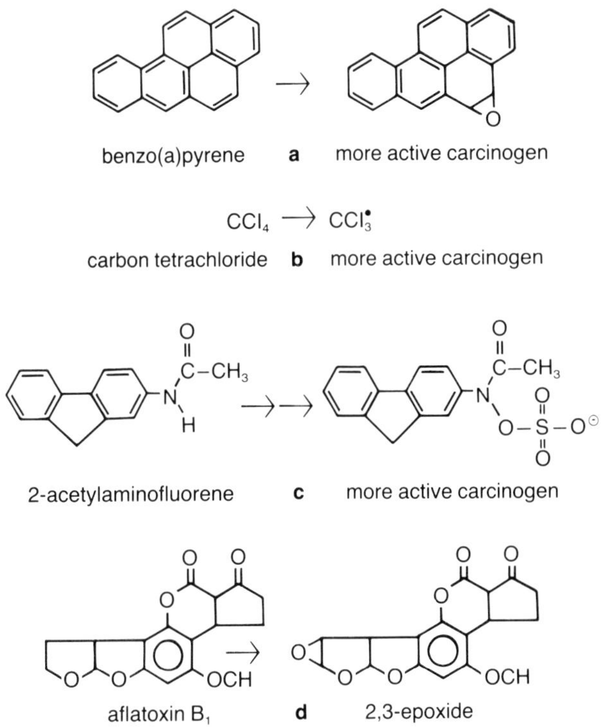

Figure 8.12 Examples of the conversion (activiation) of precarcinogens

implanted directly into the bladder. Metabolic activation provides some other important explanations.

The fact that different organisms have different arrays of metabolic enzymes and thus different metabolic capabilities provides most, if not all, of the explanation for why a chemical may be carcinogenic in one species but not in another. The aromatic amine 2-acetylaminofluorene (AAF) must be converted to a sulfate ester before it can act as a carcinogen (Fig. 8.12). Guinea pigs do not get cancer following exposure to AAF, apparently because they lack the enzymes needed to generate the ultimately carcinogenic form (Miller and Miller, 1974). Metabolic activation may well even explain such otherwise imponderable questions as "Why don't *all* two-pack-a-day smokers get lung cancer?" Some data indicate that heavy smokers with high levels of the enzyme aryl hydrocarbon hy-

droxylase in their circulating lymphocytes may be more susceptible to lung cancer (Kellermann et al., 1973). Such findings raise hope for an accurate way of identifying "high-risk populations" (Chapter 16).

Metabolic activation is no doubt an important part of the explanation for why certain carcinogens cause cancer in certain organs—enzyme arrays that do just the right thing to a precarcinogen may be found only in certain organs (see Dahl et al., 1982).

Although some of the preceding statements imply that *fixed* metabolic capabilities exist in particular organisms, people, and organs, this is not really the case. Many things can influence the course of metabolism of a compound. Some of these are previous exposure to that compound and the presence of drugs (see Faris and Campbell, 1981) or other chemicals. Figure 8.13 illustrates the generalized pathway by which a chemical causes cancer. This pathway varies with the organism, with the individual, with the organ involved, with the time of day, with age, and with the chemical environment—just to name *some* of the things that complicate chemical carcinogenesis.

Host Factors and Chemical Carcinogenesis

In the last section, we introduced the concept of "host factor." With this section still in mind, think ahead to the chapter on genetics and cancer. Imagine how differences in susceptibility to cancer might be explained, in part at least, by differences in genetic determinants of metabolism, or perhaps to differences in the genetic specification of enzymes able to repair damage to DNA. These points are emphasized here to help prepare you to understand genetic predisposition to cancer—we are not all created equal when it comes to the likelihood of dying of cancer.

Chemical Carcinogens and Oncogenes

In the last chapter we introduced the connections between the things we have considered here and the oncogene concept. Let's now list some elements of connection:

Chemical carcinogens, as mutagens, can obviously be responsible for mutation of proto-oncogenes. Some such mutations could conceivably elicit cancer by specifying a more potent oncogene *product*. Some of the mutations caused by chemical mutagens may involve key regulatory genes, impairing their regulatory functions. Chemical mutagens could, for example, be responsible for the chromosome breaks that transfer quiescent oncogenes from inactive chromosomes to activated chromosomes (see Chapter

7). It is even conceivable that a carcinogen might do its damage by reacting with a DNA-dependent, RNA-polymerase-binding site on a promoter gene (see Chapter 2) in such a way that the associated oncogene is transcribed, more rapidly yielding *more* oncogene product.

Other specific connections between oncogenes and chemicals that modify them directly or indirectly are in the process of being discovered at this very moment.

In Search of Carcinogens

The statement "Chemicals cause cancer" sounds much more profound than it really is. The first time this statement is heard, the tendency is to say, "Aha! Now that we know what causes cancer, it should be a simple matter to identify all 'bad' chemicals and get rid of them!" But there are many, many reasons why this task is far from simple. Perhaps chief among these is that every material thing in the universe is made of chemicals. There are millions of different kinds of chemicals (see Box). Thousands of different chemicals make up cigarette smoke; and several hundred may be actively used in just one plastic-making factory. The fact that particular combinations of chemicals and particular sequences of exposure may be important complicates things considerably. Just 20 different chemicals can be combined in more than one million ways—even if just one dose or level of each is considered.

The carcinogenicity of chemical compounds can be evaluated in basically three ways: (1) short-term and long-term assays involving experimental animals; (2) assays involving single cells (bacteria or mammalian cells in culture); and (3) epidemiology (systematically looking for associations between cancer and chemical exposure in human beings, particularly in occupational settings).

The standard way by which potential human carcinogens are evaluated is a bioassay de-

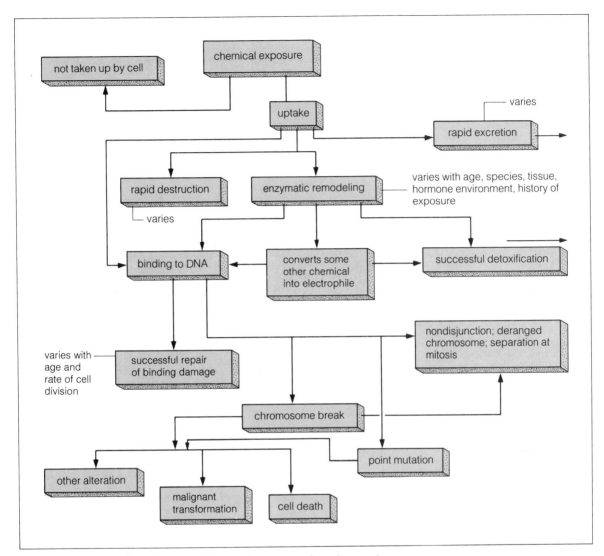

Figure 8.13 The fate of carcinogens and precarcinogens may be quite complex.

veloped at the National Cancer Institute (NCI). In this assay (see Fig. 8.15), both males and females of two kinds of animals, usually rats and mice, are given standard doses of suspect carcinogens under the same conditions. Typically, the assay involves twelve groups of 50 animals each. First, 50 males and 50 females of each species receive a previously determined **maximum tolerated dose** (the highest dose that will *not* result

in the early death of the animals from any cause other than cancer). Another such group receives half that dose; still another group serves as a control group (receives none). Where possible, the dose is administered in the same way that a human might be expected to contact the material if it were loose in the environment. Treatment is usually continued for about two years—the lifetime of a rat or a mouse. Animals that die during

How Many Different Chemicals Are There?

Although estimates vary a little, apparently just over 60,000 different chemicals are in common use. How many are there all together? Well, the American Chemical Society's Abstract Service registers somewhere between 6 and 7 million different chemicals. Some other relevant "gee whiz" facts:

More than 9 million different names are used for the more than 6 million chemicals; some have many different names.

About 97 percent of the chemicals in existence contain carbon.

More than 90 percent of the chemicals amount to exotic formulations for one-time, short-term use, synthesized by graduate students and others engaged in research.

About 1,000 new chemicals are created each day (see Maugh, 1978).

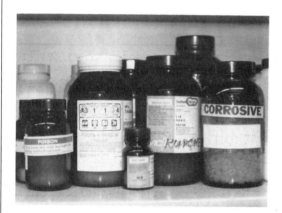 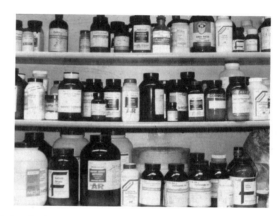

Figure 8.14 There are more than six million different kinds of chemicals.

the test are autopsied; at the end of the test, all animals are killed and their tissues examined grossly and microscopically for cancer. From start to finish, each test takes up to four years and the cost varies from $300,000 to $600,000 (*Decade of Discovery*, 1981).

Only several hundred chemicals have been tested using the NCI bioassay;* another several hundred tests are in progress at the time of this writing. According to the National Institutes of Health, of the nearly 3,000 chemicals cited in the chemical literature as carcinogenic, only about

400 have been adequately tested; reasonably solid evidence indicts a total of maybe 700 or 800 (*Decade of Discovery*, 1981). The National Research Council (1984) has determined that only a small fraction of the more than 60,000 chemicals in widespread use have been tested for toxicity *of any kind*! The NRC found that toxicity data were inadequate for two-thirds of the nearly 3,500 pesticides and pesticide carrier chemicals in use, three-fifths of some 1,800 drugs, and two-thirds of the 8,600 food additives being used.

The only problems with the NCI bioassay system are that it takes up a lot of space, involves a lot of people for a long time, and is expensive; and the results do not always gener-

---

*Gori published a review of this National Cancer Institute (NCI) Bioassay in 1980; readers interested in more detail should consult this source.

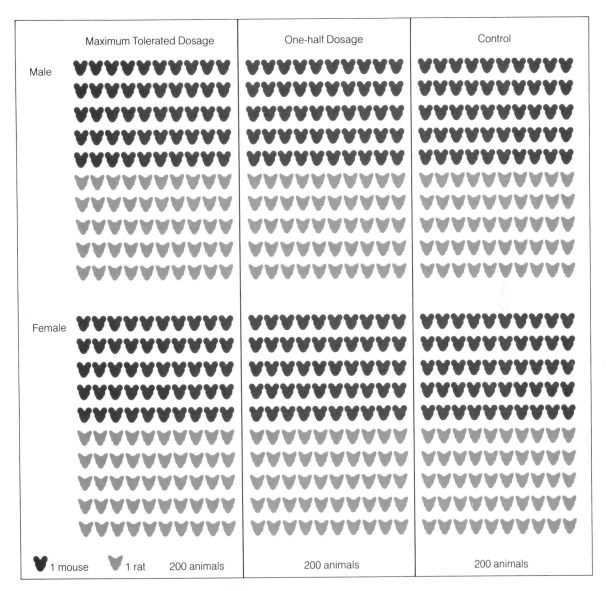

Figure 8.15 The NCI bioassay for carcinogenicity

ate crystal-clear conclusions (see Salsburg, 1983). According to the National Cancer Institute, even if all the laboratories in the world with appropriate facilities could be mobilized to conduct animal bioassays, it would still be possible to test only about 500 chemicals per year. Consider this limitation in light of the fact that somewhere between 700 and 1,000 new chemicals are introduced into common use each year—and that there are already some 60,000 chemicals in common use, most of them untested. Little wonder that *in vitro* bioassay systems involving bacteria came on with such promise in the mid 1970s (*in vitro* literally means "in glass" and refers to studies in test tubes or the like—outside the "host" of interest).

In Vitro *Bioassays of Carcinogenicity: Putting Bacteria to Work Testing Carcinogens*

If carcinogens are all (or nearly all) mutagens and if most mutagens are carcinogens, the ability of a chemical to cause a mutation (and thus cancer) should be testable with *any* living organism. This hypothesis, coupled with the facts that billions of bacteria can be housed in a single test tube and that they grow rapidly, dividing as often as every 20 minutes, suggested to Bruce Ames that test systems involving bacteria might be valid, quick, and inexpensive (Ames et al., 1975). The essence of the test system he and his colleagues developed makes use of mutants of the bacterial species *Salmonella typhimurium*. While the parent (unmutated) strain is able to make histidine, the mutant strains are unable to make this essential amino acid. Billions of *mutants* can be subjected to a test chemical in a single petri dish. If the chemical is able to change DNA, then some of the exposed mutants experience a reversal of the mutation that made them unable to make histidine. They signify that this reversal has occurred by growing on an agar medium lacking histidine. More advanced versions of the Ames test include pretreatment of carcinogens with homogenated mammalian liver—the homogenates providing enzymes that bring about something allegedly "close" to normal metabolic activation. Bacteria, after all, cannot be expected to metabolize precarcinogens in the same way as a human or other mammals.

Variations of the basic Ames test involve other tester strains and other modifications. One variation utilizes animal cells, even human cells grown in tissue culture. Another variation puts the carcinogen into an animal, and then the bacteria are put in. The bacteria are isolated from the animal and tested for mutation. This procedure presumably better mimics normal metabolic activation.

The beauty of Ames-type tests is that they are quick and cheap. A typical assay takes just a few days and might cost $500. But there are problems, too! Such tests apparently miss about 15 percent of known carcinogens presumably because of some very particular feature or features of the *in vivo* (in life) system that they fail to match. Even if this problem can be eliminated by improvements and by using *batteries* of *in vitro* tests, and even though these kinds of tests figure to play an important role in screening chemicals, the only way to determine with certainty which chemicals are carcinogenic in humans is to see if they cause cancer in humans. The only way to accomplish this ethically is to watch (using carefully executed epidemiological methods—see Chapter 13) what happens to people who are inadvertently exposed to particular chemicals in the workplace and elsewhere.

The main problem with the epidemiological approach to the identification of chemical carcinogens is that results come *after* the fact. By the time epidemiology identifies a chemical-cancer connection, a number of people already have cancer and many more are developing it.

Summary of the Problem

The first few paragraphs of this chapter amounts to a chapter summary; we will close here with a summary of the problem of dealing with cancer-causing chemicals in human beings.

For many reasons, it is extremely difficult to prevent human beings from being exposed to chemical carcinogens. One of the most important reasons is that it is extremely difficult to determine just which chemicals are carcinogenic to human beings, specifically. Despite the fact that millions of chemicals exist, thousands of which are suspect carcinogens, we have identified only about 20 human chemical carcinogens (Table 8.2). What are the main problems?

The ultimate experiments can't be done. We simply cannot ethically inject human beings with suspect carcinogens to see if cancer develops.

Experiments with animals are slow, costly, and the results are not unequivocally applicable to human beings. What happens in a rat may or

Table 8.2 Chemicals and Groups of Chemicals Causally Associated with Cancer in Humans

4-aminobiphenyl
Analgesic mixtures containing phenacetin[a]
Arsenic and arsenic compounds[a]
Asbestos
Azathioprine
Benzene
Benzidine
N,N-bis(2-chloroethyl)-2-naphthylamine (Chlornaphazine)
Bis(chloromethyl)ether and technical-grade chloromethyl methyl ether
1,4-butanediol dimethanesulphonate (Myleran)
Certain combined chemotherapy for lymphomas[a] (including MOPP[b])
Chlorambucil
Chromium and certain chromium compounds[a]
Conjugated estrogens[a]
Cyclophosphamide
Diethylstilbestrol
Melphalan
Methoxsalen with ultraviolet A therapy
Mustard gas
2-naphthylamine
Soots, tars, and oils[a,c]
Treosulphan
Vinyl chloride

Note: This table does not include known human carcinogens such as tobacco smoke or alcoholic beverages, since they have not yet been considered within the IARC Monographs.

[a]The compound(s) responsible for the carcinogenic effect in humans cannot be specified.
[b]Procarbazine, nitrogen mustard, vincristine, and prednisone.
[c]Mineral oils may vary in composition, particularly in relation to their content of carcinogenic polycyclic aromatic hydrocarbons.

Source: *Chemicals, Industrial Processes and Industries Associated with Cancer in Humans*, 1982. IARC Monographs on the Evaluation of the Carcinogenic Risk of Chemicals to Humans (1982) Chemicals, Industrial Processes and Industries Associated with Cancer in Humans, IARC monographs Vols. 1-29. Supplement No. 4, International Agency for Research on Cancer, Lyon. Used by permission of Elsevier Scientific Publishers.

may not also happen in a human being. Humans and rats may metabolize chemicals differently, and metabolism plays an important role in chemical carcinogenesis. Fortunately, humans and other mammals are enough alike that a chemical that proves to be a carcinogen in one or more mammals will very probably also be carcinogenic in humans.

There are more chemicals to be tested than there are people or facilities or money to test them.

Evidence exists that certain combinations of chemicals individually unable to produce cancer may in fact generate cancer when exposure occurs in some particular order. If the absolute number of chemicals amounts to a difficult

problem, the problem of chemical combinations is "impossible."

Cancer takes a long time to develop, and this lag obscures the connection between chemical exposures and cancer. Who remembers what he or she ate for lunch twenty-five years ago? How many people can really relate to the possibility that what they do in 1987 might mean cancer in the year 2020?

Carcinogens do not all act directly; most require metabolic activation. The complexities of metabolism and the various influences on metabolism in human beings mean that it is difficult if not impossible to look at the structure of a chemical and decide if it might be converted into an ultimate carcinogen.

References and Further Reading

Ames, B. N., et al. 1982. In T. Sugimura, S. Kondo, and H. Takebe, eds., *Environmental Mutagens and Carcinogens*. New York: University of Tokyo Press/Liss.

Ames, B. N., McCann, J., and Yamasaki, E. 1975. Methods for Detecting Carcinogens and Mutagens with the Salmonella Mammalian-microsome Mutagenicity Test. *Mutat. Res.* 31:347–64.

Arcos, J. C., Woo, Y., and Argus, M. 1982. *Chemical Induction of Cancer: Structural Bases and Biological Mechanisms. Aliphatic Carcinogens*, Vol. 3A. New York: Academic Press.

Boutwell, R. K. 1982. Inhibition of Chemical Carcinogenesis. In J. G. Fortner and J. E. Rhoads, eds., *Accomplishments in Cancer Research, 1981*. Philadelphia: Lippincott.

Cerutti, P. A. 1985. Prooxidant States and Tumor Promotion. *Science.* 227:375–81.

Chemicals, Industrial Processes and Industries Associated with Cancer in Humans. 1982. IARC Monographs of the Evaluation of the Carcinogenic Risk of Chemicals to Humans. Lyon, France: International Agency for Research on Cancer.

Committee on Chemical and Environmental Mutagens. 1983. *Identifying and Estimating the Genetic Impact of Chemical Mutagens.* Washington, D.C.: National Research Council, National Academy Press.

Cornfield, J. 1977. Carcinogenic Risk Assessment. *Science.* 198:693–99.

Dahl, A. G., et al. 1982. Cytochrome P-450-Dependent Monooxygenases in Olfactory Epithelium of Dogs: Possible Role in Tumorigenicity. *Science.* 216:57–59.

Decade of Discovery. 1981. NIH Publication No. 81–2323. Washington, D.C.: U.S. Department of Health and Human Services.

De Serres, F. J., and Hollaender, A., eds. *Chemical Mutagens.* Vol. 7: *Principles and Methods for Their Detection.* New York: Plenum.

Devoret, R. 1979. Bacterial Tests for Potential Carcinogens. *Scientific American.* 241(2) August, pp. 40–49.

Douglas, J. F., ed. 1984. Carcinogenesis and Mutagenesis Testing. *Contemporary Biomedicine.* Clifton, N.J.: Humana Press.

Everything Doesn't Cause Cancer. 1980. NIH Publication No. 80-2039. Bethesda, Md.: National Cancer Institute.

Faris, R. A., and Campbell, T. C. 1981. Exposure of Newborn Rats to Pharmacologically Active Compounds May Permanently Alter Carcinogen Metabolism. *Science.* 211:719–20.

First Annual Report on Carcinogens. 1980. Washington, D.C.: U.S. Department of Health and Human Services, Public Health Service.

Gori, G. B. 1980. The Regulation of Carcinogenic Hazards. *Science.* 208:256–61.

Grimmer, G., ed. 1983. *Environmental Carcinogens: Polycyclic Aromatic Hydrocarbons.* Boca Raton, Fla.: CRC Press.

Harris, C. C., and Cerutti, P. A., eds. 1982. *Mechanisms of Chemical Carcinogenesis.* New York: Alan R. Liss.

Harvey, R. G. 1982. Polycyclic Hydrocarbons and Cancer. *American Scientist.* 70:386–92.

Hecker, E., et al., eds. 1982. *Carcinogenesis: A Comprehensive Survey.* New York: Raven Press.

Hoel, D. G., Kaplan, N. L., and Anderson, M. W. 1983. Implication of Nonlinear Kinetics on Risk Estimation in Carcinogenesis. *Science* 219:1032–36.

Interdisciplinary Panel on Carcinogenicity. 1984. Criteria for Evidence of Chemical Carcinogenicity. *Science.* 225:682–87.

Kellermann, G., Shaw, C. R., and Luyten-Kellermann, M. 1973. Aryl Hydrocarbon Hydroxylase Inducibility and Brochongenic Carcinoma. *N. England J. Med.* 289:934–37.

Kolata, G. 1983. Clues to Cell Growth and Differentiation. *Science.* 230:291–92.

Konstantinidis, A., Smulow, J. B., and Sonnenschein, C. 1982. Tumorigenesis at a Predetermined Oral Site after One Intraperitoneal Injection of N-Nitroso-N-Methylurea. *Science.* 216:1235–37.

Kruse, L. C., Reese, J. L., and Hart, L. K., eds. 1979. *Cancer: Pathophysiology, Etiology, and Management.* St. Louis: Mosby.

Kupchella, C. E., and Hyland, M. C. 1986. *Environmental Science: Living Within the System of Nature.* Boston: Allyn & Bacon.

LeServe, A., et al. 1980. *Chemical, Work and Cancer.* New York: Van Nostrand/Reinhold.

Lewin, R. 1983. NAS Study Highlights Chemical Mutagens. *Science.* 219:1304–05.

Magee, P. N. 1982. Chemical Carcinogenesis. In J. G.

Fortner and J. E. Rhoads, eds., *Accomplishments in Cancer Research, 1981*. Philadelphia: Lippincott.

Marx, J. L. 1978. Tumor Promoters: Carcinogenesis Gets More Complicated. *Science*. 201:515–18.

Marx, J. L. 1983. Do Tumor Promoters Affect DNA after All? *Science*. 219:158–59.

Maugh, T. H. 1978a. Chemical Carcinogens: How Dangerous Are Low Doses? *Science*. 202:37–41.

Maugh, T. H. 1978b. Chemicals: How Many Are There? *Science*. 199:162.

Maugh, T. H. 1978c. Chemical Carcinogens: The Scientific Basis for Regulation. *Science*. 201:1200–05.

Miller, E. C., and Miller, J. A. 1974. Biochemical Mechanisms of Chemical Carcinogenesis. In H. Busch, ed., *The Molecular Biology of Cancer*. New York: Academic Press.

Miller, E. C., and Miller, J. A. 1980. In Search of Ultimate Chemical Carcinogens and Their Reactions with Cellular Macromolecules. In J. G. Fortner and J. E. Rhoads, eds., *Accomplishments in Cancer Research, 1980*. Philadelphia: Lippincott.

National Research Council. 1984. *Toxicity Testing: Strategies to Determine Needs and Priorities*. Washington, D. C.: National Academy Press.

National Toxicology Program. 1983. *Third Annual Report on Carcinogens: Summary*. NTP 83-101. NTS PB-83-135855. Springfield, Va.: National Technical Information Service.

Nishio, Y., et al. 1986. L-Isoleucine and L-Leucine: Tumor Promoters of Bladder Cancer in Rats. *Science*. 231:843–45.

Pitot, H. 1980. The Two-Stage Process of Carcinogenesis: Its Relevance to Human Cancer. In J. G. Fortner and J. E. Rhoads, eds., *Accomplishments in Cancer Research, 1980*. Philadelphia: Lippincott.

Powles, T. J., et al., eds. 1982. *Prostaglandins and Cancer: First International Conference*. New York: Alan R. Liss.

Pryor, W. A. 1976–1982. *Free Radicals in Biology*, Vols. 1–5. New York: Academic Press.

Ryser, H. J. P. 1974. Special Report: Chemical Carcinogenesis. *Ca-A Cancer Journal for Clinicians*. 24(6):351–60.

Salsburg, D. 1983. The Lifetime Feeding Study in Mice and Rats—An Examination of Its Validity as a Bioassay for Human Carcinogens. *Fundamental and Applied Toxicology*. 3:63–67.

Second Annual Report on Carcinogens. 1981. Washington, D.C.: U.S. Department of Health and Human Services, Public Health Service.

Searle, C. E., ed. 1976. *Chemical Carcinogens, Monograph 173*. Washington D.C.: American Chemical Society.

Selkirk, J. K., and MacLeod, M. C. 1982. Chemical Carcinogenesis: Nature's Metabolic Mistake. *BioScience*. 32(7):601–05.

Shimkin, M. B. 1977. *Contrary to Nature*. NIH Publication No. 76-720. Bethesda, Md.: Department of Health, Education and Welfare.

Shimomura, K., et al. 1983. Bromine Residue at Hydrophilic Region Influences Biological Activity of Aplysiatoxin, a Tumor Promoter. *Science*. 222:1242–44.

Singer, B., and Grunberger, D. 1983. *Molecular Biology of Mutagens and Carcinogens*. New York: Plenum.

Slaga, T. J., ed. 1983 and 1984. *Mechanisms of Tumor Promotion*. 4 vols. Boca Raton, Fla.: CRC Press.

Stich, H. F., and San, R. H., eds. 1981. *Short-term Tests for Chemical Carcinogens*. New York: Springer-Verlag.

Sugimura, T., et al. 1976. Overlapping of Carcinogens and Mutagens. In P. Magee et al., eds., *Fundamentals in Cancer Prevention*. Baltimore, Md.: University Park Press and University of Tokyo.

Suovaniemi, O., et al. 1985. An Automated Analysis System for Bacterial Mutagenicity Assays. *American Laboratory*. 17 (March):122–29.

Weisburger, J. H., and Williams, G. M. 1981. Carcinogen Testing: Current Problems and New Approaches. *Science*. 214:401–07.

9

Radiation as a Cause of Cancer

Most chapters and books on the effects of radiation manage to include the tired metaphor "Radiation is a two-edged sword" (this book can now be added to the list). The intended meaning of this phrase is that radiation is both good and bad. And, this is true! The very kinds of radiation that *cause* cancer happen to be extremely useful in diagnostic medicine (X-rays) and even in cancer therapy (see Chapter 17). Also, the phrase "Let there be light!" stated a little more generally, could have been "Let there be radiation!" Light is one kind of radiation. Thus, far from being a bad thing, radiation is absolutely essential to the existence of life on earth. The sun is a continuous nuclear reaction that bathes the earth in light and gives plants the energy they need to start food chains.

Still, some kinds of radiation cause cancer. Problem radiation is radiation that is penetrating and powerful enough to cause changes in the chemistry of the things it strikes. Cancer becomes the problem when radiation directly or indirectly causes changes in DNA.

Historical Overview

A German, Paul Unna, concluded in 1894 that there was a connection between skin cancer and sunlight; many other studies have led to the same conclusion in the years since. Human cancer from X-rays was already recognized in 1902. In 1908, seven years before Yamagiwa and Ichikawa produced cancer by painting rabbit ears with tar, cancer was induced in animals by exposing them to X-rays. In 1928, a British pathologist successfully induced skin cancer in mice by exposing them to ultraviolet radiation.

Because they didn't know much about the effects of radiation; because of indiscriminate "messing" with radiation when it was still a novelty; and probably also because of the "it won't happen to me" attitude that comes standard in most human beings, many early radiation workers—including doctors, dentists, and

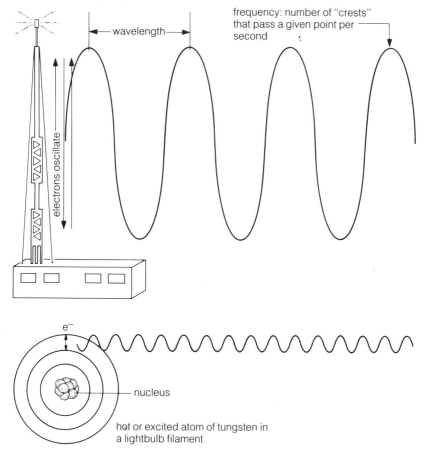

Figure 9.1 Electromagnetic radiation is an electrical and magnetic disturbance caused by the acceleration of something bearing a charge. Since these radiations are disturbances of pure energy, they can even traverse a vacuum. They travel at the "speed of light" in a vacuum, and slightly slower in air, water, and other media with which they can interact. Examples include the radio waves produced when electrons are accelerated up and down a transmitter, the light waves produced when electrons are accelerated in a heated lightbulb filament, and the X-rays produced when an electron decelerates as it strikes a target in a cathode ray tube. The differences between radio waves and X-rays are wavelength and energy content.

watch dial painters—developed cancer from radiation exposure. Radiologists in the early part of the twentieth century got leukemia at three to four times the rate of comparable nonradiologists. Dentists developed cancer of the hands and fingers from years of holding X-ray film against teeth being X-rayed. So that our grandparents could see their watches in the dark, dial

painters were employed in factories to dab radium-containing, glow-in-the-dark pigments on the "big hands" and "little hands" of watches. They used their lips to bring the tips of their tiny, radium-contaminated brushes to fine points. In this and other ways the painters absorbed radium that lodged in their bones. Years later, a significant number of these dial painters—many

Miniglossary of Radiation Terms

Alpha emitter A radioisotope that gives off alpha particle radiation when it undergoes radioactive decay.

Alpha particle A positively charged particle emitted by certain radioactive substances; consists of two protons and two neutrons (essentially, a helium nucleus). Because of their mass and charge, alpha particles are *not* very penetrating; they can be stopped by a sheet of paper.

Beta emitter An isotope that gives off beta particle radiation when it undergoes radioactive decay.

Beta particle A particle, equal in mass and charge to an electron, emitted by certain radioactive substances.

Curie (C:) An amount of a radioactive material that will undergo 37 billion nuclear disintegrations per second (this is roughly the amount of activity in a gram of radium).

Gamma ray Electromagnetic ray emitted by atomic nucleus, similar in nature to an X-ray but usually with a shorter wavelength (and therefore more energetic). These very penetrating rays are emitted in the decay of certain radioactive substances.

Half-life The characteristic amount of time it takes for half of *any* amount of a particular radioactive isotope to undergo "decay."

Ionizing radiation Radiation of sufficient energy to break chemicals into charged parts (ions).

LET, *linear energy transfer* The energy transferred or delivered per unit length of path the radiation takes through an absorbing medium. High LET particle radiation does more damage over a shorter distance in tissue than do equivalent amounts (in terms of total energy delivered) of low LET radiation such as X-rays or gamma rays.

Nuclide One of the series of atoms with different total numbers of protons and neutrons. All nuclides that have the same number of protons are **isotopes** of the same *element*. Nuclides that are unstable (they undergo spontaneous radioactive decay) are called **radionuclides** or **radioactive nuclides**. Radioactive forms (nuclides) of an element are called **radioisotopes** or **radioactive isotopes** of that element. Altogether about 1,700 nuclides are known, only 300 of which are *not* radioactive.

Rad, *radiation absorbed dose* A unit of radiation dose: 100 ergs of absorbed energy per gram of tissue.

Radium A radioactive metallic element found in pitchblende and other uranium-containing ores. Radium was discovered by Nobel Prize winners Pierre and Marie Curie.

Radionuclide See **nuclide**.

---

of them long since retired—developed osteogenic sarcoma (a form of bone cancer).

The case of the watch dial painters raises a number of interesting and important points; for example, there are two distinctively different ways of getting "radiated." One is to be hit by rays that come from some *external* source. The other is to be hit by rays emitted from some *internal* source—a radio*active* isotope that is breathed in, eaten, or absorbed through the skin. To appreciate this difference, it will be necessary to know a little bit more of the nature of radiation.

What Is Radiation?

Whenever something bearing an electrical charge is accelerated, an electromagnetic disturbance is propagated away from it at a speed around 186,000 miles per second. Except for the speed, and for the fact that the disturbance is electrical *and* magnetic, the disturbance is much like the disturbance or wave that results when a stone is thrown into a pond. As an electron moves back and forth between two energy levels in an atom or as electrons are run up and down a radio transmission tower (Fig. 9.1), the result

RBE, relative biological effectiveness A measure of the biological effect of a given type of radiation relative to the amount energy of a standard kind of radiation (200 KeV-medium-energy X-rays)* necessary to produce the same biological effect. Fast neutrons (> 0.1 MeV) have an RBE of 10 for producing cataracts. This means that 10 times the dose of medium-energy X-rays is required to equal the cataract-producing effect of a given dose of fast neutrons.

Rem, *rad* equivalent *mammal (or *man*) A rad adjusted for differences in the relative biological effectiveness of different forms of radiation; the amount of radiation that produces a biological effect equal to that of one rad of gamma radiation. A rem gives more weight to high LET radiation (radiation that delivers all its impact over a very short distance). The rad and rem values for X-rays and gamma rays are about the same. For high LET alpha particles, the rem value may be as much as 20 times the rad value. This is because the relative biological effectiveness of alpha particle radiation can be 20 times that of X-rays delivering the same amount of energy. rem = rad × rbe

Roentgen (R) A unit of radiation exposure that will produce 2.1 billion ion pairs in one cc of dry air at 760 mm Hg and at 0°C. A Roentgen is a unit of exposure to radiation without regard to how much of the dose is absorbed.

Ultraviolet radiation The region of the electromagnetic spectrum (see Fig. 9.2) just beyond the shorter wavelengths of the visible light spectrum. Ultraviolet radiation is generally nonionizing.

X-rays A region of the electromagnetic spectrum of very short wavelength radiations (see Fig. 9.2). Because X-rays rarely interact with light atoms, they can penetrate deeply into soft tissue and otherwise light solids. When they do interact, X-rays may cause chemical or biological changes.

There are essentially four fundamentally different ways of defining radiation: (1) source activity or disintegration rate (Curies); (2) exposure or the amount of radiation *reaching* a target (e.g., Roentgen); (3) the amount actually *absorbed* by the target (e.g., rad) and (4) relative biological effectiveness (RBE) further qualifies the absorbed dose in terms of specific biological effect per unit dose.

*An **electron volt** is the energy of motion (kinetic energy) acquired when a charge, e (charge on an electron) is accelerated by a potential difference of 1 volt. MeV = 1 million electron volts; KeV = 1000 electron volts.

ing disturbance takes the form of a repetitious wave, with a wavelength that varies with the frequency of oscillation of the charge being accelerated.

There is actually a spectrum of electromagnetic radiation that can be specified by wavelength or by energy content, as is depicted in Figure 9.2. The longer the wavelength, the lower the energy per packet ("packet" because the energy in electromagnetic radiation is absorbed in multiples of discrete units or packets called **photons**) and vice versa. Radio waves have very long wavelengths and carry very little energy per photon. Radiation in the gamma region of the spectrum, however, has extremely *short* wavelengths and extremely *high*-energy photons. This difference is important because the chemical and biological effects of radiation are functions of the electromagnetic radiation's energy content per photon and the number of photons absorbed.

As suggested earlier, the radiation spectrum is sometimes divided into "nonionizing" and "ionizing" regions. Ionizing radiation does the most damage. Visible light, microwave, and ultraviolet radiation do not usually cause ioniza-

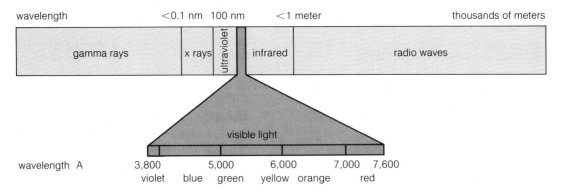

Figure 9.2 The electromagnetic radiation spectrum

tion. Ultraviolet radiation, visible light, and microwaves do, however, have sufficient energy to produce chemical changes by "exciting" molecular electrons and making the molecules more reactive. We will concern ourselves only with ionizing radiation and ultraviolet radiation here.

Generally speaking, there are two forms of ionizing radiation. The high-energy, short-wavelength *electromagnetic* radiation just described is one kind. Accelerated atomic *particles* such as protons, beta particles, and alpha particles is another kind. Both kinds of radiation are generated when atomic nuclei undergo radioactive decay.

A diagram illustrating what happens when the nucleus of an atom of uranium 235 (^{235}U) undergoes fission followed by decay is illustrated in Figure 9.3. The splitting of the uranium nucleus illustrated in the figure is called **nuclear fission**. Fission yields heat and fission fragments, which subsequently undergo radioactive decay.

Because the biological "effect" of particulate ionizing radiation depends on the mass and the charge of the particle, it makes sense to recognize four kinds of ionizing radiation:

Positive ions   Activated ions generated as a result of nuclear disintegration (Fig. 9.3); one example is the alpha particles. Alpha rays are *high* linear energy transfer (LET) radiations (see box). Although such rays are easily shielded, if alpha

emitters are swallowed or inhaled the resulting radiation can badly damage vital tissues.

Electrons (beta particles) **and positrons**   Have charges equal in magnitude to that on a proton but with almost negligible mass. They are a hundred times more penetrating than alpha particles. They tend to produce ionization along a relatively long crooked path in tissue because they are easily deflected.

Gamma rays   Electromagnetic rays *without* mass. Gamma rays do not cause ionization directly; they interact with electrons that then do the ionizing. Gamma rays are much more penetrating than beta particles.

Neutrons   Uncharged but nearly equal in mass to a proton. Neutrons in motion (fast or slow) can cause ionization *indirectly* by colliding with nuclei, causing proton and gamma ray emissions secondarily.

Generally speaking, particulate radiation doesn't penetrate very far, but it does a lot of damage along a short path. Getting hit with an alpha particle is like getting hit by a slow cannon ball; an X-ray is more like a .22-caliber bullet by comparison. The analogy holds in terms of the fact that you can be hurt badly by either one but you would be much more likely to survive a direct hit in a vital target by the latter. In real terms, we speak of particulate radiation as having relatively high LET, or linear energy transfer

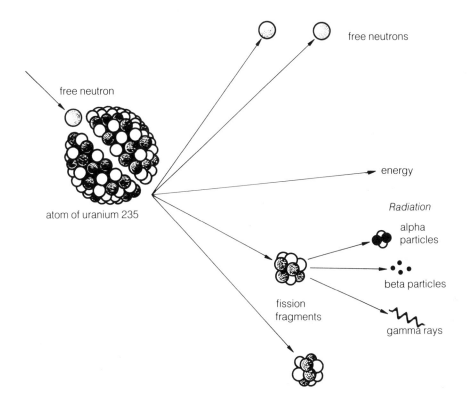

Figure 9.3 The results of the fission and radioactive decay of an atom of uranium 235. (*Source:* Kupchella and Hyland, 1986. Used with permission of Allyn & Bacon.)

(see box). High LET radiation tends to create dense clusters of ions along a short path.

Half-Life

Radionuclides have unstable nuclei. Unstable nuclei have a relatively high probability of undergoing spontaneous disintegration or decay (Fig. 9.3). The probability of undergoing decay is a very specific characteristic of each radionuclide such that a certain fraction of *any* number of atoms of a particular radionuclide will undergo radioactive decay in a fixed amount of time. The characteristic length of time required for half of a particular radionuclide to undergo decay is called that radionuclide's **half-life**.

The half-lives of radionuclides range from extremely small fractions of a second to thousands and even millions of years. A stable nuclide is essentially one with an infinite half-life. Some of the more important bone-seeking radionuclides and their half-lives are listed in Table 9.1.

Biochemistry of Radionuclides

Radioactive isotopes of carbon, hydrogen, iodine, phosphorus, and other elements behave chemically exactly like their stable counterparts. This is because chemical reactivity is a property of the electron cloud around a nucleus, while radioactivity is a property of the nucleus of an atom. Radioactive nuclides end up in tissue

Table 9.1 Some Important Bone-Seeking Radionuclides and Their Half-Lives

Radionuclide	Half-Life
Calcium 45	165 days
Strontium 89	51 days
Strontium 90	28 years
Ytrium 90	64.2 hours
Radium 224	3.64 days
Radium 226	1620 years
Radium 228	5.7 years
Thorium 228	1.91 years
Plutonium 239	24,400 years
Phosphorous 32	14.3 days

Source: Vaughn, 1976, p. 457.

wherever their nonradioactive isotopes would end up. Carbon, a constituent of all organic molecules by definition, is present in all tissues and organs; carbon 14, a radioactive isotope of carbon, distributes itself relatively uniformly throughout any living organism. The same is true of hydrogen and its isotopes. Radioactive iodine 131 is concentrated in the thyroid gland because the thyroid normally concentrates iodine. Strontium 90 concentrates in bone because strontium is chemically very similar to calcium. In living tissue, radioactive isotopes continue to undergo decay and give off radiation in a statistically predictable way specified by their half-lives; for example, half of the strontium-90 deposited in a bone decays every 28 years.

How Does Radiation Cause Cancer?

The general mechanism by which *chemicals* cause cancer is reaction with DNA leading first to distortion of DNA molecules and then to mutation. Radiation carcinogenesis probably also has a chemical basis. There appear to be several kinds of radiochemical pathways to cancer.

Ionizing radiation is a powerful mutagen. As X-rays and other forms of ionizing radiation pierce living cells, they cause electrons to be moved from their usual locations in the molecules encountered along the way. Many of the ions produced as molecules lose their electrons become extremely reactive; they become strongly electrophilic. In this respect, they are similar to electrophilic chemical carcinogens in that their potential for reaction with electron-rich macromolecules such as DNA is increased. As we have already discussed in the last chapter, such reactions in turn raise the possibility that mutations will occur.

Radiation can also distort DNA molecules directly. Although it is generally *non*ionizing, ultraviolet radiation can induce the formation of bonds between adjacent thymine residues in DNA molecules, creating what are called "thymine dimers." Although these are repaired rather efficiently in most normal cells, the existence of these dimers increases the probability of mutation. Cells undergoing DNA replication are subject to mutation as replication is attempted in a strand that has not been repaired, or in a case where thymine dimers have formed opposite one another in the same molecule. In the later case, the repair mechanisms are deprived of a normal reference point from which to make the correct repair. Ionizing forms of radiation also can change DNA directly more than likely by breaking bonds (see Fig. 8.8) rather than creating them, but in either case resulting in an increased probability of mutation.

Still another mechanism, relevant to our earlier discussion of oncogenes, is that radiation may directly or indirectly sever the sugar-phosphate backbones of DNA molecules. Subsequent breaks in chromosomes and translocation of oncogenes and/or oncogene control sequences could then lead to the kind of deranged control we have discussed already. Still other mechanisms have been suggested including one in which radiation somehow activates latent oncogenic viruses (see Chapter 10).

The Effects of Radiation: How Much Radiation Does It Take to Cause Cancer?

In 1927, the Nobel laureate H. J. Muller found that high-energy radiation could damage the chromosomes of living organisms. Most of what we have found out about the effects of radiation on humans since Muller, came (and still comes) from studies of atom bomb survivors; studies of Marshall Islanders who were exposed to radiation during atomic tests in the early 1950s; studies of patients who received high doses of therapeutic or diagnostic radiation; and data from chronic exposure of X-ray technicians and radiologists. Still other data comes from uranium miners and, of course, a considerable amount of additional basic information has come from experiments with laboratory animals.

Death *can* occur in just a few weeks from a whole-body dose of 500 rads. The dose that will kill half the people exposed to it is 400–450 rads. Just about everybody who receives more than 700 (whole-body) rads at one time or within a short period will *die* within a relatively short time.

While we know a lot about acute effects of radiation above the levels of 150 rads, we have less information about the effects of short-term radiation in smaller doses or at very low dose rates. We do know that low doses of radiation may produce genetic effects leading to birth defects and cancer.

Somewhere between 100 and 500 rems will double the risk of dying of cancer, and cancer risk is generally thought to be directly proportional to total *accumulated* dose. A small percentage of cancers is no doubt due to background radiation in the environment and the implication is that if background radiation goes up, the number of cancers induced by radiation may increase proportionately.

The importance of the radiation in medicine and in industry has made it necessary for regulatory agencies to set up standards and systems by which to monitor occupationally exposed workers and citizens at large. Present guidelines allow maximum cumulative doses of five rads per year per person or 100 millirems per week. A person occupationally exposed to radiation or to radioactive materials would be allowed to receive a lifetime dose of 25 rem. Radiation technicians wear film badges that indicate the amount of radiation they receive in their work.

The doses indicated below are **acute** (all-at-once), whole-body doses, or the equivalent. The causes of death and sickness at high doses include blood cell deficiencies (anemia, leucopenia-immune suppression-infection) and gastrointestinal problems (nausea, vomiting, fluid loss-diarrhea, hemorrhage). Most causes of death and illnesses reflect the high sensitivity of rapidly dividing (e.g., blood cell-forming) cells to radiation.

Dose	Effect
700 rads	Practically everybody dies within a month or so.
450 rads	Everybody gets sick; 50 percent die within 30–60 days.
150 rads	Half get sick.
100 rads	20 percent get sick; few deaths.
50 rads	Sickness rare; possibly some long-term risk to leukemia.

Dose	Source
1 rad over 30 years	Average exposure from man-made radiation.
0.4–0.8 rad	Upper gastrointestinal X-ray series.
0.1–0.2 rad	Mammographic series (see Chapter 16).
0.02–0.06 rad	Chest X-ray.
0.01–0.03 rad	Dental X-ray (whole mouth).

Source: Compiled from various sources, including U.S. Public Health Service, National Research Council, and National Academy of Science's Committee on Biological Effects of Ionizing Radiation (BEIR) Report, 1972.

Carcinogenesis: A Step Ahead of Repair

All cells, even those of bacteria, have a limited ability to repair damage to DNA. If direct chemical action or radiation-induced reaction causes a change in one strand of a DNA molecule, enzymes whose job it is to monitor such changes (1) cut out the affected part of the affected strand and (2) rebuild it using the "complementary" information in the opposite strand. This kind of repair in mammalian cells is very efficient and very accurate.

Even when damage extends to both strands of the double-stranded DNA molecule, there appear to be repair mechanisms—in some kinds of cells at least—that stick "something in." This kind of repair tends to be highly error-prone and is much more likely to lead to mutation.

Evidence that this finding may have some practical human importance comes from the atom bomb survivors in Japan. The Nagasaki bomb produced mostly X-rays, which tend to generate single-stranded breaks. There, cancer incidence was proportional to the *square* of the dose received. The Hiroshima bomb, on the other hand, generated neutrons, which tend to cause problems across both strands of DNA, and there is some evidence that Hiroshima cancer incidence was more *directly* proportional to dose.

Repair takes time. If radiation or chemical-induced damage to one strand of DNA can be repaired before the cell in which the damage has occurred tries to replicate its DNA during cell division, no harm done. If, on the other hand, a cell tries to replicate damaged DNA, the probability of mistakes is higher. Replicating enzymes "simply don't know what to do" when they encounter an unrepaired damaged portion of a damaged single strand of DNA! It is more likely that a mutation will occur. If the mutation occurs in a gene that remains suppressed, no harm done. If the mutation occurs in an activated gene, or if the mutation activates a gene, abnormal products will be produced by that cell and its progeny. One such abnormal cell among many normal cells may have no effect on the organisms. If the mutated cell divides many times to give rise to *many* cells carrying the same mutation, however, the organism could be harmed significantly. If the mutation involves a key oncogene, a cancer may be initiated.

If Radiation Causes Cancer, How Can It Be Used to Treat Cancer?

By causing changes in vital molecules, radiation damages cells, and at high-enough doses it kills them. In radiation therapy, the idea is to direct killing doses of radiation at cancer cells while sparing surrounding normal cells. As we will show in Chapter 17, radiation can be narrowly directed at specific locations using shielding and various other means; for example, by taking advantage of the fact that certain types of radiation exert greater killing effects at certain depths in tissue. Helping matters considerably is the fact that many types of cancer cells are more sensitive to radiation than normal cells. The reason for this is apparently related to cell division.

Proliferating cells—cells going through the cell cycle—are generally more susceptible to being killed by radiation than are nonproliferating cells. The faster cells are dividing, the more susceptible. The sensitivity of dividing cells is what apparently accounts—at least in part—for the effectiveness of radiation in treating cancer. It also accounts for the fact that proliferating *normal* tissues such as bone marrow, tissues lining the digestive tract, and the cells that give rise to hair are also particularly sensitive to radiation. Normal cells of these tissues are even more sensitive to the killing effects of radiation than are slow-growing cancers (see Chapter 17).

Sources of Radiation Exposure

Radiation comes from a number of different sources. The principal categories are (1) natural sources; (2) medical sources; (3) industrial sources, including nuclear energy; and (4) nuclear weapons testing.

On the sun, atomic fusion and other processes give rise to unstable nuclides and in other ways give off all types of electromagnetic radiation, including both ionizing and nonionizing forms. Fortunately, little harmful radiation reaches the earth's surface; most of that which does reach the earth is absorbed in the upper atmosphere. A notable exception is ultraviolet radiation.

Radioisotopes such as radium 228 and uranium 238 occur naturally and can be purified from ores. Other natural sources of radiation (e.g., radon 222 and thorium 220) can be released from soil, rocks, and from coal when it is burned (Waldbott, 1978).

Solar Radiation and Cancer

There is definitely a relationship between skin cancer and ultraviolet radiation in sunlight. The circumstantial link between skin cancer incidence and sunny climates (Fig. 9.4) makes the connection very obvious (Gordon et al., 1972; Mason et al., 1975). Skin cancer is more common among farmers, sailors, beach bums, and others who spend a lot of time outdoors.* It shows up on arms, faces, and necks and other exposed areas and is relatively less common in unexposed locations. Within the United States and Australia, the patterns of skin cancer incidence follow the patterns of "sunniness"; there is more skin cancer in the sunbelts. Fair-skinned people—"Celts," for example—are particularly susceptible. People with xeroderma pigmentosum—an inability to repair the DNA damage caused by ultraviolet radiation (Fig. 9.4)—nearly always develop skin cancer.

---

*Anaise, Steinitz, and Ben Hur (1978) evaluated solar radiation as a possible etiological factor in malignant melanoma in Israel. Israel is a sunny, subtropical country populated by many different kinds of people. The study revealed that melanoma was more common (1) in light-skinned Israelis, (2) in immigrants who stayed in Israel longer, and (3) in those who worked outdoors.

The effects of ultraviolet radiation on humans are limited to the skin because the ultraviolet (UV) region of the electromagnetic spectrum doesn't penetrate deeply into tissue. This is not to say that ultraviolet is nothing to worry about. While it is true that most skin cancers metastasize slowly and are highly curable (see Chapter 18), sunlight is also thought to induce malignant melanoma, one of the most deadly of all human neoplasms (see Chapter 18).

Melanoma is an especially deadly form of skin cancer (see Chapter 19); it is fatal in about one out of four cases. Until recently, the connection between this form of skin cancer and exposure to the sun was not clear; individuals with the greatest total exposures to the sun did not seem to have the greatest risk to melanoma. At the 28th (1986) American Cancer Society's Science Writers Seminar (held in Daytona Beach, of all places), a Massachusetts General Hospital study was reported to show that intense exposure in childhood increases one's risk to melanoma—that one or more blistering sunburns early in life doubled the risk. Melanoma was relatively rare a half century ago, but it now strikes about one in 150 people (there was a 700 percent rise between 1940 and 1980—23,000 new cases are expected this year alone). It is now one of the most common cancers among teens and young adults.

Nuclear Energy and Cancer

As the number of atomic power plants has increased, public resistance to their construction has increased because of the fear of radioactive contamination of the environment. Normally, negligible amounts of radioactivity are released into the environment from nuclear power plants. Measurements of radioactivity made in waters and areas surrounding correctly functioning nuclear power plants by state health departments and nuclear power facility operators and the EPA have nearly always revealed no measurable increase in environmental radiation. Before the accident at Chernobyl, in Russia, it

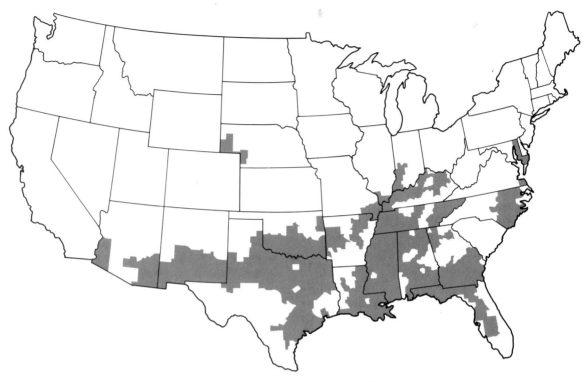

Figure 9.4 Skin cancer mortality (other than malignant melanoma) (1950–1969) in white males. The shaded areas had significantly higher death rates. (*Source:* Mason et al., 1975. Drawing from Kupchella and Hyland, 1986; used with permission of Allyn & Bacon.)

was estimated by many sources that, overall, nuclear power contributed *in*significantly to background radiation*; according to one source, nuclear power installations added no more than 0.0001 millirads per year to background radiation. But there was far from universal agreement on the nature of the radiation "leak" problem even before Chernobyl.

In 1979, two major National Academy of Sciences studies were made public (see Marshall,

1979). The studies indicated that nuclear power would account for some two thousand cancer deaths by the year 2,000 (a hundred people per year). The projection was not arrived at easily or with complete agreement; five of the sixteen commission members filed a dissenting opinion that the estimate was far too high.

The "Chronic" Problem of Radioactive Waste The word *chronic* has a special meaning used in connection with atomic wastes. Plutonium, one by-product of atomic fission, has a half-life greater than 24,000 years. Half of the plutonium in any given amount will remain after 24,000 years; half of the remaining half will be around after another 24,000. Where do you

---

*According to McBride et al. (1978), coal contains radioactive material, and radiation doses from coal-burning, electricity-generating plants may be greater than those from a properly operated nuclear plant producing similar levels of energy.

put something you want to keep safely tucked away for 100,000 years? Nuclear power proponents argue that although wastes do remain radioactive for thousands to hundreds of thousands of years, most harmful high-energy radiation will have been dissipated after a few hundred years (Hammond, 1979). Obviously, even conceding this point, the disposal of atomic waste presents a serious problem.

Nuclear Power Plant Accidents A U.S. government report (commissioned by the then Atomic Energy Commission, published in 1975, and generally known as the Rasmussen Report) concluded that there was essentially no chance of an atomic power plant accident that would lead to a disaster. In January 1979, two months before the Three Mile Island accident, the Nuclear Regulatory Commission declared that the risk was actually higher than had been thought.

It must be made clear that when nuclear accidents are discussed, it is *not* an atomic explosion, as in a nuclear bomb, that is feared. Atomic power plants cannot explode like an atom bomb. There is generally thought to be some finite possibility of a meltdown, however. A meltdown is what happens when a nuclear reactor core cooling system and all backup systems fail. The core would melt through the floor of the reactor into the ground and, if the meltdown occurred in the United States, "head in the general direction of China" (thus, **China syndrome**). The molten core would theoretically come to rest less than 100 feet down as a boiling, seething mass of molten materials. Any water coming into contact with the molten core would be converted into contaminated steam which could carry gases and particles over a wide area.

Some say that Three Mile Island came close to a meltdown. The cooling system failed, and this was followed by a compounding of human errors, mechanical collapses, bad luck, and design flaws. Although some radiation was vented into the environment, no one was seriously overexposed to radiation, injured, or killed at Three Mile Island. A major consequence was that public opinion turned against nuclear energy.

Chernobyl On April 26, 1986, an explosion and fire at the Soviet Union's Chernobyl nuclear power plant (80 miles north of Kiev in the Ukraine) sent radioactive materials into the atmosphere, and these eventually spread as fallout throughout much of the world. Although many of the details of the accident remain unclear, Chernobyl clearly surpassed Three Mile Island as the most serious accident in the 32-year history of nuclear power.

Although relatively few people were killed outright by the initial explosions, a few more were killed more-or-less immediately by exposure to high doses of radiation. Some unknown number are expected to die later as a result of delayed radiation effects, including cancer and birth defects. Although much depends on the actual pattern of distribution (wind patterns at the time of, and subsequent to, the accident), the greatest danger is to those near the plant; even within a hundred miles of the plant there will likely be significant increases in leukemia and other types of cancer over perhaps as many as 30 years. The fact that tens of thousands of people were evacuated suggests that the number of people potentially exposed to abnormally high levels of radiation may be quite high.

Radioactive materials will likely remain in the soil and water over a wide area of the Soviet Union for some time, and it is impossible to state with any certainty just how many people were, and will be, exposed to how much radiation for how long. Because of the half-lives of some of the radioisotopes released (cesium 137—30 years; strontium 90—28 years), the area immediately around the plant may have to remain uninhabited for many decades—depending on how much radioactivity in these forms was deposited and how much of it can be removed by scraping off the upper layer of soil. It will take years before the full impact of the accident, particularly in terms of cancer, are better known.

Medical X-rays, Nuclear Medicine, and Cancer

When used judiciously and discriminately, diagnostic radiation yields much more benefit than it does risk. Medical X-rays and radiopharmaceuticals are routinely used in the detection, diagnosis, and treatment of disease. In fact, 50 percent of the ionizing radiation to which the U.S. population is exposed comes from diagnostic medicine; natural background accounts for almost all of the other half (Clifton, 1983). In the past, before the dangers of radiation were appreciated, the risk of cancer from medically applied radiation was discovered after the fact.

Not long ago, thorium dioxide was used to produce diagnostic images of the liver. Thorium dioxide is an alpha particle emitter, and not surprisingly, some liver cancer has been linked to this practice.

Chest fluoroscopy was used to check the status of tuberculosis in young women when TB was common. Later studies revealed that women subjected to multiple fluoroscopy developed ten times more breast cancer than normal (Hutchison, 1977).

For several decades beginning in the early 1920s, X-ray therapy was considered good treatment for enlarged thymus glands in babies with breathing problems. Such therapy was later found to lead to thyroid cancers. X-ray therapy has also been used for deafness caused by lymphoid infiltration around the Eustachian tube (connecting the middle ear with the throat), acne, ringworm of the scalp, enlarged tonsils, and enlarged adenoids. Such practices are no longer common.

Nuclear Weapons and Cancer

When we worry about the radiation associated with nuclear war or with nuclear power plant disasters, we sometimes forget that there was a nuclear war that ended in 1945. Considerable data were collected concerning the cancer aftermath.

Following the nuclear destruction of Hiroshima and Nagasaki and the end of World War II, an Atomic Bomb Casualty Commission was set up to monitor the effects of the radiation exposure in the survivors.* Over the intervening years, epidemiological methods have been used to evaluate cancer in people of different ages in relationship to the radiation dose they received by virtue of their location and circumstance at the time of impact. Among the findings cataloged are the following:

Radiation from the bombs was found to induce several kinds of leukemia.

Even as little as 20 to 49 rads apparently increased the risk of leukemia.

Children under age 10 were the most susceptible (to leukemia).

The bombs produced an excess of thyroid cancer.

Those over age 10 when exposed showed an increased risk to *all* forms of cancer.

The total number of cancers induced by the two bombs was less than 500, but they proved that even a single significant exposure to radiation can, in fact, cause cancer.

Cancer and Atomic Testing

In the early 1950s, some hundred experimental atomic bombs were detonated above ground in central Nevada. Soldiers were exposed to radiation as a result of their participation in these exercises, and civilians were—and in fact still are—exposed to some radiation derived from fallout. In the news in recent years have been aired a number of court suits and disputed allegations regarding the connection between these

---

*Later this commission became a joint venture of the U.S. National Academy of Sciences and the Japanese National Institute of Health. In 1975 it became the Radiation Effects Research Foundation (Finch and Hamilton, 1976; Shimkin, 1977)

exposures and cancer. Because the doses received are uncertain or have remained classified, the science is not clear; epidemiology has not revealed any clear conclusions. Lyon et al. (1979), for example, reported that there was a connection between childhood leukemia death rates in southern Utah and the period of most intense testing in adjacent Nevada. Land, McKay, and Machado (1984) later disputed this study, asserting that an apparent increase in leukemia deaths reflected an abnormally *low* death rate in the 1940s, the period used for comparison by Lyon et al.

In May 1984, a federal judge ruled that the government was, in fact, negligent in the aboveground testing program and that cancers were, in fact, caused by radiation exposure. He ordered that $2.6 million be paid to 10 individuals who had lost relatives to cancer. These 10 were selected as test cases from among almost 1,200 original plaintiffs. What will happen to the others depends upon the outcome of appeals now underway with the test cases.

Imagine the difficulty in deciding, for individuals in a population in which one person in three is destined to develop some form of cancer anyway, which cancers may have been related to radiation exposure some thirty to forty years earlier! Early in 1984, President Reagan signed a measure to develop probability tables for the relation between radiation exposure and certain cancers to be used as guides in compensation cases.

Radiation Carcinogenesis from Cigarettes?

Cigarette smokers have been estimated to get up to 20 rads of polonium 210 in the lung epithelium. Little, Kennedy, and McGandy (1975) demonstrated that lung cancers could be induced in hamsters from lung doses of polonium 210 equivalent to 15 to 300 rads. Although the connection is highly speculative, polonium 210 may well contribute to the lung cancers associated with cigarette smoking.

The Problem of Low Doses Over a Long Time

Experiments in radiation carcinogenesis often (but not always) fail to show any cancer at very low doses. This absence may well reflect a limitation of experimentation rather than the harmlessness of low doses of radiation. The same kinds of limitations apply here as apply with chemical carcinogens (as discussed in the last chapter).

The reasons for the disagreement over the risks from low doses of ionizing radiation are nicely summarized by Charles Land (1980:1197), a statistician with the Environmental Epidemiology Branch of the National Cancer Institute:

> First, precise direct estimation of small risks requires impracticably large samples. Second, precise estimates of low-dose risks based largely on high-dose data . . . must depend heavily on assumptions about the slope of the dose-response curve, even when only a few of the parameters of the theoretical form of the curve are unknown.

Nevertheless, the dose response curve for the relationship between radiation exposure and human cancer is roughly depicted in Figure 9.5. It is generally believed that the form of the curve reflects repair of DNA damage at low doses and the death of injured cells at high doses. Between these plateaus is a curve reflecting enhanced transformation with increasing doses. Although such curves have been confirmed by animal data, the exact shape of the curve is not known in humans because it has been derived from uncontrolled observations of people exposed accidentally to uncertain amounts of radiation. The lower dose region of the curve has been the subject of much interest and controversy, especially as related to the exposure risk associated with nuclear power plants.

In 1943 Hanford Works, an atomic plant in Richland, Washington, began to monitor its workers. In a still disputed report issued in 1977, Mancuso, Stewart, and Kneale compared the long-term radiation exposure of the workers with their causes of death as reported on death

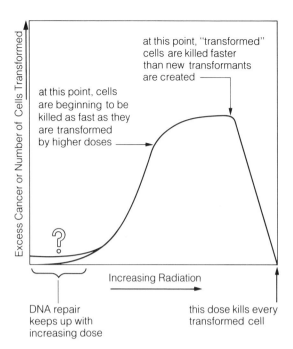

Plot axes: y-axis labeled "Excess Cancer or Number of Cells Transformed"; x-axis labeled "Increasing Radiation"

Annotations on figure:
- at this point, "transformed" cells are killed faster than new transformants are created
- at this point, cells are beginning to be killed as fast as they are transformed by higher doses
- DNA repair keeps up with increasing dose
- this dose kills every transformed cell

Figure 9.5 The general shape of the curve relating radiation dose and cancer or transformation. The lower plateau is believed to be related to repair or sublethal damage. For a while, repair keeps up with the damage. Higher doses cause carcinogenesis to run ahead of repair until they are so high that the cells are as likely to die as to become transformed by radiation damage. The question mark reflects uncertainty about the completeness of repair even at very low doses and uncertainty about the possibility that *very* low doses cause no transformation at all.

certificates. The results showed that plant workers receiving exposure rates below the annual dosage established as safe by the federal government had more than double the normal expectancy of certain types of cancer. However, this study and its methodologies have been the subject of much controversy. The reader is referred to the 1981 report *Problems in Assessing the Cancer Risk of Low Level Ionizing Radiation Exposure*, prepared by the U.S. General Accounting Office (GAO). As of the time of this writing, there really has been no generally accepted definitive

study of the impact on humans of long-term, low-level exposure to radiation. Data gathering continues as the U.S. government attempts to prescribe standards for exposure well within an "acceptable risk" level. Summaries of 52 studies involving humans are presented in the GAO report just cited.

Although we know that repair can and does take place following radiation damage, we do not know for a fact that this repair is 100 percent effective. If unrepaired cells remain, some of them could very well go on to become cancers. There is much controversy over the risk associated with low doses over long periods of time. It has also been agreed that some degree of risk will be treated as acceptable (Table 9.2) when risk-benefit considerations are favorable. ALRA (as low as reasonably allowable) is a concept now used to guide radiation exposure.

Human Neoplasms Associated with Radiation

The collective experience with Japanese atom bomb survivors, early radiologists, uranium miners, patients who developed cancers as a result of diagnostic and therapeutic uses of radiation, and Marshall Islanders exposed to fallout as a result of atomic testing indicates that many kinds of human cancer can be caused by radiation (Fig. 9.6).

The experience of watch dial painters early in this century established the relationship between radium and bone cancer in humans. Neoplasms caused by bone-seeking radionuclides include osteosarcoma (arising from the cells lining the bone surface), fibrosarcoma (tumors characterized by the proliferation of connective tissue cells and collagen synthesis), chondrosarcoma (tumors of cartilage), lymphoma (malignant blood-forming elements of bone marrow), carcinoma of the sinuses (tumors of the soft tissues of the skull), and reticulum cell sarcoma (arising from cells in the bone marrow—Vaughn, 1976).

Table 9.2 Maximum Permissible Doses (MPD) for Whole-Body Exposures as Set in 1971 by the National Council on Radiation Protection. Larger doses are permitted for some parts of the body.

	MPD
General population	
MPD for any individual[a]	500 millirems per year
Average for whole U.S. population[b]	170 millirems per year
Radiation workers	
Annual	5,000 millirems per year
3-month period	3,000 millirems per 3 months
Pregnant workers	500 millirems per 9 months

[a]Facilities using radiation may occasionally expose some individuals to this dose.
[b]This is the average for everyone, including radiation workers.

From Table 34-4, p. 607 in Kane, J. and Sternheim, M. *Physics*, 2nd Edition. Copyright © 1978 John Wiley & Sons. Reprinted by permission of the publisher.

Studies of atom bomb survivors to date have revealed an increased frequency of leukemia, thyroid cancer, breast cancer, lung cancer, and other cancers.

It became evident in the 1950s that thyroid cancers developed in some children who as infants had received radiation to the neck in the treatment of enlarged thymus glands. Thyroid tumors are also potentially environmentally important because thyroid-seeking radioiodine is a by-product of nuclear fission and is present in fallout from accidents like the one at Chernobyl and after atomic tests.

Nearly a third of the deaths that occur in uranium miners are due to lung cancer (Epstein, 1976). Presumably, this incidence is mainly a result of cigarette smoking compounded by inhaling radon and other radioisotopes. We have also learned some things about lag and about dose response, relationships between radiation and human neoplasms. Solid tumors take longer to develop from radiation exposure than do the leukemias. While thyroid tumors take from 15 to 20 years to show up, the first peak incidence of leukemia in Japanese atom bomb survivors was 4 to 8 years. The excess in leukemia in children exposed to medical X-rays as fetuses peaked between 3 and 5 years and disappeared by age seven (MacMahon, 1962).

Summary

Radiation can cause cancer. The radiation most effective in doing so is that of sufficient energy to ionize and cause radiochemical changes. It seems most likely that the most common ultimate effect is mutation. In some kinds of tissue and at some doses, radiation may induce only one of several necessary steps leading to transformation. In any case, radiation is known to be mutagenic and could thereby activate oncogenes either by direct mutation, by mutations that reduce cellular control over oncogenes or by inducing displacement of oncogenes from regions where they are relatively well controlled. The risk from actual "rays" comes mostly from medical X-rays, work with radioactive materials, and natural, background, cosmic gamma radiation. Still another part of the risk is that derived from the radioactive isotopes that contaminate the environment.

Figure 9.6 Types of human cancer associated with radiation. (*Source:* Upton, 1979. Courtesy American Cancer Society, Inc.)

	Atom Bomb Radiation			Occupational Radiation				Medical Radiation										
Type of Cancer	*Japanese atom bomb survivors*	*Marshall Islanders*	*Nuclear test participants*	*Radium dial painters*	*Radiologists*	*Uranium and other miners*	*Nuclear workers*	*Ankylosing spondylitis (X-ray)*	*Ankylosing spondylitis (radium)*	*Benign pelvic disease*	*Benign breast disease*	*Multiple chest fluoroscopy*	*Tinea capitis (fungus infection of scalp) (children)*	*Enlarged thymus (infants)*	*Thorotrast (contrast medium)*	*Thyroid cancer (Iodine 131)*	*In utero X-ray*	*Diagnostic X-ray*
Leukemia	●		◉		●		◉	●		X				X	●	◉	●	◉
Thyroid	●	X											X	●				
Female breast	●								◉		●	●						
Lung	●					●	◉	●										
Bone				●				◉	●									
Stomach	X							X										
Esophagus	X							X										
Bladder	X																	
Lymphoma (including multiple myeloma)	X				X		◉	X							◉			
Brain					X								X			◉		
Uterus										●								
Cervix	◉																	
Liver	◉														●			
Skin					●	X							X	X				
Salivary gland	◉												X	X				
Kidney								◉	◉						◉			
Pancreas							◉											
Colon	◉			◉						X								
Small intestine										◉								
Rectum										X								

Strong associations are indicated by ●, meaningful but less striking associations by **X** and suggestive but unconfirmed associations by ◉. See text for more complete explanation.

References and Further Reading

Anaise, D., Steinitz, R., and Ben Hur, N. 1978. Solar Radiation: A Possible Etiological Factor in Malignant Melanoma in Israel. *Cancer.* 42(1):299–304.

Beebe, G. W. 1982. Ionizing Radiation and Health. *American Scientist.* 70:35–44.

Blum, H. F. 1976. Ultraviolet Radiation and Skin Cancer: In Mice and Men. *Photochemistry and Photobiology.* 24:249–54.

Bond, V. P., and Thiessen, J. W., eds. 1982. *Reevaluation of Dosimetric Factors: Hiroshima and Nagasaki.* Springfield, Va.: National Technical Information Service.

Cleary, S. F. 1983. Microwave Radiation Effects on Humans. *Bioscience.* 33(4):269–73.

Clifton, K. H. 1983. Ionizing Radiation Carcinogenesis in Man. In S. B. Kahn et al., eds., *Concepts in Cancer Medicine.* New York: Grune & Stratton.

Committee for the Compilation of Materials on Damage Caused by the Atomic Bombs in Hiroshima and Nagasaki. 1981. *The Physical, Medical, and Social Effects of the Atomic Bombings.* Translated by E. Ishikawa and D. L. Swain. New York: Basic Books.

Cornforth, M. N., and Bedford, J. S. 1983. X-ray-Induced Breakage and Rejoining of Human Interphase Chromosomes. *Science.* 222:1141–43.

Epstein, S. S. 1976. *Cancer and the Environment: A Scientific Perspective, Facts, and Analysis.* Industrial Union Dept., AFL-CIO, No. 25 (February) 1–13.

Finch, S. C., and Hamilton, H. B. 1976. Atomic Bomb Radiation Studies in Japan. *Science.* 192(4242):845.

Gordon, D., Silverstone, H., and Smithhurst, B. 1972. The Epidemiology of Skin Cancer in Australia. W. H. McCarthy, ed., *Melanoma and Skin Cancer.* Sydney: NWS Government Printer.

Hall, E. J. 1984. *Radiation and Life.* Elmsford, N.Y.: Pergamon Press.

Hammond, R. P. 1979. Nuclear Waste and Public Acceptance. *American Scientist.* 67:146–50.

Hutchison, G. B. 1977. Carcinogenic Effects of Medical Irradiation. In H. H. Hiatt, J. D. Watson, and J. A. Winsten, eds., *Origins of Human Cancer.* New York: Cold Spring Harbor Laboratory.

Irradiation-Related Thyroid Cancer. NIH Publication No. 77-1120. Washington, D. C.: U.S. Department of Health, Education, and Welfare, Public Health Service.

Klement, A. W. 1982. *CRC Handbook of Environmental Radiation.* Boca Raton, Fla.: CRC Press.

Kupchella, C. E., and Hyland, M. C. 1986. *Environmental Science: Living Within the System of Nature.* Boston: Allyn & Bacon.

Land, C. E. 1980. Estimating Cancer Risks from Low Doses of Ionizing Radiation. *Science.* 209: 1197–1203.

Land, C. E., McKay, F. W., and Machado, S. G. 1984. Childhood Leukemia and Fallout from the Nevada Nuclear Tests. *Science.* 23:139–44.

Little, J. B., Kennedy, A. R., and McGandy, R. B. 1975. Lung Cancer Induced in Hamsters by Low Doses of Alpha Radiation from Polonium-210. *Science.* 188: 736–38.

Lyon, J. L., et al. 1979. Childhood Leukemias Associated with Fallout from Nuclear Testing. *New England J. Med.* 300:397–402.

MacMahon, B. 1962. Prenatal X-ray Exposure in Childhood Cancer. *Journal of the National Cancer Institute.* 28:1173–91.

Mancuso, T., Stewart, A., and Kneale, G. 1977. Radiation Exposures of Hanford Workers Dying from Cancer and Other Causes. *Health Physics.* 33:369–84.

Marshall, E. 1979. NAS Study on Radiation Takes the Middle Road. *Science.* 204:711–14.

Mason, T. J., et al. 1975. *Atlas of Cancer Mortality for U.S. Counties 1950–1969.* NIH 75-780. Washington, D.C.: U.S. Department of Health, Education, and Welfare.

McBride, J. P. et al. 1978. Radiological Impact of Airborne Effluents of Coal and Nuclear Plants. *Science.* 202:1045–50.

Norman, C. 1986. Hazy Picture of Chernobyl Emerging. *Science.* 232:1331–33.

Pochin, E. E. 1976. Some Illustrative Systems of Radiation Carcinogenesis: (3) Thyroid Neoplasia. In T. Symington and R. L. Carter, eds., 1976. *Scientific Foundations of Oncology.* Chicago: Heinemann Medical Books/ Yearbook Medical Publications.

Reif, A. E. 1981. The Causes of Cancer. *American Scientist.* 69:437–47.

Scott, D. J., Craig, A. W., and Iype, P. T. 1976. Effects of Ionizing Radiation on Mammalian Cells. In T. Symington and R. L. Carter, eds., *Scientific Foundations of*

Oncology. Chicago: Heinemann Medical Books/Yearbook Medical Publications.

Shellabarger, C. J. 1976. Radiation Carcinogenesis. *Cancer.* 37(2):1090–96.

Shimkin, M. B. 1977. *Contrary to Nature.* Washington, D.C.: U.S. Department of Health, Education, and Welfare, Public Health Service.

Upton, A. C. 1979. Low-Level Radiation. *Ca-A Cancer Journal for Clinicians.* 29(5):306–15.

Upton, A. C. 1982. The Biological Effects of Low-level Ionizing Radiation. *Scientific American.* 246:41–49.

Vaughn, J. 1976. Some Illustrative Systems of Radiation Carcinogenesis (2) Boneseeking Isotopes and Neoplasia. In T. Symington and R. L. Carter, eds., *Scientific Foundations of Oncology.* Chicago: Heinemann Medical Books/Yearbook Medical Publications.

Waldbott, G. L. 1978. *Health Effects of Environmental Pollutants.* 2nd ed. St. Louis: Mosby.

We all know viruses best as the causes of colds and flu. Most of us have also encountered them in measles, chicken pox, shingles, mumps, and fever blisters. All of us at least know of people who have experienced much more devastating viral diseases such as hepatitis, polio, genital herpes, viral pneumonia, viral encephalitis, or AIDS. Viruses get a chapter of their own in this book because viruses are one of the three most important classes of things that cause cancer.

Certain viruses cause cancer in animals, and similar viruses may also cause some cancers in human beings. We have already discussed viruses as *experimental* transforming agents (Chapter 4), and we have explored their role in defining oncogenes (Chapter 7) in cancer research laboratories. Here we give some extended coverage to viruses as carcinogenic agents in the world at large.

Since only people with electron microscopes can actually *see* viruses, we begin with a general description of viruses and how they fit into the grand scheme of life. Then we will reconsider just how viruses cause cancer. We will conclude the chapter with a review of those human cancers that have been most closely linked to viruses. Along the way we will consider the difficulty of *proving* that viruses are the causes of at least some forms of human cancer.

10

Viruses and Cancer

What Exactly Are Viruses, Anyway: What Are They Made of and What Do They Look Like?

Depending on one's point of view, viruses are either among the simplest living things or they are not living things at all.* One feature that distinguishes living from nonliving things is reproduction. Viruses cannot replicate in an independent fashion—without using the nucleic acids

---

*In the last decade or so, disease-causing agents even simpler than viruses, called *viroids*, have been discovered (see Diener, 1983). Viroids are simply "naked" molecules of RNA, and they are known to cause about a dozen plant diseases.

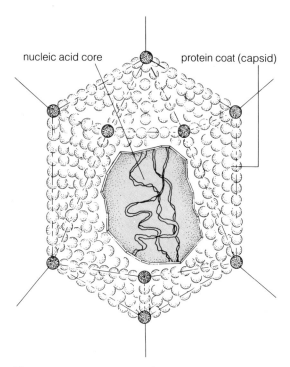

nucleic acid core   protein coat (capsid)

Figure 10.1 A human adenovirus looks something like this and has just two basic components: a (mostly) protein coat or capsid and a core of nucleic acid—DNA, in the case of adenoviruses.

and protein-synthesizing machinery in host cells of other living things—and some say that this inability disqualifies them. We won't get into the debate here.

Bacteria are very small, and viruses are much smaller. In concrete terms, viruses are ten to several hundred *nanometers* long or across—they come in various shapes. Thousands of the smallest varieties of viruses could be stuffed into the average bacterial cell. Some viruses are essentially complex molecular aggregates consisting of a few protein molecules and a few molecules of nucleic acid—DNA *or* RNA, but not both. Some cancer-causing viruses contain only four or five genes; a human cell, by comparison, contains more than 50,000 genes.

The basic "parts" of a virus are (1) a protein coat or **capsid** (sometimes containing a little lipid) and (2) a nucleic acid core (Fig. 10.1). Virus

assembly lines are very short. The parts of a virus do not even add up to a cell. Viruses are "acellular."

When they are *not* infecting something, viruses lead an unbelievably dull existence not unlike that of a crystal. They do not metabolize, they do not generate ATP, they do not respire, ferment, or conduct photosynthesis. They can't even *move* under their own power; they just drift until they happen to bump into the right kind of host cell.

When they *are* infecting something, however, viruses are far from dull. As described in detail below, when viruses get into an appropriate host cell, they literally take over the genetic machinery. Some of them shut down their host cell's normal functions and cause the cell to concentrate on making more viruses.

Viruses are "obligate intracellular parasites": each kind of virus absolutely depends on the cells of one or a few specific host species for their reproduction. If they don't run into the right kind of cell, they can't reproduce.

How Do Viruses Reproduce?

A number of movies in recent years have had plots that mimic viral reproduction. In all these movies, a creature from outer space inhabits the body of some Earth creature—a dog, a cat, or a human. The "space thing" takes over from *within*, unbeknownst to other earth creatures—except that other dogs, horses, or cats always seem to suspect that something isn't quite right. Anyway, the creature emerges at some opportune time and attacks and takes over another dog or human, and so it goes until the end of the movie. Even at the end of the movie, the whereabouts of the thing are unknown—gone until a sequel is released.

Once inside host cells, viruses disappear (as morphologically recognizable entities) but they may transform the infected cells. Viruses may also reappear and kill their host cells as they reemerge to infect and kill other cells. It is often difficult to tell if a virus, or part of a virus, is present in a cell or not.

Adhesion and Break-in

Although some viruses do attack the cells of *many* species, usually a given virus attacks just one or two species. Many viruses prefer the cells of certain tissues of certain species—hepatitis viruses attack human liver cells, human polio virus attacks human nerve cells, and so on. The basis of this specificity is a match between the viral capsid and receptor configurations particular to the target cell's cytoplasmic membrane. The binding somehow induces the cell to take in the virus by endocytosis (see Chapter 2).

Takeover and Break-out

After the host cell digests the protein capsid, the viral nucleic acid takes over, directing the host genes to make more viral nucleic acid and messenger RNA coded for viral protein. The viral protein and nucleic acid made by the host cell combines spontaneously to form new viruses that escape the host cell by exocytosis or budding, or by causing the cell to rupture.

DNA virus reproduction is different from RNA virus reproduction, but in both cancer-causing RNA and DNA viruses the formation of a double-stranded viral DNA is part of the process of viral replication. We will consider some additional features of RNA and DNA virus reproduction later, in the context of how these viruses cause cancer.

Viruses in Hiding

Viruses don't always reproduce or kill the host cell straightaway. Sometimes when a virus invades a cell, it simply incorporates itself into the genome or remains in the cytoplasm somewhere and stays there as a so-called **latent** (hidden) **virus** until something triggers its activation. All the while it is acting as a latent virus, the viral genome is replicated as the host cell divides. Each daughter cell ends up with its own latent virus.

Perhaps the most familiar example of latency is the *Herpes simplex* virus that causes cold sores or fever blisters. These herpes viruses can apparently be activated by fever, stress, and sunlight (ultraviolet radiation); they do their damage and then lie dormant only to emerge again another day. Generally speaking, hormones, radiation, stress, and temperature changes are among the things that can activate viruses; there is some evidence that chemical carcinogens *generally* have the ability to activate latent viruses.

Kinds of Viruses

Viruses can be classified in a number of ways. The most common way is to separate them according to whether their nucleic acid core is (1) RNA or DNA, and (2) double- or single-stranded. Other criteria used in classification include size, shape, and host.

Oncogenic Viruses

It has been known since just after the turn of the century that viruses initiate cancer. Ellermann and Bang (1908) succeeded in producing a form of leukemia in chickens, with a bacteria-free extract prepared from a chicken with leukemia. Peyton Rous (1911) extracted viruses from chicken sarcomas by passing tumor extracts through filters with holes too small to allow anything but viruses through. He showed that such extracts could cause sarcomas in chickens.

About the time that Ellermann, Bang, and Rous were publishing their results, chemicals and radiation were being implicated as causes of cancer and this latter finding drew much more attention. Apparently it was difficult to see what viruses had to do with either radiation or chemical-induced cancer, and it wasn't until the middle of this century that significant numbers of scientists began to believe that viruses were important general causes of cancer, despite the fact that many other animal cancers were linked to viruses throughout the 1930s and 1940s.

Viruses were implicated as the cause of rabbit papillomas in the 1930s by Richard Shope. John Bittner and his colleagues found in 1936 that mother mice could transmit a breast cancer causing virus to their daughters via milk. A turning point in thinking appeared to come at mid century when Ludwik Gross showed that mouse leukemias could be transmitted by cell-free filtrates and the powerfully carcinogenic polyoma viruses were discovered at the National Institutes of Health. The general stature of virology as a science also got a big boost during the crusade against polio fueled by the March of Dimes during the 1940s and 1950s.

Over the years it became clear that there are really two major categories of oncogenic viruses. One group contains DNA. DNA viruses carry their "plans and programs" in DNA. Oncogenic RNA viruses (sometimes called **oncoRNA viruses** or *oncorna viruses; see Table 10.1) carry their "codes for action" in RNA; they have no DNA. RNA viruses get their host cells to make DNA from RNA codes—exactly the opposite of the way the two kinds of nucleic acids usually relate (see Chapter 2)—with a special enzyme called *reverse transcriptase*. Viruses that carry this enzyme in order to replicate are called **retroviruses**. Virtually all RNA viruses that cause cancer are classifiable as retroviruses.

Oncogenic DNA Viruses

Papovaviruses are DNA viruses that cause cancer in a relatively wide variety of mammals, including primates. Viruses belonging to this group have repeatedly been isolated from human cancer cells and are suspect as human carcinogenic agents. In terms of experimental cancer research, the two most important kinds of papovaviruses are the mouse polyoma virus group and the SV-40 virus.

The prototype **polyoma virus** was isolated from a mouse salivary gland tumor. The virus was later named *polyoma* (literally, many tumors) because it was found to cause over 20 different kinds of mouse cancers originating in virtually every kind of mouse tissue. Polyoma viruses can also induce cancer in many other kinds of mammals—hamsters, rabbits, rats, and so on. There are no known polyoma virus-induced human cancers.

The **SV-40 virus** is a **simian** (monkey-ape) **virus**. Although first isolated from monkey kidney cells, it causes cancer when injected into baby hamsters and mice, but not in monkeys or in humans.* Thousands of people were inadvertently injected with SV-40 viruses between 1958 and 1961 when it was an unknown contaminant of attenuated polio vaccine. So far, no virus-related cancer patterns have emerged in these individuals.

Two kinds of papova viruses, **JC viruses** and **BK viruses**, are found in the tissues of most human beings. Both of these viruses can transform human and animal cells in tissue culture, and both can induce brain tumors in rodents. Both BK and JC viruses are therefore potential candidates as causal factors in human cancer.

Papillomaviruses infect many mammalian species, humans included. They are known to induce neoplastic lesions (warts or wartlike lesions) in skin, in the larynx, and in epithelial tissue of other organs. Most recently, **papillomaviruses** have been implicated in cervical cancer.

Adenoviruses make up a second major group of oncogenic DNA viruses. More than two dozen different adenoviruses have been isolated from human nasal washings (the name is related to *adenoid*), and about half cause cancers when injected into young rodents. Although

---

*There is apparently no natural connection between SV-40 and hamster or mouse cancer.

Table 10.1   Oncogenic Viruses

Group/Name	Species Viruses Isolated From	Cancer and Species in Which Cancer Induced
Oncogenic DNA Viruses		
Papovaviruses (Papovaviridae)		
Polyoma	Mouse	Mainly leukemias in mice and hamsters, and transforms cells in tissue culture
Papilloma	Fish and many mammals	Papillomas, sarcomas in fish and other animals; warts (benign neoplasms) and possibly cervical cancer in humans
SV-40 (Simian virus-40)	Monkey	Lymphosarcomas in hamsters and mice, and transforms cells grown in culture
Adenoviruses (Adenoviridae) (some 30 different kinds)	Monkeys, humans	Sarcomas, lymphomas in hamsters and mice, and transforms cells grown in culture
Herpes viruses (Herpetoviridae)		
Epstein-Barr virus	Human	Possibly Burkitt's lymphoma and nasopharyngeal cancer in humans
Lucké virus	Frog	Kidney carcinoma in frogs
Marek's disease virus	Chicken	Lymphoma in chickens
Herpes simplex virus 2	Human	Possibly cervical cancer in humans
Hepatitis B Virus	Human	Possibly hepatocellular cancer in humans
Oncogenic RNA Viruses (Retroviridae)		
Chicken sarcoma viruses	Chicken	Sarcomas in many fowl, hamsters, certain reptiles, monkeys, and transforms cells grown in culture
Fowl leukemia viruses	Chicken	Chicken leukemia and transforms cells grown in culture
Mammalian sarcoma viruses	Mouse, cat, dog	Sarcomas in mice, rats, cats, hamsters, cell culture, dogs, monkeys
Mammalian leukemia viruses	Mouse, cat, guinea pig	Leukemia in mice, rats, cats, hamsters, guinea pigs; also lymphoma
"B"-type viruses	Mouse	Mice mammary tumor (carcinoma)

adenoviruses can be isolated from virtually all humans, they appear to cause little more than colds in humans.

Herpes viruses have received much attention lately, not all of it because of their link to cancer. Herpes-type viruses exploit almost all vertebrate species and are linked to cancer in nearly all classes of vertebrates—for example,

amphibia: kidney cancer in frogs; aves: lymphoma in chickens; mammalia: cancer in rodents and in humans and other primates. Strong circumstantial evidence links *Herpes simplex* viruses to human cancer, but we will hold our discussion of this until later.

Oncogenic DNA viruses tend *not* to cause the production of new viruses when they are incorporated into the host genome and have transformed the host cell (see Fig. 10.2).

Oncogenic RNA Viruses

However difficult it may be to get used to the idea that there could be organisms without DNA, RNA viruses are not at all uncommon. RNA viruses are responsible for yellow fever, tick fever, polio, mumps, influenza, and many other well-known diseases. They infect a wide variety of plant and animal species. Of most direct interest to us here is that they cause animal leukemias, lymphomas, and mammary cancer. It was an oncoRNA virus that Ellermann and Bang confirmed as a cause of chicken leukemia. RNA viruses also cause leukemias in cats and apes, lymphomas in cattle and cats (see Table 10.1).

The RNA viruses that cause leukemias and lymphomas in some kinds of animals are infectious and commonly provoke outbreaks of cancer among animals that are in close proximity to one another. This fact has some important implications for human cancer now that human leukemias have fairly convincingly been linked to viruses (see below). We should say here, however, that even among cats infected with feline leukemia viruses relatively few actually develop leukemia. Also, a large fraction of cats that do develop leukemia do not shed new viruses, apparently because the viruses are unable to replicate in their cells for some reason. All these clues suggest that even though carcinogenic viruses may indeed be infectious, they are obviously nowhere near as easily spread as, say, the common cold virus among humans.

An oncoRNA virus called the **"B"-virus** or **Bittner virus** causes mammary cancer in mice. It can be transmitted from mother mouse to daughter mouse through the mother's milk with great efficiency. Particles very similar to B-viruses have also been observed in primate milk, including human milk. There is no hard evidence that viruses cause human breast cancer, but the possibility has not been ruled out.

RNA viruses are more clandestine than DNA viruses. In some species it appears that virtually every cell of every organ has latent RNA viruses in the form of a DNA copy (transcript) of the RNA genome (Fig. 10.3). Presumably this latency is a result of **vertical transmission** (from parent cells to offspring) and replication. If a fertilized egg gets an RNA virus and a DNA transcript gets into the genome, the transcript is replicated each time the egg divides, and all resulting cells will, in effect, contain RNA virus genes. RNA tumor viruses can also cause their host cells to continue to produce new RNA viruses while they are embedded in the host cell genome. They can cause host cells to steadily produce new viruses, which are shed and infect neighboring cells. Some such shed viruses can also infect other animals (**horizontal transmission**), usually of the same species.

Viruses and Oncogenes: How Do Viruses Cause Cancer?

We have already discussed the question of how viruses cause cancer in Chapter 7—when we considered virus-transmitted oncogenes. Viruses cause transformation either by bringing genes that specify "cancerness" into cells or by disrupting the control of cancer-specifying genes already present (proto-oncogenes) in a turned-off state.

As discussed in Chapter 7, oncogene-bearing viruses are believed to be have come into existence when the ancestors of these viruses took what were then normal *host cell* proto-oncogenes with them (as hitchhikers) as the ancestor viruses were being assembled during reproduction. Some such host cell oncogenes may have become permanent parts of oncogenic virus genomes during the course of evolution. Possibly because they have changed (mutated) and/or because they are inserted in such a way (see King et al., 1985) that they avoid normal host cell control (see Derse, Caradonna, and Casey, 1985), these virus-transmitted oncogenes

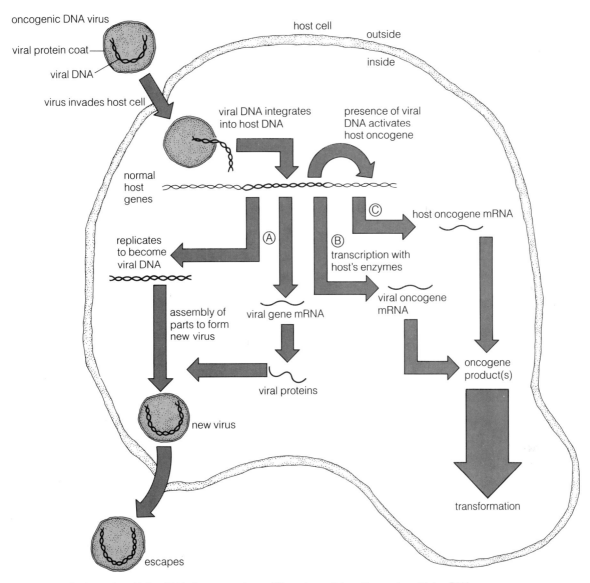

Figure 10.2 Pathway by which a DNA virus reproduces (A); and possible pathways by which a DNA virus may transform a host cell (B) and (C)

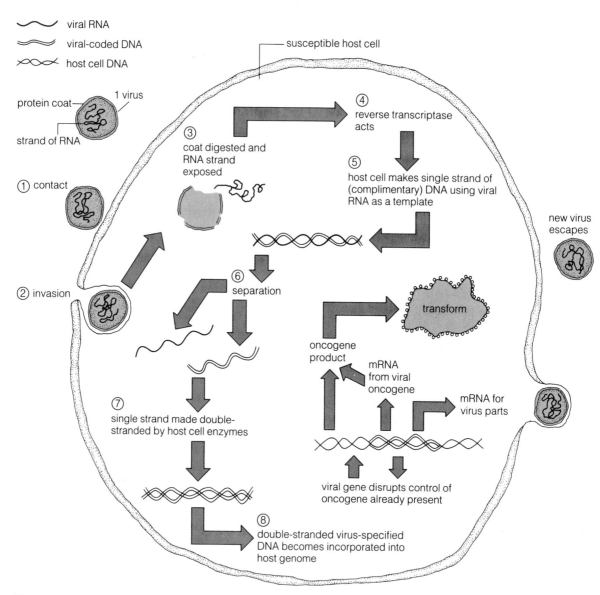

Figure 10.3 Sequence of events in an infection of a host cell by an oncogenic RNA virus (oncoRNA virus or oncogenic retrovirus), and some possible models of oncogenic transformation

elicit malignant transformation when they become incorporated into host cell genomes. Non-oncogene-bearing oncogenic viruses are believed to insert their DNA into the host genome in such a way that it physically disrupts control of normally quiet proto-oncogenes.

Viruses, Cancer, and Koch's Postulates

Almost as soon as it became clear that microorganisms could cause disease, it was recognized that proving that a particular microbe caused a particular disease would not always be easy. Simple association would not always be enough. Consider the fact that because buzzards are "always" found around dead things, it would be easy to falsely conclude that buzzards are killers.

A German physician, Robert Koch, immortalized himself in 1884 by coming up with what we now call **Koch's postulates**—rules for determining that specific infectious agents cause specific diseases. Koch's postulates are (1) the microbe must be present in every case of the disease; (2) the microbe must be isolated in pure culture from fluids or tissue of an organism with the disease; (3) on inoculation from culture into a susceptible host, the disease must reappear with *all* its symptoms; and (4) the microbe must be isolated, again, from the experimentally infected host. It should be easy to see that the application of some variation of these postulates to buzzards would quickly clear them of being killers.

Koch's postulates have been satisfied for more than one hundred different viruses causing cancer in animals. They have not been satisfied for a single human cancer-virus association. But viruses haven't been cleared of the crime of human cancer, either. Koch didn't tell us what to do if the disease in question might be specifically human and inoculation might lead to death. The problems applying Koch's postulates to viruses and human cancer are multiple, but

Postulate 3 is the crux of the problem. It is a problem because the inoculation cannot ethically or morally be done. However, some very strong circumstantial evidence exists that viruses do cause human cancer, and this type of evidence is what we will consider now.

Viruses and Human Cancer

Because literally hundreds of virus-induced cancers are documented in animals and because human beings are also animals, it is highly likely that human cancers (a few of them, at least) are also caused by viruses. Suspicious-looking viruses *have* been found in association with human cancers but, as already pointed out, these cannot be injected into normal humans to see if they do in fact cause cancer. Let's look at some of the evidence we *do* have.

Warts

Warts (papillomas) are neoplasms. Because warts are "benign," cell-free wart extracts can and have been given to human volunteers to see if more warts resulted. Cell-free extracts of human papillomas have in fact caused more papillomas. Also, electron micrographs of warts reveal viruses in what appear to be various stages of formation. Recently, certain papilloma viruses have been linked to human colon and cervical cancer (see below).

Burkitt's Lymphoma

Burkitt's lymphoma is a malignant neoplasm or cancer that researchers seem most willing to concede—even in the absence of direct proof—has at least a *partly* viral etiology.

Burkitt's lymphoma is named for a British surgeon, Denis Burkitt, who first saw this unique neoplasm in Uganda in the late 1950s.

His first case was a young boy with a very rapidly growing lymphoma of the jaw. He later found that this particular disease was the most common childhood cancer in Africa. It occurs most frequently in children 6 to 8 years old and is rare in children over 14. Burkitt's lymphoma is almost completely confined to Africa's low country and seemed to suggest an insect-borne virus (Fig. 10.4).

Epstein, Achong, and Barr (1964) later showed that a particular virus (a large, DNA-type herpes virus later named Epstein-Barr virus, or EBV) was rather consistently present in the lymphocytes that become malignant in this disease. Burkitt's lymphoma patients tend to have high titers of antibody to EBV antigens, compared to normal individuals. And malignant Burkitt's lymphoma cells have EBV genes incorporated into their genomes; EBV can transform "normal" human lymphocytes grown in culture. All these things amount to highly convincing circumstantial evidence that EBV causes Burkitt's lymphoma.

The fact that EBV is found throughout the world while Burkitt's lymphoma is practically restricted to central Africa amounts either to a nagging contradiction or suggests that the virus is just one of two or more cofactors. It may be that the malarial parasite, also endemic in central Africa and also having B-lymphocytes as a target, is the other—or one other—cofactor.

Nasopharyngeal cancer has also been linked to EBV. Nasopharyngeal cancer patients also tend to have elevated titers of antibodies to EBV antigens.

At the time of this writing, a vaccine for Epstein-Barr virus was being tested in monkeys, but not yet in humans.

Cervical Cancer

It has been known for some time that the incidence of cervical cancer is positively correlated with low socioeconomic status, early indulgence in sexual activity, and promiscuity (multiple sexual partners). Also, it has been shown rather recently that women who marry men whose first wives developed cervical cancer are three to four times more likely to develop cervical cancer than similar women who marry men whose wives did not develop cervical cancer (Rapp, 1978). All these clues give cervical cancer *some* of the character of an infective venereal disease—although this is certainly *not* to say that the monogamous, the virtuous, the chaste, and the celibate never get cervical cancer. The suspect infectious agents in cervical cancer include (1) one of the *Herpes simplex* viruses, *Herpes simplex* Virus 2 (HSV 2)—Herpes 1 is the cold sore virus, and (2) human papillomavirus (HPV).

Cervical cancer patients tend to have higher antiherpes antibody titers than women who do not have cervical cancer (Rapp, 1978). Also, professional prostitutes have a higher incidence of cervical cancer and a greater likelihood of having anti-HSV 2 antibodies than nuns or even the general population of women. It has been suggested that if, in fact, Herpes 2 virus is a causal factor in cervical cancer, the patterns of cervical cancer should follow the patterns of genital herpes infections. In the early 1980s, the incidence of cervical cancer was falling while the incidence of genital herpes was rising. But if there is a lag of, say, 20 years in the generation of a cervical cancer from a virus infection, we could well see an epidemic of cervical cancer in the mid 1990s—as a consequence of the relaxed sexual mores that brought the genital herpes epidemic of the 1970s and 1980s. Rapp (1978) points out that Marek's disease, a virally induced malignancy in turkeys, can be prevented with a vaccine. The Marek's disease virus is also a herpes virus, suggesting that there may one day be a vaccine against both genital herpes and cervical cancer, together. Wentz et al. (1983) have already shown that an inactivated herpes virus can be used to protect mice from herpes virus-induced cervical carcinoma.

More recently, papillomaviruses have been linked to cervical cancer (see Reid et al., 1984; Boshart et al., 1984; Prakash et al., 1985; and Schwartz et al., 1985). Most of the connection is based on the relatively common occurrence of papillomavirus in cells and tissue isolated from cervical neoplasms. Some of this evidence indicates that the link between cervical cancer and papillomavirus (Types 16 and 18) may be even stronger than that for herpes virus (Prakash et al., 1985).

Recently, human papillomavirus DNA has been found in the semen of three patients, two of whom had severe wart disease (see Ostrow et al., 1986). These findings suggest that human papilloma viruses may be transmitted sexually.

Other cancers, such as penile and vulval cancers, have also been linked to papilloma virus.

Liver Cancer

Patterns like those just discussed also implicate a virus in the etiology of liver cancer. Although liver cancer is rare in the United States, worldwide some 300,000 to 1.2 million cases of primary hepatocellular cancer are reported each year. It is an important form of cancer particularly because it is almost always fatal. Blumberg and London (1982), and others, hypothesize that liver cancer can be caused by the Hepatitis B virus; Blumberg cites nine pieces of incriminating circumstantial evidence:

1. Where there is a lot of hepatocellular cancer, there is also a lot of hepatitis; where there is little hepatitis, there is little hepatocellular cancer.

2. People with hepatocellular cancer—in areas where the hepatitis is endemic *and* in areas where it is rare—almost all have the Hepatitis B antigen or antibodies to the antigen in their blood; significantly *fewer* of those *without* the cancer have the antigen or the antibody.

3. Most hepatocellular cancer occurs in livers already affected by hepatitis, cirrhosis, or both.

4. Proteins characteristic of Hepatitis B virus can usually be found in hepatocellular cancer tissue.

5. In a Taiwanese study involving some 22,000 men (Beasley et al., 1981), over four years of

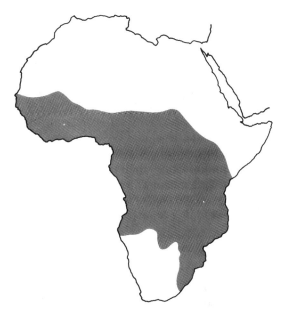

Figure 10.4 Distribution of Burkitt's lymphoma in Africa. (Drawing from Kupchella and Hyland, 1986; used with permission of Allyn and Bacon.)

observation, nearly all cases of hepatocellular cancer arose in a group of 3,500 asymptomatic, chronic carriers of Hepatitis B virus.

6. A Japanese study (Obata et al., 1980) showed that after four years of observation, significantly more hepatocellular cancer appeared in a group of patients with liver cirrhosis who were also Hepatitis B antigen-positive than in a similar group of cirrhotics who did not have the antigen.

7. Studies in several countries indicate that the mothers of those who get hepatocellular cancer are significantly more likely to be Hepatitis B virus carriers.

8. Hepatitis B virus DNA can be found in hepatocellular cancer cells, and there is some indication that the process of integrating hepatitis virus genes is slow—the longer one has carried the virus, the more likely the virus is to have been incorporated, even in people free of hepatocellular cancer.

9. Woodchucks, at least in Pennsylvania, have a high frequency of hepatocellular cancer, and

they also have a high frequency of infection with a virus very similar to the human Hepatitis B virus.

Moriarty et al. (1985) recently reported that a Hepatitis B gene product correlated highly with hepatocellular cancer.

Blumberg and London (1982) suggest that, taken together, these facts amount to strong evidence that the Hepatitis B virus is one cause—and an important cause—of human hepatocellular cancer. (Such are the lengths that have to be gone to when Koch's postulates cannot be tested.)

There have already been some successful trials of Hepatitis B vaccine with respect to preventing hepatitis (see Goodfield, 1984). Also, as we went to press, efforts were underway in China to mount a large-scale vaccination trial designed to see if a Hepatitis B vaccine can block liver cancer.

Leukemia

Robert Gallo and his coworkers at the National Cancer Institute have accumulated some relatively convincing evidence that a "C-type" oncoRNA virus (retrovirus) causes human T-cell leukemia (See Gallagher and Gallo, 1975; Poiesz et al., 1980; and Guroff et al., 1982). Initially, this group of investigators found a "reverse transcriptase" in the cells of patients with acute leukemia. Later, in the same laboratory, it was reported that budding Type C virus was continually released by cells of peripheral blood leucocytes taken from a patient with acute myelogenous leukemia. Still later, a virus later named "human T-cell leukemia virus" (HTLV) was isolated from the cells of patients with T-cell lymphoma and patients with T-cell leukemia. In a study done still later, high titers of antibodies to HTLV were found in the serum of a group of patients with adult T-cell leukemia but not in the serum of normal controls.

In 1977, a group of Japanese investigators reported the isolation and characterization of an adult T-cell leukemia virus (ATLV) associated with a type of adult T-cell leukemia (ATL) common to an area of southwestern Japan. Another group of Japanese workers later showed that antibodies to the virus were common in the serum of patients with this form of leukemia—but not in those free of the disease. Cultures have been established from peripheral leukemic cells from patients with ATL, and both viral antigens and virus particles have been detected in such cultures. Although efforts to transform normal human leukocytes with cell-free virus preparations so far have been unsuccessful, Yamamoto and coworkers (1982) have reported that they were able to transform normal cells by cocultivating them with cell lines carrying the virus—apparently through direct cell to cell infection. It is now agreed that HTLV and ATLV are virtually identical (see Homma et al., 1984), and all researchers have agreed to call the virus HTLV. There is actually a family of HTLV-like viruses (see Guo, Wong-Staal, and Gallo, 1984). Two of them, HTLV I and HTLV II, are unique in their ability to transform human T-cells *in vitro* and their association with T-cell leukemias and lymphomas (see Slamon et al., 1984).

Retroviruses are known to cause leukemia in chickens, many kinds of rodents, cattle, cats, and monkeys. It seems very likely that the viruses now linked to some human leukemias will in fact be shown more conclusively to cause these diseases.

Acquired Immune Deficiency Syndrome (AIDS)

Some History

In the summer of 1981, the Center for Disease Control noted an outbreak of rare cancers and rare lung infections among homosexuals in Los Angeles and other cities. Later in the year the same syndrome was also reported among intravenous drug abusers. Because the principal characteristic features of the syndrome were a greatly compromised immune system and some degree of contagiousness, the syndrome was called, *acquired immune deficiency syndrome*—or more commonly, "**AIDS**." It soon became apparent that AIDS is almost inevitably fatal—85 percent mortality three years after diagnosis (Osborn, 1986). Since 1981, AIDS has been seen all over the United States and the rest of the world; by early 1986 there had been more than 17,000 cases in the United States alone—with half of the victims already dead—and there were projections of 40,000 U.S. cases by the end of 1986. Through 1985, the number of cases roughly doubled every year (Norman, 1985a). So far, no effective way has been found to cure AIDS. A transmissible, fatal, incurable disease that moves incredibly fast, AIDS has understandably caused alarm.

What Causes AIDS?

Nearly all available evidence indicates that AIDS is caused by a virus known as **human T-lymphotropic virus III** or **HTLV III**. It is also known as **lymphadenopathy/AIDS virus (LAV)** and **AIDS-associated retrovirus (ARV)**. Recently, a new name, **human immunodeficiency virus (HIV)**, has been proposed.

The evidence for an HTLV III–AIDS connection is very strong if not overwhelming (see Shaw et al., 1984, 1985; Gallo et al., 1984; Alter et al., 1984; Arya et al., 1984; Culliton, 1984; and Marx, 1984). Although other HTLVs have been found in association with AIDS, it is now clear that HTLV I and HTLV II have little to do with AIDS. It appears that HTLV I and HTLV II transform T-cells, causing various types of T-cell cancers (see above), while HTLV III destroys the same subset of T-cells.

The evidence? First of all, the HTLV III virus has been isolated from hundreds of AIDS patients. Indeed, it is found in virtually all AIDS patients tested and in only 1 percent of nonhomosexuals without AIDS. Second, AIDS is common in regions of the Caribbean and Africa where HTLV III is prevalent. Third, HTLV III attacks T-cells, which are also the cells primarily affected by AIDS. Also, neither AIDS nor HTLV III are transmitted easily; apparently, intimate contact is required in both cases. Finally, it is well established that certain other related viruses (e.g., feline leukemia virus) cause immune suppression. Although HTLV-specified DNA has not been found in the T-cells of very many cases of AIDS (see Gallo et. al., 1983), this may be a result of the rapid demise of virus-infected cells.

What Is AIDS—And Why Now?

The principal features of the AIDS syndrome are a greatly compromised immune system and resultant opportunistic infections. The compromised immunity is a direct consequence of the fact that the principal target of the AIDS virus is a group of T-lymphocytes that normally play a key role in fighting off infection (see Chapter 14). A variety of infections appear as the T-cells are wiped out. Symptoms usually begin with some combination of the following: night sweats, sustained fever, chronic diarrhea, weight loss, and lymph node enlargement, followed by oral yeast infection, and/or Kaposi's sarcoma (a malignant neoplasm marked by purplish skin lesions) (Osborn, 1986), and/or unusual chronic pneumonias. This course is often followed by neurologic degeneration. Recent evidence indicates that the AIDS virus attacks cells other than T-cells—the brain and other tissues of the central nervous system, for example. It is now known that 60 percent of adult AIDS victims will develop dementia ("madness"); even a greater percentage of children with AIDS develop neurological problems (Barnes, 1986).

Where did the AIDS virus come from and why did it wait until now—or did it wait until now? As far as we know, AIDS is relatively new. One idea is that it came originally from other primates (monkeys), where it may have been relatively harmless, and that it somehow made the species-cross into humans, where it now causes AIDS—possibly through a relatively recent mutation (Norman, 1985b). The species-cross is believed to have first occurred in Central Africa (Osborn, 1986; see also Kanki et al., 1986).

The Cancer Connection

Of chief interest to us in this book is the impact of AIDS upon cancer. The most notable association is with Kaposi's sarcoma, but increased incidence of other cancers have also been reported among AIDS patients. We know very little about the connection thus far; the cancers may or may not be induced by the AIDS virus; some may well be the consequence of impaired immune defense.

The HTLVs offer some promise of helping us to come to a better understanding of cellular growth-control. HTLV I and HTLV II viruses somehow cause T-cells to grow uncontrollably, while HTLV III kills them. More might be learned about growth control in trying to answer the question: Why these dramatically opposite effects? All three types of viruses apparently generate proteins that stimulate the expression of viral genes. Possibly some of these proteins also stimulate the expression of cellular oncogenes, thus producing T-cell cancers in the cases of HTLV I and II; perhaps the HTLV III version of these so-called trans-acting proteins somehow interferes with T-cell division.

Who Gets AIDS?

Although we are not exactly sure just who, doing what, is at risk of getting AIDS, the pattern so far almost restricts AIDS to several high-risk groups. Of all victims in the United States over the past four years or so, 73 percent are homosexual or bisexual men, 17 percent are intravenous drug users, 3 percent were infected via blood transfusions, and 6 percent don't fit any of these categories (Norman, 1985a). Apparently AIDS is not easily contagious; infection re-

quires direct insertion of the virus into the blood stream. The risk to health-care workers and even family members of AIDS victims is minimal to non-existent (Friedland et al., 1986). At the time of this writing, there were no known cases of spread of the AIDS virus through casual contact.

Since it has become possible to test for the presence of AIDS antigen in blood samples, it has become clear that many more people have the virus than have the disease. What percentage of these will eventually develop disease? We don't know yet. The **incubation interval** (time between exposure and the onset of disease) may be as long as 5 years. It is not expected that all or even a very large fraction of those with a history of virus exposure will develop the disease, but presumably they can all act as carriers. Some of these may express lesser forms of the disease, e.g., **lymphadenopathy syndrome (LAS)**. By some estimates, at a time when there were 14,000 cases of AIDS, there were 70,000 cases of LAS and 700,000 people infected (see Osborn, 1986). It has been estimated that between 5 and 20 percent of those infected will eventually develop the disease (Marx, 1986).

Prospects for the Future

AIDS as an Epidemic   How bad will the AIDS epidemic get? It's hard to say, for several reasons. It is not clear yet what percentage of those infected with the virus will actually come down with the symptoms of the disease; only recently have we been able to test people for the presence of the virus. Not enough people have been tracked long enough yet, and the testing and tracking is fraught with sociological and ethical problems. Since the availability of tests for antibodies to the AIDS virus (indicating exposure to the virus and presumably its presence in some cells), it has become apparent that high percentages of high-risk groups *have* such antibodies— 73 percent of one homosexual/bisexual group in San Francisco; 53 percent of a group of 66 homosexuals in New York; 25–30 percent of a group of drug users in New York; 90 percent of hemophiliacs—have been found to carry the antibody (Osborn, 1986). The Public Health Service now estimates that there will be over a quarter of a million new cases of AIDS over the next five years (Barnes, 1986b).

Although the experts agree that there is some danger that AIDS will become more of a *hetero*sexual disease in the United States, we really don't know how readily the AIDS virus is transmitted sexually from women to men (although the virus has recently been isolated from vaginal secretions). It is interesting that AIDS does not appear to be transmitted in this manner in the United States, but in Africa, AIDS affects men and women in equal numbers, indicating that it can.

Prospects for Control and Treatment Strategies to deal with AIDS include: (1) the use of drugs that would interfere with the virus's life cycle—e.g., 3'-azido-3-deoxythymidine (AZT), which inhibits viral DNA synthesis, and HPA-23, an inhibitor of reverse transcriptase; (2) immune-system stimulants such as the interleukins (see Chapter 14); and (3) vaccines directed at viral antigens. It is too early to tell just how effective these strategies will be.

Recently, AIDS investigators in this country and others were beginning to speak optimistically of being able to exploit neutralizing antibodies against AIDS. Healthy carriers of the AIDS virus apparently have several times as much of the antibody as do persons with disease symptoms. This suggests the possibility of passive immunization using the antibody—assuming that it can be made by recombinant gene technology (see Chapter 14).

Is Viral Carcinogenesis Accidental?

If viruses could think, they would surely realize that it is *not* in their best interest to cause cancer in humans—or in any other living thing, for that matter. When living things get cancer, they tend to die and practically all the viruses present in the host at that time die with them. It would make more sense if the causing of cancer by viruses were accidental.

Viruses, like all living things, have just one principal biological objective, namely, reproduction. It could be that viral carcinogenesis is relatively directly related to the ability of viruses to turn host genes on. Maybe they aren't very selective about which genes they turn on, and perhaps some of them accidentally turn oncogenes on! It could also be that viral carcinogenesis derives from the accidental ability of viruses to take copies of host cell genes with them when they "go." Perhaps, in becoming incorporated into host cell genomes, viruses accidentally activate proto-oncogenes by physically or otherwise disrupting controls.

There is some evidence that viral genes characteristically become incorporated into host genomes adjacent to oncogenes and take the oncogenes or parts of oncogenes with them when they go. The notion that such oncogenes could be taken into other cells by viruses is not so far out. Nor, as we have already discussed, is it such a remote possibility that when such genes are introduced to another cell they don't function quite right.

If Viruses Cause Certain Cancers, Are These Cancers Contagious?

Cancer is not contagious, but the viruses that cause some forms of cancer in some animals, including humans, may very well be. Viruses are known to cause leukemia in cats, and feline leukemia is indeed contagious. One cat can get leukemia from viruses from another cat in some of the same ways that humans "catch" colds. Mice, on the other hand, cannot "catch" leukemia virus from another mouse. Mice inherit virus-induced leukemia from their parents if the parents belong to a leukemic strain of mice. Leukemia virus in cows and in chickens is also contagious. What about the transmission of leukemia from one human to another?

Dozens of epidemiological studies have been made all over the world, but none turned up any solid evidence for the transmission of leukemia by contact. Most leukemics are isolated cases within their familial or social groups. Suspicious clusters of cases are believed to be a result of chance distribution and/or to be related to genetic factors—but maybe not. As we have just seen, viruses that go by the names EBV, HTLV I, and Hepatitis B virus are strongly linked to human cancers, and they are indeed contagious.

Viruses and Interferon

Interferon is a family of chemical substances produced by cells when they are infected by a virus. Interferon production is a defense mechanism; it influences neighboring cells to produce antiviral enzymes that work by blocking the translation of viral messenger RNA into viral protein. Interferon has been found to act as an anticancer agent in a manner that goes beyond its antiviral activity. We will consider interferon in more detail in the chapter on treatment (Chapter 17).

Other Biological Causes of Cancer

Viruses are apparently not the only biological causes of cancer. A parasite called *Spirocerca lupi* is associated with sarcomas of the dog esophagus. Another parasite, strobilocercous, has been linked to hepatic sarcomas of the rat. A bacteria, *Agrobacter tumifaciens*, causes crown gall tumors in plants. The most thoroughly documented relationship between parasitic infection and cancer in humans is the link between bladder cancer

and *Schistosoma haematobium* infection found in Egypt and other African countries. The mechanism(s) of cause and effect is (are) unknown.

Summary

There are two kinds of viruses, RNA and DNA viruses, and both groups have cancer-causing members. RNA-directed DNA synthesis is a unique and critical feature of RNA oncogenic viruses; a special enzyme called *reverse transcriptase* makes this possible. RNA viruses rarely kill their host cells, and it is not unusual to find animals with virtually every cell carrying RNA-directed genes. The oncogenes carried by certain oncogenic viruses were apparently derived from historical recombination with normal host cell genes, specifically the host cell proto-oncogenes.

More than one hundred different viruses have been shown conclusively to cause cancer in animals and plants. Although it is highly likely that some human cancers involve viruses as causal factors, we may always be just a bit short of definitive proof. Part of the problem is that suspect viruses simply cannot (ethically) be given to humans to see if cancer does indeed develop. In most cases, even circumstantial evidence isn't all that strong, because it is difficult to find viruses that have become incorporated into cancer cell genomes. Among human cancers almost certainly caused (at least in part) by viruses are hepatocellular cancer (Hepatitis B virus), Burkitt's lymphoma (EBV), some types of leukemia and lymphoma (HTLV I and HTLV II), and cervical cancer (Herpes Virus 2 and papilloma viruses).

Viruses remain interesting to cancer researchers mostly because they greatly aid in the study of general mechanisms of carcinogenesis. It does *not* seem likely—for the moment, anyway—that very many human cancers will ultimately be shown to be caused by viruses.

References and Further Reading

Alter, H. J., et al. 1984. Transmission of HTLV III Infection from Human Plasma to Chimpanzees: An Animal Model for AIDS. *Science*. 226:549–52.

Andrews, C., and Pereira, H. G. 1972. *Viruses of Vertebrates*. Baltimore: Williams & Wilkins.

Arya, S. K., et al. 1984. Homology of Genome of AIDS-Associated Virus with Genomes of Human T-Cell Leukemia Viruses. *Science*. 225:927–30.

Baltimore, D. 1976. Viruses, Polymerases, and Cancer. *Science*. 192:632–36.

Barnes, D. 1986a. Brain Function Decline in Children with AIDS. *Science*. 232:1196–.

Barnes, D. 1986b. Grim Projections for AIDS Epidemic. *Science*. 232:1589–90.

Beasley, R. P., Lin, C. C., Hwang, L. Y., and Chien, C. S. 1981. Hepatocellular Carcinoma and Hepatitis B Virus. A Prospective Study of 22,707 Men in Taiwan. *Lancet*. 2(8256):1129–33.

Bishop, J. M. 1985. Viruses, Genes, and Cancer II. Retroviruses and Cancer Genes. *Cancer*. 55:2329–33.

Blumberg, B. S., and London, W. T. 1982. Hepatitis B Virus Pathogenesis and Prevention of Primary Cancer of the Liver. In J. G. Fortner and J. E. Rhoads, eds., *Accomplishments in Cancer Research, 1981*. Philadelphia: Lippincott.

Borden, E. C., Steeves, R. A., and Hogan, T. F. Infectious Carcinogenesis: Viruses and Human Neoplasia. In S. B. Kahn, et al., eds., *Concepts in Cancer Medicine*. New York: Grune & Stratton.

Boshart, M., et al. 1984. A New Type of Papillomavirus DNA, Its Presence in Genital Cancer Biopsies and in Cell Lines Derived from Cervical Cancer. *EMBO J*. 3(5):1151–57.

Burke, D. C. 1977. The Status of Interferon. *Scientific American*. 236(4) March:42–50.

Butler, P. J. G., and Klug, A. 1978. The Assembly of a Virus. *Scientific American*. 39(5) November:64–69.

Chiu, I., et al. 1984. Major *pol* Gene Progenitors in the Evolution of Oncoviruses. *Science*. 223:364–70.

Culliton, B. 1984. Crash Development of AIDS Test Nears Goal. *Science*. 225:1128–31.

Derse, D., Caradonna, S. J., and Casey, J. W. 1985. Bovine Leukemia Virus Long Terminal Repeat: A Cell Type-Specific Promoter. *Science*. 227:317–20.

DeVita, V., et al. 1985. *AIDS: Etiology, Diagnosis, Treatment, and Prevention*. Philadelphia: Lippincott.

Diener, T. O. 1983. The Viroid: A Subviral Pathogen. *American Scientist*. 71:481–89.

Ellermann, V., and Bang, O. 1908. Experimentelle Leukamie Bei Huhnern. *Centralbl, f. Bakteriol*. 46:595–604.

Epstein, M. A., Achong, B. G., and Barr, Y. M. 1964. Virus Particles in Cultured Lymphoblasts from Burkitt's Lymphoma. *Lancet*. 1:702.

Fields, B. N., ed. 1984. *Virology*. New York: Raven Press.

Folks, T., et al. 1986. Induction of HTLV-III/LAV from a Nonvirus-Producing T-Cell Line: Implications for Latency. *Science*. 231:600–02.

Fraenkel-Conrat, H., and Wagner, R., eds. 1974. *Comprehensive Virology*. Vols. 1-4. New York: Plenum Press.

Friedland, G. H., et al. 1986. Lack of Transmission of HTLV III/LAV Infection to Household Contacts of Patients with AIDS or AIDS-Related Complex with Oral Candidiasis. *N. Engl. J. Med*. 314(6):344–49.

Gallagher, R. E., and Gallo, R. C. 1975. Type-C (RNA) Tumor Virus Isolated from Cultured Human Acute Myelogenous Leukemia Cells. *Science*. 187:350–53.

Gallo, R. C., et al. 1983. Isolation of Human T-cell Luekemia Virus in Acquired Immune Deficiency Syndrome (AIDS). *Science*. 220:865–67.

Gallo, R. C., et al. 1984. Frequent Detection and Isolation of Cytopathic Retroviruses (HTLV III) from Patients With AIDS and at Risk for AIDS. *Science*. 224:500–03.

Goedert, J. J., et al. 1986. Three-Year Incidence of AIDS in Five Cohorts of HTLV-III Infected Risk Group Members. *Science*. 231:992–95.

Goodfield, J. 1984. Vaccine on Trial. *Science 84*. 5(2) March pp. 79–84.

Guroff, M., et al. 1982. Natural Antibodies to Human Retrovirus HTLV in a Cluster of Japanese Patients with Adult T-Cell Leukemia. *Science*. 215:975–78.

Guo, H., Wong-Staal, F., and Gallo, R. 1984. Novel Viral Sequences Related to Human T-Cell Leukemia Virus in T Cells of a Seropositive Baboon. *Science*. 223:1195–96.

Henle, W. 1981. Search for Human Cancer Viruses. In J. G. Fortner and J. E. Rhoads, eds. *Accomplishments in Cancer Research, 1980*. Philadelphia: Lippincott.

Henle, W., Henle, G., and Lennette, E. 1979. The Epstein-Barr Virus. *Scientific American.* 241 (July):48–59.

Homma, T., et al. 1984. Lymphoma in Macaques: Association with Virus of Human T Lymphotrophic Family. *Science.* 225:716–18.

Howley, P. M., and Broker, T. R., eds. 1986. *Papillomaviruses: Molecular and Clinical Aspects.* New York: Alan R. Liss.

Jonsen, A. R., Cooke, M., and Koenig, B. A. 1986. AIDS and Ethics. *Issues in Science and Technology.* 2(2) Winter: 56–65.

Karpas, A. 1982. Viruses and Leukemia. *American Scientist.* 70:277–85.

Kanki, P. J., et al. 1986. New Human T-Lymphotropic Retrovirus Related to Simian T-Lymphotropic Virus Type III (STLV$_{AGM}$). *Science.* 232:238–43.

King, W., et al. 1985. Insertion Mutagenesis of Embryonal Carcinoma Cells by Retroviruses. *Science.* 228:554–58.

Klein, G. 1981. Viral Oncology. In J. G. Fortner and J. E. Rhoads, eds., *Accomplishments in Cancer Research, 1980.* Philadelphia: Lippincott.

Klein, G., ed. 1985. *Viruses as the Causative Agents of Naturally Occurring Tumors.* New York: Raven Press.

Kulstad, R. 1985. *AIDS: Papers from Science, 1982–1985.* Washington D.C.: American Association for the Advancement of Science.

Lewin, R. 1981. New Reports of a Human Leukemia Virus. *Science.* 214:530–31.

Lewis, A. M., and Cook, J. L. 1985. A New Role for DNA Virus Early Proteins in Viral Carcinogenesis. *Science.* 227:15–20.

Lonberg-Holm, K., and Philipson, L. 1980. *Virus Receptors.* Part II: *Animal Viruses, Receptors and Recognition Series B.* Vol. 8. New York: Chapman and Hall.

Maramorosch, K., and Koprowski, H., eds., 1984. *Methods in Virology.* Vol. 8. Orlando, Fla.: Academic Press.

Marx, J. L. 1974. Viral Carcinogenesis: Role of DNA Viruses. *Science.* 183:1070–112.

Marx, J. L. 1983. Human T-Cell Leukemia Virus Linked to AIDS. *Science.* 220:806–09.

Marx, J. L. 1984. Strong New Candidate for AIDS Agent. *Science.* 224:475–77.

Marx, J. L. 1986. The Slow Insidious Natures of the HTLV's. *Science.* 231:450–51.

Maugh, T. H. 1974. RNA Viruses: The Age of Innocence Ends. *Science.* 183:1181–85.

Maugh, T. H. 1975. Leukemia: A Second Human Tumor Virus. *Science:* 187:325–26.

Moriarty, A. M., et al. 1985. Antibodies to Peptides Detect New Hepatitis B Antigen: Serological Correlation with Hepatocellular Carcinoma. *Science.* 227: 429–32.

Norman, C. 1985a. AIDS Trends: Projections from Limited Data. *Science.* 230:1018–19.

Norman C. 1985b. Africa and the Origin of AIDS. *Science.* 230:1141.

Obata, H., et al. 1980. A Prospective Study on the Development of Hepatocellular Carcinoma from Liver Cirrhosis with Persistent Hepatitis B Virus Infection. *Int. J. Cancer.* 25:741–47.

Osborn, J. E. 1986. The AIDS Epidemic: An Overview of the Science. *Issues in Science and Technology.* 2(2) Winter: 40–55.

Ostrow, R. S., et al. 1986. Detection of Papillomavirus DNA in Human Semen. *Science.* 231:731–33.

Pitot, H. 1978. *Fundamentals of Oncology.* New York: Dekker.

Poiesz, B. J., et al. 1980. *Proc. Natl. Acad. Sci. USA.* 77:7415.

Prakash, S. S., et al. 1985. Herpes Simplex Virus Type 2 and Human Papillomavirus Type 16 in Cervicitis, Dysplasia, and Invasive Cervical Carcinoma *Int. J. Cancer,* 35(1):51–57.

Rapp, F. 1978. Herpesviruses, Venereal Diseases, and Cancer. *American Scientist.* 66:670–74.

Rapp, F. 1984. *Herpesvirus.* New York: Alan R. Liss.

Reid, R., et al. 1984. Genital Warts and Cervical Cancer III: Subclinical Papillomaviral Infection and Cervical Neoplasia Are Linked by a Spectrum of Continuous Morphologic and Biologic Change. *Cancer.* 53(4): 943–53.

Rigby, P. W. J., ed. 1985. *Viruses and Cancer.* New York: Cambridge University Press.

Rous, P. 1911. A Sarcoma of the Fowl Transmissible by an Agent Separable from the Tumor Cells. *J. Exptl. Med.* 13:397.

Schwartz, E., et al. 1985. Structure and Transcription of Human Papillomavirus Sequences in Cervical Carcinoma Cells. *Nature.* 314(6006):111–14.

Scolnick, E. M., and Levine, A. J., eds. 1983. *Tumor Viruses and Differentiation*. New York: Alan R. Liss.

Shaw, G. M., et al. 1984. Molecular Characterization of Human T-Cell Leukemia (Lymphotropic) Virus Type III in Acquired Immune Deficiency Syndrome. *Science.* 226:1165–71.

Shaw, G. M., et al. 1985. HTLV III Infections in Brains of Children and Adults with AIDS Encephalopathy. *Science.* 227:177–81.

Slamon, D. J., et al. 1984. Identification of the Putative Transforming Protein of the Human T-Cell Leukemia Viruses HTLV I and HTLV II. *Science.* 226:61–65.

Smith, K. M., and Ritchie, D. 1980. *Introduction to Virology.* New York: Chapman and Hall.

Sodroski, J., et al. 1985. *Trans*-Acting Transcriptional Regulation of Human T-Cell Leukemia Virus Type III Long Terminal Repeat. *Science.* 227:171–73.

Temin, H. M. 1977. The Relationship of Tumor Virology to an Understanding of Nonviral Cancers. *Bioscience.* 27(3):170–76.

Thomas, D. B., and Rawls, W. E. 1978. Relationship of Herpes Simplex Virus Type-2 Antibodies and Squamous Dysplasia to Cervical Carcinoma in Situ. *Cancer.* 42(6):2716–25.

Tooze, J., ed. *Molecular Biology of Tumor Viruses.* Part 2, *DNA Tumor Viruses.* 2nd ed. Cold Spring Harbor, N.Y.: Cold Spring Harbor Laboratory.

Weinberg, R. A. 1983. A Molecular Basis of Cancer. *Scientific American.* 249(5)November:126–42.

Viral Oncogenes. 1980. *Cold Spring Harbor Symposium of Quantitative Biology.* 44 (Entire Volume).

Wentz, W. B., et al. 1983. Effect of Prior Immunization on Induction of Cervical Cancer in Mice by Herpes Simplex Virus Type 2. *Science.* 222:1128–29.

Wong-Staal, F., et al. 1985. Genomic Diversity of Human T-Lymphotropic Virus Type III (HTLV III). *Science.* 229: 759–62.

Wyke, J., and Weiss, R., eds. 1984. *Viruses in Human and Animal Cancers.* Oxford University Press.

Yamamoto, N., et al. 1982. Transformation of Human Leukocytes by Cocultivation with an Adult T Cell Leukemia Virus Producer Cell Line. *Science.* 217:737–39.

Cancer is a genetic disease in the sense that the things that cause cancer do so by influencing genes. In this chapter, we will look at genetics and cancer in two *other* ways. First, we will pick up where we left off in Chapter 7, looking at the notion that some cancers may be the result of the abnormal expression of perfectly *normal* genes. We will then look at the ways in which humans and other animals actually *inherit* the tendency to develop certain cancers.

Cancer as an Accident in the Unfolding of the Genetic Program

It could be said that the genetic program unfolds. All the genes needed to specify the construction of a human being are present in the fertilized egg. But the egg does *not* contain a tiny human being. The human form emerges gradually, its parts appearing in a highly ordered *sequence*. The genetic program first gives rise to germinal tissue and then to more specialized stem cells that give rise to ever increasingly differentiated cells, tissues, and organs. All this development occurs as a result of the highly ordered activation and deactivation of genes. The genes expressed at any one moment create the microchemical environment that determines the array of genes to be activated and deactivated at the *next* moment.

There is evidence that some forms of cancer amount to problems of development. They appear to be departures from the normal program of genetic expression.

Oncogenes and Proto-oncogenes Revisited

The oncogene concept encompasses all the ways in which cancer can arise from the "failure of normal development." Oncogenes are apparently supposed to be suppressed in an adult. Among the factors that can cause this plan to fail and that we have discussed thus far are (1) mutations in the oncogene itself, or in genes that

11

Cancer, Genetics, and Heredity

control the expression of oncogenes, (2) chromosome breaks in which oncogenes are translocated to "active" locations, and (3) the introduction of new genetic material—abnormal oncogenes or other genetic material that disrupts the control of normal oncogenes.

There is at least one other possibility. Cancer may be a result of a reversible mixup or derangement in the control of expression of otherwise normal genes in their usual locations. This mixup is sometimes called **epigenetic carcinogenesis**. The principal evidence in support of an epigenetic mechanism of oncogenesis is that some kinds of cancer appear to be *reversible*! A discussion of this idea follows.

Cancer Cells with Normal Genes?

Many cancer cells retain the ability to be normal; that is, they can give rise to normal cells. Under one set of circumstances, they behave like *cancer* cells; under other circumstances, they behave like *normal* cells. Examples include teratocarcinomas in mice and teratomas in plants, plant crown gall tumor cells, transformed plant cells that develop from normal cells grown in tissue culture, human skin cancer cells, cells isolated from patients with acute myelocytic leukemia, neuroblastoma cells in several species, and kidney adenocarcinoma cells in the frog. Space limitations permit expanded discussion of only a few of these examples here; other examples are discussed elsewhere in the book (see also Ruddon, 1981).

Mouse Teratocarcinomas The bizarre neoplasms called mouse teratocarcinomas consist of mixtures of variously differentiated cells including bone cells, hair cells, muscle cells, epithelial cells, and other kinds of cells—14 different cell types in all. One of the fourteen is clearly malignant, an undifferentiated cell type called an **embryonal carcinoma cell**.

· Teratocarcinomas are more like the pellets that owls spit up, or like what one would get if a mouse were placed in a blender, than they are like other neoplasms. They apparently arise—in all their confused complexity—from a single embryonal carcinoma cell. If just one such cell is placed in the abdomen of a normal mouse, the embryonal cell gives rise to a teratocarcinoma (Fig. 11.1). But that's not all!

If teratocarcinoma cells are placed inside a very early mouse embryo, teratocarcinoma cell progeny end up in all the tissues of a *normal mouse*—you get, not a tumor, not a mouse with a tumor, but a perfectly normal mouse! (Illmensee and Mintz, 1976; see also Illmensee and Stevens, 1979). The *early* embryo environment apparently causes teratocarcinoma cells to give up their malignant ways and to join in the making of a mouse! Could it be that a teratocarcinoma is derived from a cell that skips or misses a key step during embryogenesis—and that if that cell or one of its derivatives is put back on the other side of the step that was missed, it gets the procedure right the second time?

Neuroblastoma One of the more common malignancies afflicting preschool children is neuroblastoma. Neuroblastoma cells arise from pre-nerve cells called **neuroblasts**. Although neuroblastomas are normally highly malignant and offer a poor prognosis, there have been cases in which the tumors spontaneously (meaning the real reason is not known) quit their malignant ways and became benign. This event suggests that neuroblastomas are made up of cells that get off the track of normal differentiation without surrendering the ability to get back on. Mouse neuroblastoma cells give rise to cells that behave much like normal nerve cells; they can conduct nerve impulses, for example. Work with mouse neuroblastoma has also revealed that the tendency of the malignant neuroblasts to revert to normal can actually be *increased* by exposing the cells to certain drugs and chemical agents that inhibit DNA synthesis or increase cyclic AMP levels (see Chapter 4).

Etcetera Other examples such as the preceding exist, all suggesting that cancer cells can have normal genes and that the chemical environ-

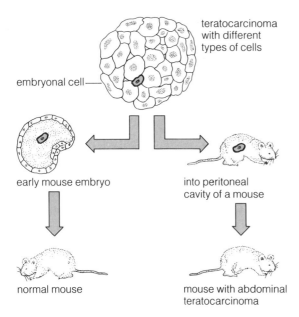

embryonal cell

teratocarcinoma with different types of cells

early mouse embryo

into peritoneal cavity of a mouse

normal mouse

mouse with abdominal teratocarcinoma

Figure 11.1 Malignant embryonal carcinoma cells apparently give rise to all the many differentiated kinds of cells found in a teratocarcinoma. But embryonal carcinoma cells are developmental "chameleons"; if placed inside a mouse, they develop into an unmistakable teratocarcinoma; if placed inside a very early mouse embryo, they become part of a "normal" mouse.

ment in which otherwise normal genes operate can be the cause of the malignant condition. The chemical microenvironment can apparently influence genes in ways more subtle than the induction of mutations. If the nucleus is taken from a **Lucké (kidney) adenocarcinoma** cell of a leopard frog and put inside a frog egg from which the nucleus has been removed, the egg goes on to become a normal tadpole—not a tumor, not a tadpole with a tumor, but a normal tadpole (McKinnell, Deggins, and Labat, 1969). Conclusion: the kidney **cancer cell nucleus must contain a set of normal genes.** When human acute myelocytic leukemia (AML) cells are grown in tissue culture, they can be restored to normal by adding a particular protein. The pro-

tein presumably removes whatever it was that was blocking normal differentiation (see Price et al., 1974).

We don't know what all this means yet, but it does suggest that cancer can be caused by something *other than* a permanent genetic change, something other than a mutation.

The picture that seems to be emerging relates to the general trend in the development of a human being that all cells divide rapidly in the early stages of life but that only a small fraction divide regularly in a fully mature adult. The highly ordered shutdown of cell division is apparently orchestrated by chemicals—each stage of development sets up a uniquely complex three-dimensional chemical environment that turns on and off the genes that specify the *next* stage. If cell division can be turned down in this way, it certainly seems possible that cancer (uncontrolled growth) might result from a cell failing to get the right chemical message at the right time. Cancer could be a snag in the unfolding of the genetic program. This hypothesis is intriguing, because it suggests that cancer cells might be converted back into normal cells *if only we knew what to do!*

Now let's turn more directly to the question, "What does it mean to inherit the tendency to develop cancer?"

We have just reconsidered *one* way in which cancer can develop. In the next section, we will be interested in *all* the ways cancer can develop—including mechanisms yet to be discovered. In essence, we will be looking at the inheritance of tendencies to have things go wrong that result in cancer and that show up as a greater risk of developing cancer. The following list shows some kinds of things one could *conceivably* inherit that could have some bearing on cancer risk:

1. Defective genes that normally serve some function in the control cell division

2. Features that make it easier for carcinogenic agents to get at genetic material—light skin, for example

3. Defective mechanisms by which genetic damage is repaired

4. A faulty immune system

5. A set of metabolic enzymes that tend to convert noncarcinogens into carcinogens

6. A set of endocrine glands that generates a hormone environment that makes it more likely for cancer to develop

7. Cancer-causing viruses (virus genes imbedded in sperm or egg genetic complements)

8. A built-in blockage of normal differentiation or development

Some things on this list *are known for a fact* to be at the roots of the inherited tendency to develop cancer; others are unproven possibilities.

The Inheritance of Cancer in Flies, Fish, and Mice

Because it is extremely difficult to study heredity in humans, much, if not most, of what we know about the inheritance of cancer and cancer tendencies has been learned from work with experimental animals. Fruit flies, fish, and mice are good subjects for this kind of work because (1) they can be inbred so as to produce pure strains; (2) they have relatively short life spans, and whatever happens, happens fast; (3) they can be raised in big batches in a little space; and (4) their breeding is easy to control. Biology and ethical considerations rule out these advantages with human beings.

Fruit Flies, Brain Cancer, and "Anti-oncogenes"

To make a long story short, somebody doing a microscopic examination noticed a brain tumor in a laboratory strain of fruit fly, and the tumor turned out to be a result of a single gene muta-

tion. Further investigation revealed that the altered gene *normally* serves to regulate the expression of *other* genes and controls the rate of division in brain cells. The gene is a lethal recessive gene, a gene that kills any offspring that carry *two* such genes*—one from Mom and one from Dad. Apparently, only one good gene is necessary to hold the reproduction of brain cells in check during early development. It should be noted that this concept is different from (actually the inverse of) the oncogene concept. Murphree and Benedict (1984) suggest that the very same sorts of **suppressor** or "regulatory" genes amount to one class of *human* cancer genes—genes that allow cancer to happen when they are suppressed or are *non*functional! This class is distinguished from the class of "expressor" genes—oncogenes—that cause cancer when they are expressed. Let's look at another nonhuman suppressor gene-related cancer before we look at human retinoblastoma.

Cancer without Carcinogens—In Fish

Tropical fish fanciers know that "platys" are elongated diamond-shaped fish with a couple of dark spots on their dorsal fins. Swordtails have no such spots, but when swordtails and platys are crossbred, the result is a fish with bigger dark spots. If the hybrid is mated with a pure-bred swordtail, some of the offspring develop spots that really get out of hand—in fact, they become malignant melanomas. Notice that no mutagens or carcinogens of any kind have been mentioned. The melanomas appear to be the result of the cross breeding-induced loss of the control of cell division.

---

*The body cells of fruit flies and humans *each* have two genes for every trait. The two genes are not necessarily the same. When they are not the same, sometimes the affected trait is a blend of the influence of the two genes; sometimes one gene is **dominant** (is the one expressed) and the other is masked (and is called a **recessive gene**). Recessive genes express themselves only when matched with another such gene.

Purebred platys have dark-spot-producing pigment cells but they apparently also have genes that control the division of these cells; hence, two dark spots, no melanoma. Swordtails have neither the pigment cells nor the controller genes; hence, no dark spots, no melanoma. A hybrid that inherits the ability to make pigment cells but not all the controlling genes ends up with a very large dark spot, but still no melanoma. Some of the progeny of the cross between the hybrid and a pure swordtail apparently get the codes for pigment cells but very few, if any, controlling genes. The result: uncontrolled growth of melanotic pigment cells, or malignant melanoma.*

Mice

Certain strains of rats and mice are either highly susceptible or highly resistant to developing cancer, apparently because of an inherited susceptibility or resistance to relevant virus infections. Some strains of mice are so susceptible to mouse leukemia viruses that virtually all the members of the strain get infected with the virus and develop leukemia. Also, some inbred strains of mice develop breast cancer with a high frequency—in this case, because of a susceptibility to a mouse breast cancer virus (see Chapter 10).

In each of these cases involving mice, fish, and fruit flies, the story is a little different. The common thread is of course a defective cell growth-control *system*. Note that in the cases of the fruit fly and the platy, the faulty control system is inherited *directly*; in effect, cancer is inherited. The mouse, however, inherits increased susceptibility to an environmental carcinogen; the cancer follows indirectly.

---

*An interesting note: Within the last ten years, it has become apparent that there are malignant melanoma-prone human families. The pattern of inheritance is such that it appears that a dominant, autosomal (that is, not on a sex chromosome) gene is inherited, having 90 percent penetrance (probability of producing a melanoma) (see Greene et al., 1985; Kolata, 1986). Perhaps controller genes similar to those in platys are involved.

The Inheritance of Cancer and the Tendency to Develop Cancer in Human Beings

Inheritance of a Genetic Defect in Which Cancer May Be the Whole Story: Retinoblastoma

A certain human neoplasm involves a suppressor gene very similar in nature to the one described earlier in fruit flies. The name of the human neoplasm is retinoblastoma. **Retinoblastoma** is a childhood cancer that usually appears before age three (Fig. 11.2). The cell of origin is a cell in the retina of the eye, hence "**retino-**." The "**-blast-**" comes from the fact that the retinal cell of origin is not fully differentiated. And "**-oma**" *incorrectly* implies that the neoplasm is benign. Although retinoblastoma can arise *de novo*— from causes unknown—many victims have a family history of the disease.

To understand what happens in retinoblastoma, it must *first* be appreciated that, except for sperm and eggs, all human cells have a double set of genes. One of each set of two genes (called **alleles** of one another) came from Mom's egg and the other came from Dad's sperm cell. It must also be understood that sperm and eggs are produced through a process called **meiosis**, in which only one set of genes ends up in a sex cell—explaining how we get one set from each parent. Keep in mind also that all the cells in any one body, including retinal cells, are derived from the *same* fertilized egg. A copy of every gene and any gene mutation that occurred in, or was carried in, the egg, the sperm, or the fertilized egg is present in all resultant body (somatic) cells. It may actually be expressed in relatively few cells, but it is present in all body cells.

As with the fruit fly brain tumor described earlier, it is believed that retinoblastoma involves a regulatory gene or genes that control the rate of proliferation of retinal cells during differentiation. Normal persons have two normal regulatory genes (Rb+/Rb+)—one from Mom and one from Dad, one normal gene is enough to effect control—to keep cancer from arising.

Suppose both parents were heterozygous; that is, they *both* had one normal gene and one defective gene (Rb+/rb−). Any fertilized egg that such a couple produces would have a one in four chance of getting *two* defective genes, one from each parent. There would be a 1-in-4 chance that the egg would get two *normal* genes, and a 50 percent chance that the egg would get one normal gene and one defective gene.

An egg with two defective genes (rb−/rb−) would permit uncontrolled growth of retinal cells from the beginning. Presumably, any such fetus would cease developing very early and would likely be naturally aborted. An egg with two good genes will, of course, direct the development of a normal individual. Such an individual would have to get mutations in both normal genes of at least one retinal cell very early in life before the retinal cells became fully mature. The odds of this happening are very long, and even if it did happen, such individuals would not transmit the tendency to develop retinoblastoma to their offspring because the genes in their germ cells would presumably still be normal.

It is also possible that mutated retinal cell regulatory gene may arise in a germ cell (precursor to sperm, or precursor to egg). An individual in whom this happened would not get retinoblastoma, but could give the tendency to get retinoblastoma to offspring.

Familial (inherited) retinoblastoma is believed to arise from individuals who develop from eggs having one normal and one defective regulatory gene (Rb+/rb−) and in whom mutations* develop in the "good" gene in one or more retinal cells in early life. Although the mutation may well be caused by some environmental factor, such cancers would clearly have been set up by genetics. A genetic heritage of only

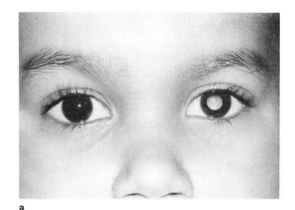

a

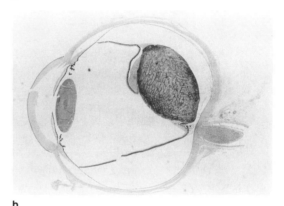

b

Figure 11.2 Retinoblastoma as seen through the pupil of the left eye (**a**) and in cross section, showing the tumor mass and retinal detachment (**b**). (Photos courtesy of Dr. Jerry Shields, Director of the Oncology Service, Wills Eye Hospital, Philadelphia. Photo (**a**) used by permission of C. V. Mosby Company.)

one good gene makes it much more likely that the cancer will appear—assuming random mutations. Clearly, if the defective retinal cell regulatory gene was present in the egg, all the cells derived from that egg will carry the defective gene. This fact is of potential consequence in only two kinds of cells, however—retinal cells and germ cells. The germ cell consequence is that half of all offspring (on the average) will get a defective gene from a mother or father with such a germ cell line. If the mate is normal, half of all children produced will be abnormally susceptible to retinoblastoma.

---

*Actually, mutation is only one of several ways in which control might be lost. Gene inactivation, chromosome deletion, and other ways in which a cell could be left without any Rb+ are described by Murphree and Benedict (1984).

Retinoblastoma and the "Odds"

If, in fact, hereditary retinoblastoma amounts to the inheritance of a pair of retinal-cell-growth-regulating genes, only one of which is defective (Rb + /rb −), why does the malignancy appear to be a *dominant* trait? Why is the malignancy so highly likely to appear in both eyes if the one gene is normal?

The answer apparently lies in the fact that, on the average, the odds of a mutation occurring in any given gene are roughly one in a million (10^6). It so happens that somewhere between 1 million and 10 million retinoblasts exist in *each* developing eye. Statistically speaking, if there are a million cells, each with a one-in-a-million chance of experiencing a critical hit, one will be hit—on the average. Some groups of one million will have two, some three, some even more hits; some such groups will have none. What this means, of course, is that a fetus that starts out life with one gene already defective is fairly certain to develop a retinoblastoma, and probably in both eyes.

Actually the "penetrance" of retinoblastoma in individuals carrying one defective gene from the start is about 95 percent for developing at least one tumor. This rate compares to the odds of 1 in 30,000 of developing retinoblastoma in a person with two normal genes from the start.

That the inheritance of a defective control gene along with a normal gene may be a pattern *common* in heritable cancer is suggested from the observation that the *same* kind of "multiple primary" pattern seen in retinoblastoma is seen in many other kinds of heritable cancers (see Fig. 11.3; also see Murphree and Benedict, 1984).

In what may be a related phenomenon, it has recently been found that tumor cells of patients with Beckwith-Wiedermann syndrome (a condition in which a child has a high risk of developing Wilms' tumor, liver cancer, or a muscle cell cancer), both pairs of chromosome 11 bear the same mutation. Since the normal cells of such patients bear the mutation only on one of the chromosome pair, it looks like the tumors develop wherever a mutation occurs in the one good gene and this gene must have a supressor function (see Marx, 1986). This is doubly significant in light of the following observations: Some transformed cells can be rendered unable to produce a neoplasm in immunodeficient mice if the transformed cells are first fused with normal cells—suggesting that the transformed cell picks up a missing control element when it fuses with a normal cell. Human HeLa cells can be rendered nontumorigenic when fused with human fibroblasts in this way, and it has been found that chromosome 11, alone, can do the job—offering more evidence that there may be a tumor supressor gene somewhere in chromosome 11.

Inheritance of a Less Fail-Safe System of Growth Control Involving More Than One Gene? Breast Cancer

The inheritance of tendencies to develop certain types of cancer is much less clear-cut for most cancers than it is for retinoblastoma.

You may have heard that the odds of a woman getting breast cancer are 1 in 14 (1 in 10, in the United States) and that if her mother or one of her sisters have it or have had it, the odds go up to 1 in 8 (1 in 5 in the United States). These odds define the degree to which the tendency to get breast cancer "runs in families" but we have no idea, in this case, *what* is actually "running" in such families!

We don't know what normally causes breast cancer. In Chapter 9, we saw that radiation can cause it, but it is unlikely that radiation is responsible for very many cases. Viruses can cause breast cancer in mice, but we don't know if viruses are involved in human cancer. We do know that breast cancer is five times more common in the United States than in Japan, that it is

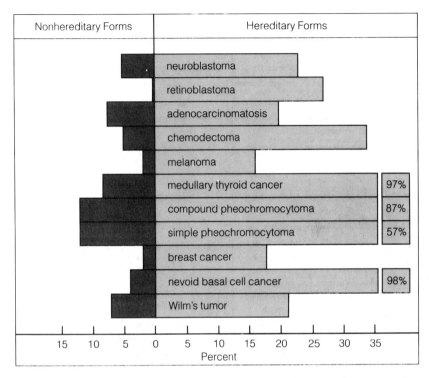

Nonhereditary Forms	Hereditary Forms

neuroblastoma

retinoblastoma

adenocarcinomatosis

chemodectoma

melanoma

medullary thyroid cancer — 97%

compound pheochromocytoma — 87%

simple pheochromocytoma — 57%

breast cancer

nevoid basal cell cancer — 98%

Wilm's tumor

15 10 5 0 5 10 15 20 25 30 35

Percent

Figure 11.3 The relative frequencies of occurrence of more than one primary cancer in hereditary and nonhereditary forms of the same kinds of malignant neoplasms. It is believed that in the hereditary forms, one of two genes that must be defective before a malignancy can develop is defective from the beginning (inherited) in *all* cells and therefore it is much more likely that neoplasms will appear more than once. (Adapted from Anderson, 1974. Used by permission of the author and the American Cancer Society.)

more common among women who bear children late or not at all, and that it is related to fat consumption and obesity. Some of these things suggest that hormones may be involved.

The picture is clouded somewhat because of a different hereditary character for premenopausal and postmenopausal "forms" of breast cancer. The incidence of breast cancer among the relatives of *pre*menopausal breast cancer patients is three times higher than in the population at large. No such pattern appears for postmenopausal breast cancer patients.

Genes are the primary determinants of circulating estrogen levels *and* of the degree to which tissues respond to the presence of hormones. Perhaps any number of the genes in-

volved in regulating breast tissue cell division are involved in the development of breast cancer. Breast cancer may result from the same sort of problem described earlier for retinoblastoma, but in a more complicated way because more than one or two genes are involved.

The bottom line? We know that a familial (inherited) dimension exists in breast cancer risk, but it remains to be defined.

Colon Cancer, Lung Cancer, and Leukemia Tendencies

Another common cancer that exhibits some inherited tendency is colon cancer. Here again, the patterns are complicated, and suggest a **polygenetic** connection (more than one pair of genes are involved or could be involved).

Lung cancer tendencies are also at least partly inheritable in a complex way such that a smoker with a close relative with lung cancer is much more likely to get lung cancer than smokers without such relatives.

The degree to which certain forms of *leukemia* tend to follow patterns of heredity is illustrated in Table 11.1. Roughly, a 20 percent correlation exists for leukemia in identical twins, but none in fraternal twins. The increased risk of leukemia in Down's syndrome and Bloom's syndrome (Table 11.1) introduces another dimension of the connection between cancer and genes.

Syndromes Associated with a Higher Risk of Cancer: Inheritance of Gene Defect in Which Cancer Is Just One of Many Problems

A number of genetic disorders are associated with increased risk to particular kinds of cancer (Table 11.2). Among these are Down's syndrome (leukemia), familial polyposis (colon), xeroderma pigmentosum (skin), Fanconi's anemia (leukemia), Bloom's syndrome (leukemia), and ataxia telangiectasia (lymphoma and leukemia).

Down's syndrome is a genetic disorder related to the presence of an *extra* copy of chromosome 21 in all cells. The risk of leukemia in those afflicted by Down's syndrome is 20 times higher than in normal children. The reason for this is not known, although the nature of the chromosome abnormality suggests that a good possibility is the "extra" expression of a gene on chromosome 21.

Familial polyposis was considered in Chapter 5, where it was described as an inherited premalignant condition in which the mucosa of the colon and other parts of the intestine is covered by benign polyps. Clinical experience has shown that malignant neoplasms are almost certain to arise from the benign lesions, given enough time. The nature of the specific defect in this case is not known, although defective

growth control is clearly the hallmark of the entire syndrome.

Other cancer syndromes are listed in Table 11.2.

Inheritance of Defective DNA Damage Repair Mechanisms

Xeroderma pigmentosum is a very rare disorder in which cells have a nonfunctional enzyme for the repair of UV-induced damage to DNA. In such individuals, exposure to direct sun means skin cancer—possibly because some of the unrepaired mutations occur in growth-regulating genes.

The inheritance of faulty repair mechanisms also appear to be the underlying reason for the increased risk to malignancy associated with Bloom's syndrome, Fanconi's anemia, and the Louis-Barr syndrome (see Table 11.2).

Inheritance of Anatomical Features That Influence Susceptibility to Cancer Indirectly: Skin Cancer

The genetics of skin cancer risk are relatively simple and straightforward. Skin cancers are nearly all produced by the action of UV radiation on the stem cells of the epidermis. Other things being equal, the amount of radiation that reaches these cells is a function of the amount of pigment (melanin) in the skin. The more melanin, the less radiation reaches the stem cells. A more or less obvious consequence of this rule is that dark-skinned people get much less skin cancer than do light-skinned people. Skin color is genetically determined. Genetics also determine the *thickness* of the epidermis shielding the basal layer of epidermal cells and the thicker the epidermis, the less UV that reaches the stem cells and the less skin cancer.

Other Aspects of the Inheritance of a Greater Than Normal Risk of Cancer

The immune system undoubtedly plays some role in protecting against cancer, and later we

Table 11.1 The Overall Risk of Leukemia in Normal 15-Year-Old Caucasian Children and in Genetically Defined Subgroups

Group	Approximate Risk	Time Interval to Onset
Identical twin of children with leukemia	1 in 5[a]	Weeks or months
Radiation-treated polycythemia vera	1 in 6	10–15 years
Bloom's syndrome	1 in 8[b]	30 years of age
Hiroshima survivors who were within 1,000 meters of the hypocenter	1 in 60	12 years
Down's syndrome	1 in 95	10 years of age
Radiation-treated patients with ankylosing spondylitis	1 in 270	15 years
Sibs of leukemic children	1 in 720	10 years
U.S. Caucasian children 15 years of age	1 in 2,880	10 years

[a]Of 22 sets of identical twins with leukemia, the cotwin was affected in five instances.
[b]Three leukemics among 23 people with Bloom's syndrome.

Source: From p. 59 of Pitot, H., 1978 *Fundamentals of Oncology*. Used by permission of Marcel Dekker, Inc.

Table 11.2 Some Genetically Inherited Syndromes That Include Increased Risk to Cancer

Condition	Underlying Defect	Type of Cancer
Familial polyposis coli*	Development of multiple polyps	Colon carcinoma
Gardner's syndrome*	Cutaneous cysts, polyps, etc.	Colon carcinoma, osteomas
Peutz-Jeghers syndrome*	Abnormal pigmentation of skin and mucous membranes, gastrointestinal (GI) polyps	GI carcinoma
Basal cell nevus syndrome*	Multiple nevi, bone defects	Basal cell carcinoma of skin, epidermoid cysts of jaw
Bloom's syndrome**	Increased chromosomal breakage *in vitro* and *in vivo*, increased sister chromatid exchange, defect in DNA repair	Acute nonlymphocytic leukemia; GI tumors
Fanconi's anemia**	Increased chromosomal breakage *in vitro* and *in vivo*, increased sensitivity to carcinogens, defect in DNA repair	Acute nonlymphocytic leukemia
Ataxia telangiectasia (Louis-Barr syndrome)**	Defective immune system, increased chromosomal breakage in cultured lymphocytes	Lymphoma, lymphocytic leukemias, reticuloendothelial (R. E.) cell tumors
Xeroderma pigmentosum**	Inability to repair UV-damaged DNA	Basal and squamous cell cancer of skin

*Dominantly inherited (see text) genes associated with specific risk to cancer.
**Recessive (see text) conditions associated with increased neoplasia and chromosomal instability.

Source: Meisner, 1983 (pp. 167, 168); adapted with permission of Grune & Stratton, Inc. and the author.

will consider how the immune system actually works both ways, for and against cancer. Here, it is important to appreciate that the immune system, like any other feature of a living organism, is specified by genes. It is conceivable—indeed, likely—that some immune systems are better at snuffing out incipient malignancies than are other immune systems. All in all, inheritance bears on the cancer problem in many and varied ways. Genes are partly responsible for hormone levels, psychological makeup, and metabolic competence, all of which have some bearing on the likelihood of developing cancer. All these things can be lumped together as "endogenous" factors contributing to the probability of getting cancer. Endogenous factors are contrasted to "exogenous" factors such as those covered in Chapters 8, 9, and 10.

Cancer and Chromosomes: Deranged Genetics in Micro "Graphic" Form

In Chapter 7, it was pointed out that chromosomal abnormalities are a common feature of malignant neoplasms; most human tumors have characteristic chromosomal defects (see Yunis, 1983, and Yunis and Soreng, 1984). It was also noted that chromosome breaks followed by translocations amount to one of the ways in which oncogenes can be turned on. We close this chapter by noting that chromosome problems such as breaks, **polyploidy** (having *more than* the normal number of complete sets of chromosomes—and therefore possibly multiple copies of "oncogenes"), and **aneuploidy** (having something other than the normal number of chromosomes—and thus the possibility of mismatched regulator and regulated genes), could obviously all be the manifestations of abnormal genes or the cause of abnormal gene expression. Chromosomal abnormalities can be the *causes* of deranged control (see Chapter 7), or they could be indications of damage that might also include mutations. The significance of chromosomal abnormalities in detection and diagnosis of cancer is covered in Chapter 17.

Summary

The relationship between genes and genetics, and cancer has at least two dimensions—maybe three. The first is that genes are the targets of mutagens, and some of the mutations that result from hits result in deranged control and cancer. A second dimension derives from the fact that normal growth and development depends on a highly orderly sequence of genes being shut down and turned on and turned up. The possibility that some cancers are a result of nonmutational accidents in the unfolding of the genetic program is real. A third dimension, which is really derived from the first two, is that some kinds of cancer have an hereditary character. This character probably amounts to the inheritance of increased likelihood of sustained mutations and/or other gene control accidents.

Cancers with a definite genetic connection are rare. Some of the more familiar are retinoblastoma, intraocular melanoma, and medullary thyroid carcinoma. Inherited precancerous conditions with an associated higher risk to cancer are also rare, but give a definite hereditary character to cancer of the colon, leukemias, and skin cancer, among others.

The key distinction between a "regular" cancer and one that has an hereditary connection is that in a "regular" cancer the gene problem occurs originally in a somatic (body) cell and not in a reproductive or reproductive stem cell. In such a case, the cancer that results is a one-time deal having no direct impact on the likelihood of cancer in any offspring. If a gene control defect arises in a reproductive cell and ends up in an egg or sperm that gives rise to a new organism, however, the defect will be present in all of the new organism's body cells. In such a case, related neoplasms would not appear in the organism in which the mutation first occurred, but would "tend" to appear in the tissues in which that gene happens to be important. The consequence of greatest significance is that the offspring will also have a certain probability of transmitting the trait to its offspring and so on.

Beyond the few cancers that have a more or

less *distinct* hereditary connection, certain common cancers appear to have a much more *diffuse* hereditary connection. Breast cancer is perhaps the best example.

Many traits, all inherited, can and probably do influence the risk to malignancy even more indirectly. We mentioned some skin features that predispose to skin cancer indirectly, and we alluded to the possibility that certain yet unknown features of the immune system, the endocrine system and other physiological systems may influence the likelihood of cancer appearing.

To conclude this chapter and introduce the epilog to Part III, note that it is *impossible* to separate genetic factors from environmental factors completely. Families tend to be exposed to the same environment as well as to carry common genetic characters. The facts presented in this chapter notwithstanding, it will become clear in the epilog following this chapter that environmental factors are actually *much more* important than genetics and inheritance when it comes to the risk of getting cancer.

References and Further Reading

Anders, A., and Anders, F. 1978. Etiology of Cancer as Studied in the Platyfish-Swordtail System. *Biochim. Biophys. Acta.* 516:61–95.

Anderson, D. E. 1974. The Role of Genetics in Human Cancer. *Ca-A Cancer Journal for Clinicians.* 24(3):130–36.

Bodmer, W. F., ed. 1983. *Inheritance of Susceptibility to Cancer in Man.* New York: Oxford University Press.

Croce, C. M., and Koprowski, H. 1978. The Genetics of Human Cancer. *Scientific American.* 238(2):117–25.

Fraumeni, J. F., et al. 1975. Six Families Prone to Ovarian Cancer. *Cancer.* 36:364–69.

Gateff, E. 1978. Malignant Neoplasms of Genetic Origin in *Drosophila melanogaster. Science.* 200:1448–59.

Gelboin, H. V. et al., eds. 1980. *Genetic and Environmental Factors in Experimental and Human Cancers.* Tokyo: Japan Scientific Press.

German, J., ed. 1974. *Chromosomes and Cancer.* New York: Wiley.

Greene, M. H., et al. 1985. High Risk of Malignant Melanoma in Melanoma-Prone Families with Dysplastic Nevi. *Ann. Intern. Med.* 102:458–65.

Huebner, K., et al. 1985. The Human Gene Encoding GM-CSF Is at 5q21-q32, the Chromosome Region Deleted in the 5q- Anomaly. *Science.* 230:1282–85.

Illmensee, K., and Mintz, B. 1976. Totipotency and Normal Differentiation of Single Teratocarcinoma Cells Cloned by Injection into Blastocysts. *Proc. Natl. Acad. Sci.* 73:549–53.

Illmensee, K., and Stevens, L. C. 1979. Teratomas and Chimeras. *Scientific American.* 240:121–29.

Kahn, S. B., et al., eds. 1983. *Concepts in Cancer Medicine.* New York: Grune & Stratton.

Knudson, A. G. 1974. Heredity and Human Cancer. *Am. J. Pathol.* 77:77–84.

Knudson, A. G. 1978. Retinoblastoma: A Prototypic Hereditary Neoplasm. *Seminars in Oncology.* 5:57–60.

Kolata, G. 1986. Researchers Seek Melanoma Gene. *Science,* 232:708–09.

Lynch, H. T. 1981. *Genetics and Breast Cancer.* New York: Van Nostrand Reinhold.

Lynch, H. T., and Guirgis, H. A. 1984. *Biomarkers, Genetics and Cancer.* New York: Van Nostrand Reinhold.

Lynch, H. T., Rozen, P., and Schuelke, G. 1985. Hereditary Colon Cancer: Polyposis and Non Polyposis Variants. *Ca-A Cancer Journal for Clinicians.* 35(2):95–115.

Lynch, P., and Lynch, H. T., eds. 1984. *Colon Cancer Genetics.* New York: Van Nostrand Reinhold.

Marcus, M. G. 1976. Cancer and Character. *Psychology Today.* 10(6) June: 52–54.

Mark, J. 1977. Chromosomal Abnormalities and Their Specificity in Human Neoplasms: An Assessment of Recent Observations by Banding Techniques. *Advances in Cancer Research.* 24:165–222.

McKinnell, R. G., Deggins, B. A., and Labat, D. D. 1969. Transplantation of Pluripotential Nuclei from Triploid Frog Tumors. *Science.* 165:394–96.

Meisner, L. F. 1983. Genetic Factors in Human Cancer. In S. Kahn et al., eds., *Concepts in Cancer Medicine.* New York: Grune & Stratton.

Mintz, B., and Illmensee, K. 1975. Normal Genetically Mosaic Mice Produced from Malignant Teratocarcinoma Cells. *Proc. Natl. Acad. Sci.* 72:3585.

Mitleman, F., ed. 1985. *Catalog of Chromosome Aberrations in Cancer.* 2nd ed. New York: Alan R. Liss.

Müller, H., and Weber, W. 1985. *Familial Cancer.* New York: Karger.

Murphree, A. L., and Benedict, W. F. 1984. Retinoblastoma: Clues to Human Oncogenesis. *Science.* 223:1028–33.

Nagley, P., et al., eds. 1983. *Manipulation and Expression of Genes in Eukaryotes.* New York: Academic Press.

Nowell, P., and Finan, J. 1978. Chromosome Studies in Preleukemic States. IV: Myeloproliferative vs. Cytopenic Disorders. *Cancer.* 42(5):2254–61.

Pierce, G., and Wallace, C. 1971. Differentiation of Malignant to Benign Cells. *Cancer Research.* 31:127–34.

Pitot, H. 1978. *Fundamentals of Oncology.* New York: Dekker.

Price, G., et al. 1974. Heterogeneity of Molecules with Low Molecular Weight Isolated from Media Conditioned by Human Leucocytes and Capable of Stimulating Colony Formation by Human Granulopoietic Progenitor Cells. *J. Cell Physiol.* 84:383–96.

Rowley, J., and Ultman, J. E., eds., 1983. *Chromosomes and Cancer.* Orlando, Fla.: Academic Press.

Ruddon, R. W. 1981. *Cancer Biology.* New York: Oxford University Press.

Shannon, R. S., et al. 1982. Wilm's Tumor and Anridia: Clinical and Cytogenetic Features. *Archives of Disease in Childhood.* 57:685–90.

Siddiqui, M. A. Q., ed. 1983. *Control of Embryonic Gene Expression.* Boca Raton, Fla.: CRC Press.

Therman, E. 1980. *Human Chromosomes.* New York: Springler-Verlag.

Yunis, J. J. 1983. The Chromosomal Basis of Human Neoplasia. *Science.* 221:227–36.

Yunis, J. J., and Soreng, A. L. 1984. Constituitive Fragile Sites and Cancer. *Science.* 226:1199–1203.

Dramatically different patterns of cancer incidence and mortality appear throughout the world, patterns that line up with places more than they do with races. The environmental importance of this patterning is highlighted by the way in which place-related differences in cancer incidence and mortality become apparent in people who move from one part of the world to another (see below). Higginson and Muir (1979) and others have argued that the lowest death rates for each type of cancer represent a baseline and that the extremes of incidence and mortality from place to place offers a plausible basis for the deduction that cancer is 90 percent environmental. Theoretically, if the world cancer death rate for each specific type of cancer could be reduced to the level found in the country where it is presently the lowest, cancer mortality could be reduced tenfold.

Table E.1 shows the range of variation in cancer mortality for certain kinds of cancer in selected countries whose registries have comparable, reliable data. Note that the ranges of variability are large. Patterns of wide variation can even be found within a single country; wide variation in cancer death rates are found in the United States, for example (see Mason et al., 1975). Typical of studies showing what happens to immigrants, a study of Japanese Hawaiians showed that they died of the same kinds of cancer as other Hawaiians—cancers different from those killing Japanese back in the "homeland" (Table E.2). Similarly, black Americans have been shown to die of cancer more like white Americans than they do like West Africans (Table E.3).

The human environment can be defined in terms of habit or lifestyle as well as in terms of geography. Studies of Seventh Day Adventists and Mormons (Fig. E.1)—groups of people who share some definitive elements of lifestyle—have shown such groups to have characteristic cancer mortality patterns that differ from those of otherwise similar people living in the *same* places.

Epilog to Part Three

Heredity or Environment?

Looking Ahead to Prevention

This epilog adapted from Kupchella, 1986 with permission of Grune and Stratton, Inc.

Table E.1   Range of Incidence Rates for Common Cancers

Site of Origin of Cancer	High-Incidence Area	Low-Incidence Area	Sex	Ratio of Highest Rate to Lowest Rate
Skin (chiefly nonmelanoma)	Australia: Queensland	India: Bombay	M	200
Esophagus	Iran: northeast	Nigeria	M	300
Lung and bronchus	England	Nigeria	M	35
Stomach	Japan	Uganda	M	25
Uterus (cervix)	Colombia	Israel: Jewish	F	15
Prostate	United States: blacks	Japan	M	40
Liver	Mozambique	England	M	100
Colon	United States: Connecticut	Nigeria	M	10
Uterus (body)	United States: California	Japan	F	30
Buccal cavity	India: Bombay	Denmark	M	25
Rectum	Denmark	Nigeria	M	20

Note: At ages 35–64 years.

Adapted from Doll and Peto, 1981. Reprinted from Kupchella, 1986; used with permission of Grune & Stratton, Inc.

Statements to the effect that most cancer is linked to environmental factors give rise to several possible misconceptions, namely, (1) we know exactly what these factors are, (2) they are mainly synthetic chemicals and pollutants, and (3) a 1-to-1 correspondence exists between the environmental connection and prevention potential. Actually, the notion that cancer is mostly environmental in origin is derived mostly from indirect lines of evidence, such as described above, and from only limited *direct* knowledge. Pollutants amount to a relatively small part of the problem, and not all environmentally derived cancers are preventable. The reader should be aware that the environment includes *everything* from the skin out and everything from the lining of body cavities open to the outside, in. Also, environmental "factors" are not restricted to carcinogens; the term "environmental factor" encompasses cocarcinogens, promoters, immune system suppressors (see Sklar and Anisman, 1979, and Riley, 1981) and other host-modifying agents, as well as carcinogens and procarcinogens.

The two most important categories of environmental factors causing cancer are diet and tobacco. Other categories of environmental factors involved in cancer causation include reproductive behavior, occupation, medical drugs and radiation, infection, background radiation, alcohol, sunlight, and pollution. A summary showing the relative importance of each of these categories is given in Table E.4. Much of the basis for this table is given in Chapters 13 and 15.

Linking Cancer to Specific Environmental Factors: The Difficulty

There are only about 40 chemicals, practices, and circumstances fairly conclusively linked to human cancer thus far. Throughout Part III, we

Table E.2 Comparison of Cancer Incidence Rates in Japan for Japanese and Caucasians in Hawaii

Primary Site of Cancer	Patient's Sex	Annual Incidence per Million People		
			Hawaii, 1968–1972	
		Japan[a]	Japanese	Caucasians
Esophagus	M	150 112	46	75
Stomach	M	1,331 1,291	397	217
Colon	M	78 87	371	368
Rectum	M	95 90	297	204
Lung	M	237 299	379	962
Breast	F	335 295	1,221	1,869
Uterus (cervix)	F	329 398	149	243
Ovary	F	51 55	160	274

Note: Ages 35–64, standardized for age as in IARC (1976).
[a]For each type of cancer, upper entry shows incidence in Miyagi prefecture, 1968–1971; lower entry shows incidence in Osaka prefecture, 1970–1971.

Source: Rates from International Agency for Research on Cancer 1976; table adapted from Doll and Peto, 1981.

have discussed many of the reasons why it is difficult to link specific environmental factors to specific kinds of cancer; some of the more important reasons might be summarized as follows:

1. Environments are usually complicated combinations of *many* factors; it is practically impossible to isolate the effects of any *one*.

2. Some 6 million chemicals already exist, 60,000 are in common use, and over 1,000 new chemicals come into common use each year.

3. The results of animal testing are not unequivocally applicable to human beings (see Brown and Kozoil, 1983; Salisbury, 1983). Animal testing is expensive, and it simply logisti-

cally cannot get at the questions having to do with very *low* doses.

4. People move around and change habits.

5. We generally don't keep records of who, dying of what, was exposed to what for how long.

6. There may be 30 or even 40 or more years of lag separating exposure and cancer.

7. More than one factor may conspire to "cause" cancer.

All these things suggest that despite the fact that nearly all cancer can be linked to the environment (see Table E.4), there will always be doubt about the identity of at least some factors.

Table E.3 Comparison of Cancer Incidence Rates for Ibadan, Nigeria, and for Blacks and Whites in the United States.

Primary Site of Cancer	Patient's Sex	Ibadan, Nigeria, 1960–1969	United States[a] Blacks	United States[a] Whites
Colon	M	34	349 / 353	294 / 335
Liver	M	272	67 / 86	39 / 32
Pancreas	M	55	200 / 250	126 / 122
Lung	M	27	1,546 / 1,517	983 / 979
Breast	F	337	1,268 / 1,105	1,828 / 1,472
Uterus (cervix)	F	559	507 / 631	249 / 302
Lymphosarcoma at age 15[b]	M	133	10 / 5	4 / 3

Note: Ages 35–64, standardized for age as in IARC (1976).

[a]For each type of cancer, upper entry shows incidence in San Francisco Bay area, 1969–1973; lower entry shows incidence in Detroit, 1969–1971.

[b]Including Burkitt's lymphoma. The cited rates are the average of the age-specific rates at ages 0–4, 5–9, and 10–14.

Source: Rates from International Agency for Research on Cancer (IARC), 1976; table adapted from Doll and Peto, 1981.

Implications for Prevention

Obviously, it is very difficult to devise a cancer prevention-avoidance strategy for unknown environmental factors. But that is not to say that avoidance is "easy" or even *possible* for factors that are well-known carcinogens. Factors such as background radiation are practically impossible to avoid. Other factors such as tobacco and sunlight are *not* avoided very well, for behavioral-motivational reasons we will explore in the context of prevention, later.

References and Further Reading

Ames, B. N. 1979. Dietary Carcinogens and Anticarcinogens. *Science.* 221:1256–64.

Antunes, C. M., and Stolley, P. D. 1977. Cancer Induction by Exogenous Hormones. *Cancer.* 39:1896–1989.

Becker, C. E., ed. 1984. *Recent Advances in Occupational Cancer.* Proceedings of the Annual Conference on Recent Advances in Occupational Cancer, San Francisco, 21–22 October, 1983. *J. Toxicol.: Clin. Toxicol.* 22(3): whole issue.

Brown, C. C., and Kozoil, A. 1983. Statistical Aspects of the Estimation of Human Risk from Suspected Human Carcinogens. *SIAM Review.* 25(2):151–81.

Committee on Diet Nutrition and Cancer, National Research Council. 1982. *Diet, Nutrition, and Cancer.* Washington D.C.: National Academy Press.

Crump, K. S., and Guess, H. A. 1982. Drinking Water and Cancer: Review of Recent Epidemiological Findings and Assessment of Risks. *Ann. Rev. Public Health.* 3:339–57.

Doll, R., and Peto, R. 1981. The Causes of Cancer: Quantitative Estimates of Avoidable Risks of Cancer in the United States Today. *JNCI.* 66(6):1192–1308.

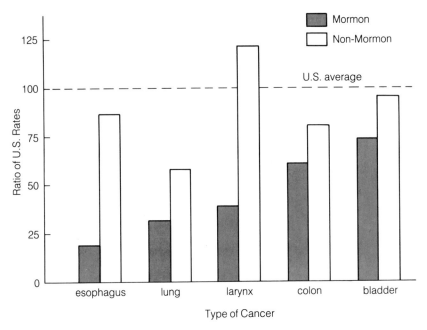

Figure E.1 Cancer in Mormons and non-Mormons in the state of Utah, 1966–1970. Note that while incidence rates are generally higher for non-Mormons, they are much higher for those cancers (esophageal and laryngeal) associated with alcohol and tobacco. Mormons do not use either of these substances. (Adopted from Lyon, 1976 (p. 131), with permission of the New England Journal of Medicine; reprinted from Kupchella and Hyland, 1986, with permission of Allyn & Bacon.)

Epstein, S. S. 1976. *Cancer and the Environment: A Scientific Perspective.* Facts and Analysis Occupational Health and Safety, Industrial Union Department AFL/CIO No. 25, February, pp. 1–13.

Gordon, D., Silverstone, H., and Smithhurst, B. A. 1972. The Epidemiology of Skin Cancer in Australia. In W. H. McCarthy, ed., *Melanoma and Skin Cancer.* Sydney, Australia: Government Printer.

Harris, R. H. 1976. *The Implications of Cancer Causing Substances in Mississippi River Water.* Washington D.C.: Environmental Defense Fund.

Higginson, J., and Muir, C. S. 1979. Environmental Carcinogenesis: Misconceptions and Limitations to Cancer Control. *JNCI* 63:1291–98.

International Agency for Research on Cancer. 1976. Cancer Incidence in Five Continents (Vol. III). In J. Waterhouse, C. Muir, P. Correa et al., eds. *IARC Sci. Publ.* 3:1–584.

Kirsh-Volders, M., ed. 1984. Mutagenicity, Carcino-

genicity, and Teratogenicity of Industrial Pollutants. New York: Plenum Press.

Kraybill, H. F. 1983. Assessment of Human Exposure and Health Risk to Environmental Contaminants in the Atmosphere and Water with Special Reference to Cancer. *J. Environ. Sci. Health.* C1(2):175–232.

Kupchella, C. E. 1986. Environmental Factors in Cancer Etiology. *Seminars in Nursing Oncology.* 2:161–69.

Lyon, J. L., et al. 1976. Cancer Incidence in Mormons and Non-Mormons in Utah, 1966–1970. *New England J. Med.* 294:129–33.

Mason, T., et al. 1975. *Atlas of Cancer Mortality for U.S. Counties, 1950–1969.* DHEW, PHS No., NIH 75-780. Department of Health, Education, and Welfare, National Institutes of Health: Bethesda, Md.

Merletti, F., et al. Target Organs for Carcinogenicity of Chemicals and Industrial Exposures in Humans: A Review of Results in the IARC Monographs on the

Table E.4 Summary of Cancer-Associated Environmental Factors

relative importance (handwritten annotation)

Factor	Sites Considered in Drawing the Estimates	Range of Estimates Associated with Factor[a]
Diet	Digestive tract, breast, endometrium, ovary	35–50 percent (35)
Tobacco	Upper respiratory tract, bladder, esophagus, kidney, pancreas	22–30 percent (30)
Occupation, all exposures	Upper respiratory tract, others	4–38 percent (4–10)
Alcohol	Upper digestive tract, larynx, liver	3–5 percent (3)
Infection	Uterus (cervix), prostate, and other sites	1–15 percent (10)
Sexual development, reproductive patterns, and sexual practices	Breast, endometrium, ovary, cervix, testis	1–13 percent (7)
Pollution	Lung, bladder, rectum	1–5 percent (2)
Medical drugs and radiation	Breast, endometrium, ovary, thyroid, bone, lung, blood (leukemia)	1–4 percent (1)
Natural radiation	Skin, breast, thyroid, lung, bone, blood (leukemia)	1–3 percent (1)
Consumer products	Possibly all sites	Less than 1 percent
Unknown associations	All sites	1–10 percent

[a]Most commonly cited "best" estimate given in parentheses.

Source: Compiled from Doll and Peto, 1981; Higginson and Muir, 1979; Wynder and Gori, 1977; and Office of Technology Assessment, 1981. Reprinted from Kupchella, 1986; used by permission of Grune & Stratton, Inc.

Evaluation of the Carcinogenic Risk of Chemicals to Humans. *Cancer Research.* 44:2244–50.

Office of Technology Assessment. 1981. *Assessment of Technologies for Determining Cancer Risks from the Environment.* Washington, D.C.: U.S. Congress.

Oftedal, P., and Brogger, A. 1986. *Risk and Reason: Risk Assessment in Relation to Environmental Mutagens and Carcinogens.* New York: Alan R. Liss.

Peto, R., and Schneiderman, M., eds. 1981. *Quantification of Occupational Cancer.* Banbury Report 9. New York: Cold Spring Harbor Laboratory.

Riley, V. 1981. Psychoneuroendocrine Influences on Immunocompetence and Neoplasia. *Science.* 212: 1100–09.

Salisbury, D. 1983. The Lifetime Feeding Study in Mice and Rats—An Examination of Its Validity as a Bioassay for Human Carcinogens. *Fundamental and Applied Toxicology.* 3:63–67.

Samuels, S. W., ed. 1986. *The Environment of the Workplace and Human Values.* New York: Alan R. Liss.

Sklar, L. S., and Anisman, H. 1979. Stress and Coping Factors Influence Tumor Growth. *Science.* 205(4405):513–15.

The Smoking Digest. 1979. NIH Publication No. 79-1549. Bethesda, Md.: National Cancer Institute.

Upton, A. (in press.) *Radiation Carcinogenesis.* New York: Elsevier.

Wynder, E. L., and Gori, G. B. 1977. Contribution of the Environment to Cancer Incidence: An Epidemiologic Exercise. *JNCI.* 58(4):825–32 (editorial).

PART FOUR
THE IMPACT OF CANCER

Now that we have considered the "genesis" of cancer and the nature of the cancer cell, we can finally get down to what cancer actually does to people.

"It kills them," you may say.

Yes, it kills some of us. But the story is actually nowhere near that simple. For one thing, cancer is the underlying cause of death for less than one out of five people. But nearly one out of three people get cancer. So it doesn't kill everybody that it afflicts. Also, different kinds of cancer kill people in different parts of the world. For another thing, even the people who die of cancer rarely *literally* die of cancer itself. They die of hemorrhages, neurological complications, indirect blockages, infections, blood clots, impaired liver function, and other "complications."

The overall purpose of Part IV is to consider the *impacts* of cancer on people. In Chapter 13 we will look at the things that neoplasms do to the bodies of the individuals afflicted, and at the ultimate causes of cancer death. Chapter 14 examines the impact of cancer on groups of people, picking up where we left off in Part III with the observation that cancer patterns differ throughout the world. Chapter 14 also outlines the methods of epidemiology. Chapter 15 deals with the specific effects of cancer on the immune system, offering a logical transition to the chapters on detection and treatment to follow in Part V. Cancer has an impact on the immune system, but the immune system offers ways of detecting cancer and the immune system has an impact on cancer. One of the most intriguing anticancer strategies is to find ways to make the immune system's impact on cancer even greater.

12

The Impact of Cancer on Normal Body Functions

Except for the fact that all living things eventually die, there is nothing inherently deadly about cell division. "Obviously," you say. But would you believe that there is likewise nothing inherently deadly about cancer cell division, at least up to a point?

Human beings can carry *some* neoplasms around for 20 years or longer without even being aware that they have cancer. During this period they aren't sick, they don't feel bad, and the neoplasm may not even be detectable using sophisticated instruments. Apparently, only when particular kinds of neoplasms reach characteristic stages in their development do they begin to have the overt effects on the body that eventually lead (if unchecked) to death.

The purpose of this chapter is to outline the "effects" of malignant neoplasms on the bodies that bear them. These effects are summarized in Table 12.1.

As with discussions of other aspects of the cancer problem, some details are missing. Again, this patchiness is not because of the author's disinterest or because of space limitations. It is certainly not because "host effects" are unimportant. Cancer is such a problem partly because key pieces of the puzzles presented here are still missing; we simply don't know the details. The reader is warned to be prepared to deal with incomplete sequences of cause and effect and with "nonexplanations" ascribed to "mystery factors."

An Arbitrary Classification of Effects

The direct effects of neoplasms on hosts fall into two general classes, physical and chemical. There are emotional effects that form still another category but we deal with these separately in a later chapter. Some authors classify the direct effects as local and systemic, but all classification schemes are arbitrary. In this book, physical impacts include the consequences of growth or expansion *and* local extension or infiltration, and are subdivided—again, arbitrarily—into three categories:

Table 12.1 Some Effects of Cancer on Host Function

Symptom/Effect	Some (Not All) of the Causes
Cachexia (weight loss)	Anorexia, abnormal energy metabolism, digestive system involvement (malabsorption), chemical imbalances; metabolic demands of tumor; and unknown factors.
Anorexia (loss of appetite)	Anxiety, changes in taste, chemical imbalances; nausea; and possibly other factors.
Hormone excess	Cancers of hormone-secreting tissue lead to increased numbers of hormone-secreting cells; ectopic hormone production by tumors in tissues that do not normally secrete hormones.
Hypercalcemia (high calcium levels)	Tumor invasion of bone, parathyroid hormone production by tumor, other factors (prostaglandins) produced by, or because of, tumors that cause calcium to be released from bone.
Hypoglycemia (low blood sugar)	Impaired liver function resulting from cancer involvement of the liver; hypersecretion of insulin; malnutrition.
Blood coagulation defects	Platelet deficiency secondary to invasion of bone marrow and to radiation or chemotherapy; chemical imbalances.
Anemia (low red blood cell count)	Invasion and crowding of bone marrow; immune reaction against red cells; chronic hemorrhage; impaired red blood cell production resulting from therapy.
Hemorrhage	Disseminated intravascular clotting depletes platelet count; erosion of blood vessel walls.
Intravascular blood clot formation	Stasis, chemical imbalances.
Polycythemia (excess red blood cells)	Erythropoietin production by kidney tumor; inappropriate erythropoietin production.
Leucopenia (too few white blood cells)	Invasion of bone and crowding out of normal bone marrow stem cells.
Leucocytosis (excess white blood cells)	Infection, necrosis.
Pain	Infection, pressure on nerves and other tissue, tissue destruction, ischemia.
Other neurological complications	Tumor invasion of brain and spinal cord.
Fever	Infection and possibly unknown factors released or induced by tumor tissue.
Immune system defects	Bone marrow invasion, other unknown factors.
Infection	Immune deficiency, impaired circulation and oxygenation; impaired GI tract motility; fistulas.
Skin changes	Excess hormone production; subdermal hemorrhage; direct invasion; unknown factors.
Kidney complications	Complication of autoimmune reaction; kidney stones associated with hypercalcemia.
Bone degeneration	Decalcification, direct invasion.
Joint inflammation	Autoimmune reaction.
Fluid accumulation (in tissue and in body cavities)	Impaired lymphatic drainage.
Obstruction of tubes and channels and consequent complications, e.g. uremia from blocked ureters	Compression and direct invasion.
Dysfunction of individual organs	Normal tissue is replaced with cancerous tissue; blood supply shut off because of compression or blockage.

1. *Compression.* Normal tissues impaired by compression, such as blood vessels and various other tubes, tracts, tissue spaces, and ducts, are squeezed shut so that things can no longer pass through them. Nerves under compression or tension are common sources of pain associated with cancer. When blood vessels are compressed, downstream tissues can be deprived of oxygen and nutrients; in turn, resulting in cell death and tissue ulceration.

2. *Infiltrative or direct blockage.* Ducts, tubes, and tracts may become filled with cancer cells, which blocks the passage of secretions, and so on.

3. *Destruction of boundaries as a result of invasion.* For example, the destruction of a blood vessel wall leads to "holes" and hemorrhages that often amount to the fatal episode in cancer.

Some effects of cancerous infiltration and growth show up as impairment of the organ in which the growth is taking place. Primary or metastatic cancer of the lung often reveal themselves as impaired respiration, cancer of the liver or metastasis to liver become manifest as impaired liver function, and so on. Other effects of infiltration and growth are more *generally* felt. Blockage of a vein or a lymph vessel, for example, can retard drainage and lead to fluid accumulation in a limb or body cavity. **Uremia** (high levels of urea in the blood) can result from compression of the **ureters** (tubes that conduct urine from the kidneys to the bladder), retarding the excretion of urine.

While the physical effects of cancer are nearly all straightforward and relatively easy to understand, many *chemical* effects of cancer elude explanation. Loss of appetite, weight loss, immune system suppression, and certain blood-clotting abnormalities associated with cancer are among the principal chemical effects of malignant neoplasms. None of these have been completely explained. Among the more straightforward chemical impacts of cancer are those that result from excess hormone secretion from neoplasms of endocrine glands.

Certain effects of cancer may result from either physical or chemical factors—or both. Anemia, for example, may be caused by erosion-induced hemorrhage and/or by disruption of delicate balances between procoagulation and anticoagulation "forces" in favor of anticoagulation. Complicating matters still more is the fact that physical effects may *lead to* chemical problems. Blockage, for example, can lead to the death of cells, and **necrotic** (dead and disintegrating) tissue may release "factors" that impair the immune response, impair appetite, and/or cause fevers.

Typically, advanced cancer is accompanied by an intensifying combination of physical and chemical effects on the host, amounting to an advanced cancer "syndrome." In the following pages, we look at the principal components of this syndrome one at a time, even though they almost never occur that way.

Cachexia

Cancer patients often appear to wither away. With some malignancies, the wasting occurs gradually (unexplained weight loss is sometimes the *first* sign of cancer); with others, it occurs more abruptly near the very end. The clinical term for this process is **cachexia**, as in "cachexia of cancer syndrome." This syndrome includes loss of appetite (**anorexia**), weight loss, pallor or anemia, apathy, malnutrition, and general weakness.

There is no clear explanation for cachexia. While it is obvious that the loss of appetite (see the next section) could be a major cause, along with such equally obviously, directly related things as blockages or other involvement of the gastrointestinal (GI) tract, cachexia occurs in patients even with good nutrition and without GI complications. Furthermore, the degree of cachexia does not correlate with the size of a neoplasm and the metabolic demands of the tumor alone. Several research studies have suggested that there may be a "factor" or factors—released in different amounts and at different times by different neoplasms and that this factor accounts for cachexia (see "TNF/Cachectin" section in Chapter 14).

We will consider the following possible causes of cachexia, individually or in combination: (1) general disruption in body chemistry, brought on by cancer; (2) the release of toxic products from cancer cells; (3) the generally wasteful energy metabolism of neoplasms (see Chapter 4); (4) the trapping of nutrients by malignant neoplasms; and (5) progressive deterioration of vital functions. Let us now take a closer look at these under the symptomatic headings "loss of appetite" and "weight loss."

Anorexia

By itself, the word **anorexia** means "loss of appetite." Anorexia is perhaps the most common symptom of cancer and is the most clear-cut cause of cachexia, if not the whole story. Anorexia nervosa is an aversion to food and is derived from an abnormal, unexplained fear of getting fat. It reportedly took the life of singer-celebrity Karen Carpenter, thus underscoring the power of mind over matter—even when the mind doesn't have everything in the right perspective. Every reader is no doubt already aware that mental state and appetite are closely related. When the mind is "in neutral," say, during a relaxed week at the lake, or whenever the mind otherwise has control of the world, appetite is good. Most people under stress lose their appetites. (In keeping with the general "truth" that there are few, if any, absolutes connected with cancer, some people overeat when they are stressed.) Cancer is a source of stress, and a loss of appetite should be expected in cancer patients. But apparently only *some* of the appetite loss results from the worry and distress of cancer.

Anorexia can be present when a neoplasm is still the size of a pea before the host knows that he or she has cancer. What then? Perhaps the brain is being influenced by something. The appetite control center is located in the hypothalamus, a small part of the brain located in the center of the skull just above the pituitary gland. Perhaps hunger is suppressed there, or the sense of fullness (**satiety**) stimulated there by a powerful factor released by the neoplasm or possibly by normal tissue in response to the presence of the neoplasm. Perhaps the appetite control center is influenced by *normal* appetite control factors in abnormal amounts. Impaired liver and the destruction of cells in and around a neoplasm are known to be able to raise the level of circulating fatty acids and amino acids—both of which are known to be able to suppress appetite.

Still another possibility, based on some evidence, is that the presumed hunger-inhibiting material may act by altering the sense of taste such that food becomes unappetizing (Bondy, 1976). Cancer patients often develop a dislike for certain foods, the smell of which can even induce nausea or the feeling of being full. A whole spectrum of taste and smell disorders have been linked to malignancy, and some of these in turn have been linked to chemical imbalances involving trace metals such as zinc and copper (Schein et al., 1975). Greater sensitivity of taste to certain things, such as urea, and decreased sensitivity to others, such as sugar, have been documented, and these changes could obviously influence the way food tastes.

It should be mentioned here that chemotherapy and radiation therapy sometimes have negative impacts on the gastrointestinal tract and these and other side effects of therapy can also result in loss of appetite. We consider this problem together with other side effects of therapy in Chapter 17.

Malaise

Cancer patients often don't feel well. Malaise is another complex symptom with many contributing causes. Malnutrition, pain, impaired function of particular organ systems, and the mental state that comes with knowing one has cancer may provide much of the explanation. But here again, even after these factors are accounted for a good portion of the problem remains. Maybe some kind of unknown systemic "factor" released by the cancer is at work here also. In any case, the somewhat subjective sensation of not feeling well could certainly be another reason for loss of appetite.

Weight Loss

Experimental animals made to carry tumors become cachexic even if they are force-fed. Likewise, cancer patients that eat very well or that receive a near perfect diet intravenously (IV), sometimes still lose weight. Even under such circumstances, the organs that lose weight (and that particularly lose nitrogen) are the *very same* ones (mainly muscle) that lose weight and nitrogen during starvation. Clearly, loss of appetite isn't the whole weight-loss story. If "all the right stuff" is going in and weight is still being lost, there are only two possible explanations: (1) the food isn't being absorbed, or (2) it isn't being used properly by the body once it *is* absorbed. The fact that IV feeding *bypasses* absorption and puts the "right stuff" directly into the blood indicates by default that the improper use of foodstuffs must be at least *part* of the story.

Malabsorption can be the ultimate result of several conditions, one of which is a hypermotile GI tract. Quite simply, if the contents of the GI tract move through too quickly, there isn't enough time for digestion or absorption, *both* of which result in diminished absorption. Certain kinds of cancer *are* associated with increased GI motility "possibly" related to imbalances in blood-borne chemicals that influence motility.

Certain neoplasms impair lymphatic drainage from the GI tract, and the lymphatics are the principal route by which *fats* are removed from the digestive tract. But even malignancies *not* involving the GI tract directly and not causing increased GI motility are known to be associated with malabsorption of fats, sugars, and other substances. The mechanisms are unknown.

In Chapter 4 we considered the tendency of malignant neoplasms to engage in a highly wasteful mode of energy metabolism; cancer cells tend to oxidize sugar only partially—anaerobically, instead of using oxygen to oxidize sugar completely. As a result, they get only a small fraction of the energy that they would if they used sugar normally. Another consequence of this anaerobic mode of metabolism is that lactic acid and other partially oxidized sugar products are formed and may cause some of the other problems we attribute to "metabolic changes" throughout this chapter. Another matter may make the energy situation even worse. Whenever lactic acid* and other organic acids accumulate, these organic acids are cycled to the liver (called the Cori Cycle) to be made into glucose once again. This recycling requires the host to use energy to make up for the metabolic mistakes of the tumor.

Another possible problem is that cancer cells, and maybe even normal cells of the tumor-bearing host, burn off energy rather like oil companies do when they flare off the natural gas from oil wells. There is some evidence that cancer cells are somehow less able to couple reactions that give off energy to those that require energy, resulting in a higher proportion of metabolic energy being given up directly as waste heat. In any case, tumor-bearing humans and other animals typically exhibit an increased basal metabolic rate. They burn up more energy at rest than do normal animals, in a manner analogous to automobiles with their "idles" turned up.

Starving animals, in sharp contrast, generally exhibit a *de*creased basal metabolic rate. This fact has suggested that the tumor possibly influences host tissue to engage in energy-inefficient

---

*In vigorous exercise, muscles short of oxygen will *also* engage in anaerobic metabolism, building up what is known as "oxygen debt"; that is, incompletely oxidized products of the breakdown of glucose.

activities. It has been suggested, for example, that selective removal of certain key metabolites by the tumor forces normal tissues to engage in more energy-costly metabolism. Because they don't have the "right" starting materials, they can't do things the "easy" way, so they do them the "hard" way. Although he admitted that experimental evidence was yet to come, Theologides (1972) hypothesized that cancer may induce cachexia by upsetting the metabolism of the host by producing chemical substances that turn various normal biochemical pathways on and off without purpose. The neoplasm makes normal host cells do useless things, while itself being relatively immune to these influences because of its near total commitment to growth.

As if all this chaos were not enough, experiments with animals (several decades ago) showed that malignant neoplasms are apparently somehow able to grow and accumulate nitrogen at the expense of the host tissues (Mider, Tesluk, and Morton, 1948). When nutrition is poor, the neoplasm gets served first; indeed, tumors are able to accumulate protein nitrogen faster than it is delivered by the diet—the difference coming from other host tissues.

In summary, cancer patients lose weight because they lose their appetite, because they don't absorb well what they do eat, because malignant neoplasms waste energy, and possibly because they induce normal host tissues to waste energy.

Hormonal Effects

Hormones from Neoplasms Originating in Hormone-Secreting Tissue

A neoplasm (benign or malignant) that arises from tissue (endocrine or placental) that *normally* secretes a particular hormone may retain the ability to secrete that hormone and may cause its levels to rise. Quite naturally, the body responds as if it had too much of that hormone—that is, it exhibits a characteristic syndrome from this *otherwise* "appropriate" hormone secretion. The effects of hormone elevations are often the first sign of an endocrine gland neoplasm. Such neoplasms are so frequently the cause of hormone elevations that when a physician sees evidence of an abnormal hormone elevation, the next step is to rule out or to confirm the presence of a neoplasm! Malignancies of each endocrine tissue can cause the syndrome associated with overproduction of the hormone normally produced. This pattern includes a wide variety of syndromes associated with neoplasms of the pituitary gland (**hypophysis**) that regulate many other endocrine glands. Complicating matters for patients and their physicians is the fact that tumors arising in tissue thought to have no business secreting hormones, do in fact sometimes secrete them.

Hormones from Tissues That "Apparently" Have No Business Secreting Them

Another way of saying that cancer cells tend to be relatively undifferentiated is to say that they really have no "clear" identity. Since all cells contain *all* the genes present in the original fertilized egg, a cell in a state of abnormal differentiation is technically capable of doing just about anything that *any* other cell can do. Many tumors arising in the lung and in other nonendocrine hormone-secreting tissue secrete hormones. Sometimes the hormones are the "real thing." Sometimes they are "near hormones," substances that have hormonelike effects. These substances may be partially active subunits (parts) of their normal, more complex counterparts. The term **paraneoplastic syndrome** is used to describe those symptoms of cancer that cannot be explained by local or distant spread of cancer or by the secretion of hormones *normally* produced by the tissue from which the cancer arose (Robbins and Cotran, 1979). Syndromes produced by the **"inappropriate" (ectopic) se-**

cretion of hormones would be included in the group of paraneoplastic syndromes.*

How is it that cancer cells *not* originating in hormone-producing tissue make hormones or "near hormones"? We don't know. Simple explanations such as the "accidental" turning on of genes normally turned off cannot explain why certain kinds of neoplasms tend to produce certain hormones and not others (although some neoplasms can produce several different hormones), or why not *all* neoplasms produce hormones. One possibility is that neoplasms arise from primitive cells normally very few in number present in all or many tissues and which already have—even before malignant transformation—the ability to produce hormones.

According to Rees and Landon (1976), the actual extent of the association of ectopic hormone production with cancer is unknown. The reason is that hormone levels may be high but not high enough to produce clinically obvious symptoms in many cases. A partial list of some of the more important ectopic hormone syndromes is given in Table 12.2.

Metabolic Complications

A number of metabolic changes are associated with cancer. Many of these are linked to other complications such as blockage of ureters, hormone imbalances, and gastrointestinal changes. Two of the most notable metabolic complications are hypercalcemia and hypoglycemia.

Malignancy is actually *the* most common cause of **hypercalcemia**, or high levels of calcium in the blood (Besarab and Caro, 1978). Hypercalcemia is associated with cancer for several different reasons. First of all, cancer associated with bone can result in the dissolution of bone and release the calcium—a primary structural component of bone. This most common cause of hypercalcemia in cancer is now believed to in-

volve prostaglandins as the agents that stimulate bone cells to release calcium. Another cause of hypercalcemia stems from the fact that tumors of the parathyroid glands can result in high levels of parathyroid hormone. **Parathyroid hormone** normally regulates blood calcium levels; it is released in response to low blood calcium levels and acts by causing calcium to be released from bone. Hypercalcemia can also result from the production of the inappropriate secretion of a parathyroid hormone-like substance (or substances) by some neoplasms. The symptoms of hypercalcemia progress from achiness, malaise, and depression to severe psychoses, coma, and, in the extreme, death.

Hypoglycemia (low blood sugar) associated with cancer may likewise have several origins, the most common being the impaired liver. The liver normally serves as a blood sugar bank, accepting "deposits" and allowing "withdrawals" so as to keep blood sugar levels *constant*. The liver normally does this so well that even after weeks of starvation it can still effectively keep blood sugar levels normal by making sugar from other things (**gluconeogenesis**). The impaired liver is unable to deal with the combined ravages of not eating and the high sugar demand of a malignant neoplasm. Hypoglycemia can also be caused by insulin-secreting tumors of the pancreas (certain cells of which normally secrete insulin) and other (ectopic) insulin-secreting tumors; it can also be caused by various other metabolic imbalances in ways that are not yet clear.

Blood Changes

Blood changes associated with cancer are derived from such *other* complications as hemorrhage, hormonal imbalances, malnutrition, autoimmune reactions to blood cells, and bone marrow infiltration. Some of the more profound blood changes associated with cancer are increases and decreases in numbers of the various types of blood cells and other forms of alteration in the clotting mechanism.

---

*Some authors use the term *paraneoplastic syndrome* in a more general way, to mean all the systemic effects cancer might have on the host.

Table 12.2 Some Ectopic Hormone Syndromes Associated with Cancer

"Hormone" and (Normal Tissue of Origin)	Some of the Neoplasms Involved	Syndrome
ACTH (Adrenocorticotropic Hormone) (adrenal cortex)	Oat cell carcinoma of the lung, pancreatic cancer, carcinoid tumors of lung	Cushing's syndrome (obesity, muscle-wasting diabetes, hypertension, edema, body hair in females)
Sex hormones; e.g., lutinizing hormone (pituitary gland/placenta)	Carcinomas of the liver and lung	Precocious puberty in young girls, breast development in older men
Antidiuretic hormone (posterior pituitary gland)	Lung carcinomas	Weakness, confusion, and coma
Parathyroid hormone (parathyroid glands)	Lung, liver, colon	Hypercalcemia leading to mental confusion, coma, death
Thyroid-stimulating hormone (pituitary gland)	Placental tumors	Hyperthyroidism, weight loss, accelerated heart rate, etc.
Insulin (pancreas)	Carcinoid tumors of lung	Hypoglycemia
Erythropoietin (kidney)	Hepatomas, pheochromocytoma	Polycythemia

Blood-Clotting Abnormalities

Malignant neoplasms sometimes produce and secrete coagulation factors into the blood. This production alone, or together with (1) other unknown "factors," (2) the retardation of blood flow (**stasis**) that results from cancer blockages or prolonged confinement to bed, and (3) an excess of **platelets** (see Chapter 3) seen in some cancer patients, can result in an *increased* tendency of the blood to clot. These things explain why—if not exactly how—some cancer patients develop blood clots (**thromboses**) in their deep veins. Such clots can become fatal problems if they break loose and lodge in a vital organ (lung, heart, or brain) causing an **infarction** (deprivation of oxygen and nutrients from tissues that critically need them). Infarctions secondary to blood clots and other causes are one of the main reasons for organ failure as a terminal event in cancer (see discussion of ultimate causes of death below). Ironically, *hyper*coagulability can lead to *hypo*coagulability with progressive consumption of platelets during coagulation.

If, over a period of time, more platelets are "used up" in clots than are generated from bone marrow, the point will eventually be reached where the blood will not clot normally, because of a critical shortage of platelets (**thrombocytopenia**). Actually the most common cause of platelet deficiency in cancer is diminished production of the bone marrow cells (**megakaryocytes**) that "break up" during maturation to form platelets. The basis of the decreased production of blood cells in bone marrow is described below under "anemia." Other causes of platelet deficiency include the abnormal *destruction* of platelets by the spleen secondary to autoimmune reactions to antigens on the surface of platelets, the reactants marking them for destruction—*by* the spleen.

Hemorrhage

Infiltrating cancer can erode the walls of a blood vessel anywhere in the body. If the vessel is large enough, and particularly if the vessel is a high-pressure artery, this process can end—along with the life of the cancer patient—as a massive hemorrhage. Hemorrhages are more likely in patients with blood-clotting problems secondary to platelet deficiency. Gradual blood loss from multiple or slow, chronic hemorrhages from small blood vessels can lead to other complications such as anemia.

Anemia and Polycythemia

Anemia is the most common complication of cancer involving the blood itself. Infiltration of bone by cancer can "crowd out" the normal blood cell production machinery and cause a decrease in circulating blood cells. Decreases in *some* kinds of blood cells can be the result of the expansion of *other* bone marrow cells, such as the increase in leukemic cells in leukemia. Infiltration can also be a result of metastasis to bone, most commonly from cancers of the breast, lung, prostate, or kidney. Whatever the source of the invading cells, marrow infiltration can result in several different kinds of blood cell deficiency problems: (1) **anemia** (decreased red blood cells and hemoglobin, and thus impaired tissue oxygenation); (2) **thrombocytopenia** (decreased platelets, and thus impaired blood coagulation); and (3) **leukopenia** (decreased white cells, and thus impaired immune competence). **Pancytopenia** is a condition in which all blood cells are reduced to critically low numbers.*

As pointed out earlier, anemia can also result from the chronic loss of blood—if red blood cells are lost faster than they can be replaced by even a *normal* bone marrow. Still another cause of anemia in cancer is the suppressive effect of many anticancer drugs and radiation therapy on the cells that generate red blood cells in the bone marrow. Nutritional deficiency resulting from either not eating or from malabsorption can be another underlying cause of cancer-associated anemia. Some specific nutritional deficiencies that retard the maturation of red blood cells in-

clude folic acid deficiency, iron deficiency, and vitamin B-12 deficiency. Still other forms of cancer-associated anemia include "**autoimmune hemolytic anemia**" most commonly associated with leukemias and lymphomas. In this form of anemia, the body develops antibodies against its own red blood cells causing the red cells to be prematurely lysed (destroyed) and removed from the circulation by the spleen.

At the other end of the spectrum, *in*creased numbers of red blood cells (**polycythemia**) can result from kidney carcinomas when the cancer cells secrete **erythropoietin**, a hormone normally secreted by the kidney serving to regulate red blood cell production. Sometimes polycythemia is a result of *ectopic* erythropoietin production by neoplasms of the lung and other organs. An increase in the number of white blood cells (other than in leukemia) is sometimes seen in cancer patients, but this is almost always a normal reaction to infection or inflammation.

Neurological Complications

The nervous system can be affected in a number of ways by malignant disease but by far the most common is the direct impact of expanding cell masses—primary tumors or metastasis—on neural tissue. A whole spectrum of abnormal behavioral effects is associated with cancer in the brain, the effect depending on the location and the extent of the impact. By causing chemical imbalances—excessively high sodium (**hypernatremia**) or calcium (**hypercalcemia**) levels, for example, neoplasms can induce psychoses and other, sometimes severe, psychotic symptoms indirectly. Pain is a special kind of neurological complication.

Pain

The first thing one usually hears about pain in cancer is that cancer patients have such severe pain that they have to take narcotics. Although pain is very commonly associated with cancer

---

*According to Fabian and Hoogstraten (1977), anemias associated with chronic diseases including cancer are usually only mild to moderate. Normally the **hematocrit** (percent of the blood that is packed red blood cells) is about 45 percent; in moderate anemia, the percentage is down around 30 percent.

(roughly a third of all cancer patients experience significant pain), its degree and impact are actually highly variable. It could actually be argued—in all seriousness—that the problem with cancer is that it doesn't cause pain soon enough. It is the *lack* of pain in malignancies of digestive organs (stomach, liver, colon) that allows cancer to grow to large size before the host suspects something is wrong.

The early growth of neoplasms causes pain only when the growth is situated so as to cause increasing tension or pressure in tissues such as connective tissue that are relatively inelastic. Neoplasms—benign or malignant—of the brain, for example, cannot expand very much at all without putting pressure on the membranes of the confining cranial cavity, causing headaches.

Pain associated with advanced cancer may result from (1) growth that leads to stretching of connective tissue, such as the periostium of bone or the capsules that surround internal organs, or even the scar tissue derived from surgery; (2) the compression (stimulation) of nerves directly; (3) compression that results in **ischemia** (diminished blood flow or oxygen); (4) direct infiltration of nerve bundles or the spinal cord by cancer cells; and (5) cancer-related infection and inflammation. The facts that nerves whose job it is to deliver pain information to the brain can be stimulated by any point along the way to the brain, and that "uncommon" pain signals can enter the spinal cord so as to be confused with more common pain signals entering the cord at the same level sets up the possibility of referred pain. **Referred pain** appears to be coming from a place other than the one where the damage is taking place. As with all kinds of pain, cancer pain perception varies with mental state.

Fever

Almost three-quarters of all cancer patients experience bouts with fever sometime during the course of their disease. Fever is more commonly associated with certain types of cancer; leukemias, Hodgkin's disease, and other lymphomas top the list. Most often, when cancer patients develop fevers it's because of an infection (Yates, 1973, claims that 75 percent of the fevers in leukemia and lymphoma patients, and virtually *all* the fevers associated with *solid* tumors, are the result of underlying infection). Sometimes fevers only *appear* not to be associated with an infection because the infection is isolated and not apparent. But apparently some cancer-associated fevers are not derived from infection, particularly in certain forms of kidney cancer. What then? Well, here once more, we have the specter of some mysterious body thermostat-resetting factor, a **pyrogen** (fever-causing substance) possibly produced by a neoplasm or by the body in response to the presence of one.

There is considerable disagreement about the degree of noninfectious fever. Some believe that *all* cancer-related fever is associated with an infection, however latent. Others believe that as many as 40 percent of cancer patients have *non*infectious fever at some time during the course of their disease (see Bondy, 1976). Although it contributes to energy depletion and weight loss, fever is a relatively unimportant component of the cancer syndrome.

Immune Suppression and Infection

Many infections associated with cancer are caused by microorganisms that are normally harmless (for example, *Escherichia coli*, a normal inhabitant of the lower GI tract). Such infections are related to impaired immune function, to antibiotic-induced upsets in normal microbial balances, and to other complications that loosen controls on microbes. Several factors in cancer compromise immune systems. Many chemotherapeutic drugs suppress immunity by killing the normally actively dividing cells that underpin the immune system (Chapter 3). Also, cancer, itself, has an immunosuppressive effect on the host.

Table 12.3 Some of the More Important Immune Defense-Compromising Cancers and the Specific Defects Associated with Each

	Decreased Number of Granulocytes[a] (granulocytopenia)	Altered Granulocyte Function	Altered Humoral Immunity	Altered Cellular Immunity
Leukemia				
Lymphocytic				
Acute	+ + + +	+ +	+ +	+
Chronic			+ + + +	+ +
Myelocytic				
Acute	+ + + +	+ +		+
Chronic		+ +		
Hodgkin's disease		+	+	+ + + +
Lymphosarcoma			+ +	+ + +
Multiple myeloma			+ + + +	
Advanced neoplasms				+ + +

Note: Degree of impairment: +, Minimal; + +, Minor; + + +, Moderate; + + + +, Severe.
[a]See Chapter 3.

Source: Yates, 1973. Reprinted by permission of Grune and Stratton and the author.

Many leukemias and lymphomas, particularly, suppress the normal immune response. This suppression is probably somehow related to the fact that these malignancies involve the lymphoid tissues. A summary of the immune system defects induced by cancer is given as Table 12.3.

Infection is also made more likely in cancer patients because of malnutrition, impaired circulation, **fistulas** (openings that connect cavities that are not normally connected, such as the GI tract and the peritoneal cavity), impaired lymphatic drainage, and impaired movement of material through the lower digestive tract. Bacteria normally reside in the lowest parts of the GI tract, and the analward movement of GI tract contents normally sweeps these microbes out about as fast as they reproduce, creating a dynamic balance. If movement of GI contents is retarded, the balance can be upset, allowing the microbes to get out of control.

Skin Changes

Skin is affected by cancer in a number of ways. One form of **acanthosis nigricans** (a disease marked by increased thickness and pigmentation of the skin of the armpit and the back of the neck) is so highly associated with neoplasms that its appearance in mid-life or later *demands* a search for an underlying cancer. **Dermatomyositis**, a nonspecific, probably autoimmune-induced inflammation of skin and muscle (see section on "other host effects" below) is also associated with cancer. The skin changes in this condition amount to a rash over parts of the head, neck, chest, and limbs. Cancer-associated skin "reddening" and/or "thickening" are associated with breast cancer, lung cancer, and cancer of various internal organs (see Bondy, 1976). For reasons unknown, some cancers are associated with itching. For a good recent review (with 29 full-color photographs) of the dermatological manifestations of internal cancer, see Thiers (1986).

Reproductive Function

Because cancer predominantly afflicts those *past* their reproductive years, the impact of cancer on psychosexual dysfunction receives far more attention than any impact it has on reproduction per se. Cancer-associated sexual problems derived from self-image and states of mind are considered, together with other psychological impacts, in Chapter 19. We will concern ourselves here only with cancer's direct impacts on reproductive organs.

First of all, cancer can obviate reproduction by directly impairing the reproductive organs or through surgical treatment. In women, removal of both ovaries (**bilateral oophorectomy**) prevents reproduction except via embryo transplant. **Hysterectomy** (removal of the uterus) obviously precludes pregnancy. Reproductive function in males can be impaired by surgery that prevents ejaculation or erection—including (1) surgery that affects nerves and blood vessels supplying the reproductive organs; (2) the effects of drug and hormone (such as estrogen) therapy and radiation therapy on spermatogenesis; and (3) surgical **castration** (removal of the testes) in testicular cancer. Impotence can also be secondary to cancer-associated psychosexual problems as well as to uremia and other metabolic complications. Malignancies of the pituitary and adrenal glands can upset the hormone balances that control reproductive function in either sex.

One final note: fetuses are, in terms of cell growth, much like neoplasms—strictly speaking, fetuses are indeed "neo" plasms, new growths (see Chapter 1). This point is raised to call attention to the fact that chemotherapeutic drugs have a devastating effect on an embryo. This is why women undergoing chemotherapy or radiation therapy are advised to avoid pregnancy during treatment.

Other Host Effects

Cancer has other complications of which we *also* know woefully little. Cancer patients show an increased tendency to develop immune reactions against "self"—called *autoimmune disease*. An otherwise rare disease mentioned earlier, dermatomyositis (nonspecific inflammation of muscle and skin tissue), is relatively commonly associated with cancer, affecting some one-fourth to one-third of all cancer patients; it is believed to be the result of an **autoimmune reaction** (immune system attacks other normal host tissue). In some cases only muscle is involved, and the condition is called **polymyositis**. This condition is marked by soreness and weakness in certain muscles, histological appearance of inflammation, and autoimmune reactivity to muscle. Anti-inflammatory agents give relief, as does complete removal of the cancer.

Bone and joint problems resembling symptoms of arthritis are not unusual in cancer patients. These symptoms are also thought to be related to autoimmune reaction (rheumatoid arthritis, itself, is an autoimmune problem). Skeletal problems also include fractures linked to the dissolution of bone by infiltrating cancer cells. Bones may also be weakened by various hormone imbalances caused by ectopically produced hormones with **osteolytic** (bone-dissolving) activity. Being confined to bed contributes to decalcification of bone for the same reason that decalcification is a problem for astronauts during periods of weightlessness—calcium is deposited in bone partly in response to local stress and when structural stress is reduced, calcium is lost.

Kidney disease is associated with some forms of carcinoma and with some sarcomas. Some of the problems result from an immune reaction—complexes between antibodies and antigens affecting the membranes of the filtering apparatus of the kidney. The most common cause of kidney failure in cancer is obstruction of the ureters or urethra; hypercalcemia is the second most common cause. Excessively high calcium levels in the urine causes a form of diuresis that eventually destroys the kidney's ability to concentrate urine, and this leads to water loss and dehydration.

Ultimate Causes of Death

According to Bondy (1976) and Inagaki, Rodriguez, and Bodey (1974), infection—usually in the form of **septicemia** (pathogenic bacteria in the blood) or pneumonia—is the cause of the ultimately fatal episode in about one-third of all cancer deaths. It is a major factor in about *half* of all cancer deaths. Following infection as the major cause of death are organ failure, infarction (blockage of a blood vessel), and hemorrhage (see Table 12.4).

According to Saunders (1976; see also Klastersky, Daneau, and Verhest, 1972, and Inagaki et al., 1974) terminal infections most commonly involve the normal bacterial inhabitant of the lower digestive tract, *Escherichia coli*, and various species of the genera *Klebsiella* and *Pseudomonas* (see Table 12.5). Blood infections in acute leukemia sometimes involve fungi, such as *Candida albicans*. It is interesting that before the age of antibiotics, a different set of microbes caused *most* of the terminal infections in cancer. The so-called gram-negative microorganisms listed above are relatively resistant to antibiotics.

Inagaki et al. (1974), in a study of 816 cancer deaths at the M.D. Anderson Hospital in the late 1960's, reported that organ failure was attributable—in order of importance—to failures of the lungs, heart, liver, brain, and kidney. Infarction as a specific cause of organ failure ranked third as a separate category.

Ultimately fatal hemorrhages most frequently occur in the brain or GI tract (see Table 12.6). In more than half of such cases in the study by Inagaki and colleagues, the massive bleeding was caused by the neoplasm directly; platelet deficiency was responsible for about another one-fifth.

The ultimate cause of death in many cancer patients cannot be pinned down because many factors contribute at the same time. Such deaths are attributed to **carcinomatosis**.

Table 12.4 The Most Common Ultimate Causes of Death from Cancer in a Study of 816 Cancer Deaths

Primary Cause	Number	Percent
Infection	380	47
Organ failure	201	25
Infarction	90	11
Hemorrhage	62	7
Carcinomatosis	83	10
Total	816	100

Source: Inagaki, Rodriguez, and Bodey, 1974. Reprinted by permission of J. B. Lippincott Co. and the author.

Summary

Because it is out of control in terms of its impact on the host via both growth and secreted products, cancer has a devastating impact on nearly all normal bodily functions. Cancer "squeezes" and "blocks," causing a host of local and systemic effects. Cancer cells secrete products including hormones, hormonelike substances, and possibly other "mystery substances" that powerfully influence normal metabolic function and wreak havoc with normal physiological control. Physical and chemical effects of cancer account for such seemingly different kinds of problems as immune suppression, infection, fever, chemical imbalances such as hypercalcemia, cachexia, loss of appetite, anemia, polycythemia, and psychoses.

The ultimate causes of death in cancer patients, in order of importance, are (1) infection, (2) impairment of key vital organs (the brain, the lungs, and the liver), and (3) hemorrhage, followed by (4) various metabolic complications and chemical imbalances lumped under the label **carcinomatosis**. All these impacts must be considered along with the underlying malig-

Table 12.5 Infections Causing Death in Cancer Patients (see Table 12.4)

Type of Infection	Number of Patients	Percent of Infections	Percent of All Patients
Septicemia (bacteria in the bloodstream)	147	38	18
Pneumonia	192	51	24
Peritonitis (infection of the abdominal cavity)	25	6	3
Other	16	5	2
Total	380	100	47

Organisms Causing Fatal Infections in a Group of 221 Cancer Patients in Whom the Fatal "Event" Was an Infection

Type/Species	Percent of the 221 Patients
Single, gram-negative organism	68
E. coli	23
P. aeruginosa	11
Klebsiella spp.	9
Proteus spp.	8
Other gram-negative	17
Single, gram-positive organism	9
Staph. aureus	4
Clostridia spp.	2
Other gram-positive	3
Multiple organisms	15

Adapted from Inagaki, Rodriguez, and Bodey, 1974. Reprinted by permission of J. B. Lippincott Co. and the author.

nancy in the medical management of cancer, which we will consider in Chapter 17.

Having considered the impact of cancer on the *individual*, we now turn to the impact of cancer on *populations*. There is far more to the impact of cancer on populations than the simple sum of its impacts on individuals.

References and Further Readings

Bernstein, I. L., and Sigmundi, R. A. 1980. Tumor Anorexia: A Learned Food Aversion. *Science*. 209: 416–18.

Besarab, A., and Caro, J. F. 1978. Mechanisms of Hypercalcemia in Malignancy. *Cancer*. 41(6):2276–85.

Bondy, P. K. 1976. Systemic Effects of Neoplasia. In T. Symington and R. L. Carter, eds., *Scientific Foundations of Oncology*. Chicago: Heinemann Medical Books/ Yearbook Medical Publishers.

Botsford, T. W., and Cady, B., eds. 1978. *Cancer: A Manual for Practioners*, 5th ed. Boston: American Cancer Society, Massachusetts Division.

Costa, G. 1977. Cachexia, the Metabolic Component of Neoplastic Disease. *Cancer Research*. 37: 2327–35.

Costa, G., and Donaldson, S. S. 1979. Effects of Cancer and Cancer Treatment on the Nutrition of the Host. *New England J. Med*. 300:1471–74.

Table 12.6 Some Common Sites of Ultimately Fatal Hemorrhages in Cancer Patients

Site	Number of Patients	Percent
Gastrointestinal	19	31
Brain	15	24
Rupture of major blood vessel	12	19
Lung	7	11
Other[a]	9	15
Total	62	100

[a]Includes peritoneal (6), pleural (2), and ventricular wall (1).

Source: Inagaki, Rodriguez, and Bodey, 1974, Table 9. Reprinted by permission of J. B. Lippincott and the author.

Deftos, L. J., and Neer, R. 1974. Medical Management of the Hypercalcemia of Malignancy. *Ann. Rev. Med.* 25:323–31.

Fabian, C., and Hoogstraten, G. 1977. Differential Diagnosis of Anemia and Cancer. *Ca-A Cancer Journal for Clinicians.* 27(2):88–99.

Fenninger, L. D., and Mider, G. B. 1954. Energy and Nitrogen Metabolism in Cancer. *Advances in Cancer Res.* 2:229–53.

Guillemin, R., et al. 1982. Growth-Hormone-Releasing Factor from a Human Pancreatic Tumor That Caused Acromegaly. *Science.* 218:585–87.

Holland, J. F., and Frei, E., eds. 1982. *Cancer Medicine.* 2nd ed. Philadelphia: Lea & Febiger.

Inagaki, J., Rodriguez, V., and Bodey, G. P. 1974. Causes of Death in Cancer Patients. *Cancer.* 33: 568–73.

Klastersky, J., Daneau, D., and Verhest, A. 1972. Causes of Death in Patients with Cancer. *European J. Cancer.* 8:149–54.

Lynch, H. T., and Fusaro, R. M. 1982. *Cancer-Associated Genodermatoses.* New York: Van Nostrand Reinhold.

Mathews, G. J., Zarro, V., and Osterholm, J. L. 1973. *Cancer Pain and Its Treatment, Seminars in Drug Treatment.* 3(1):45–53.

Mider, G. B., Tesluk, H., and Morton, J. J. 1948. Effect of Walker Carcinoma 256 on Food Intake, Body Weight, and Nitrogen Metabolism of Growing Rats. *Acta. Un. Int. Cancer.* 6:409–20.

Rees, L. H., and Landon, J. 1976. Biochemical Abnormalities in Some Human Neoplasms: (5) Inappropriate Biosynthesis of Hormones by Tumors. In T. Symington and R. E. Carter, eds., *Scientific Foundations of Oncology.* Chicago: Heinemann Medical Books/ Medical Yearbook Publishers.

Robbins, S. L., and Cotran, R. S. 1979. *Pathologic Basis of Disease.* Philadelphia: Saunders.

Saunders, C. M. 1976. The Challenge of Terminal Care. In T. Symington and R. E. Carter, eds., *Scientific Foundations of Oncology.* Chicago: Heinemann Medical Books/Medical Yearbook Publishers.

Schein, P. S., et al. 1975. Nutritional Complications of Cancer and Its Treatment. *Seminars in Oncology.* 2(4): 337–47.

Sylven, B., and Holmberg, B. 1965. On the Structure and Biological Effects of a Newly-Discovered Cytotoxic Polypeptide in Tumor Fluid. *European J. Cancer.* 1:199–203.

Thiers, B. H. 1986. Dermatologic Manifestations of Internal Cancer. *Ca-A Cancer Journal for Clinicians.* 36(3):130–48.

Theologides, A. 1972. Pathogenesis of Cachexia in Cancer. A Review and a Hypothesis. *Cancer.* 29(2): 484–88.

Yates, J. W. 1973. Problems of Neoplastic Disease: Infections. *Seminars in Drug Treatment.* 3(1):27–35.

Ecologists take great pains to point out that populations are not simply the sum of the individuals that make them up. First of all, populations, in the ecological sense and in the sense we will use the term here, are geographically (and in other ways) *defined* groups of individuals of the same species. The black bass in Golden Pond, the robins of Warren County, the squirrels in the Daniel Boone National Forest, the people of Iowa, the people of France, the Catholics in the Archdiocese of New York, the people of London with incomes of more than £30,000, and the people of Spanish descent in Los Angeles County—all qualify as populations.

Any population is more than the sum of its parts because, as a specific and unique level of biotic organization, populations have features and characteristics that individuals do not have. Populations have "densities," "patterns of distribution," "age profiles," "birth rates," "death rates," and average incomes and patterns of health and disease, to name just *some* examples.

Not only is it possible to learn things about disease by studying it at the population level, but some of the most important things to be learned about disease can be learned *only* at the population level. Almost everything we know for *sure* about the causes of human cancer, the impact of cancer, the effectiveness of cancer treatment, we learned through epidemiology.

13
The Epidemiology of Cancer

Epidemiology: A Population-Based Approach to Medicine

The Place of Epidemiology in Understanding Disease

As pointed out by Mausner and Bahn (1974), there are three fundamental ways of studying human disease, including cancer. They are (1) the basic science approach, (2) the clinical approach, and (3) the epidemiological approach.

The basic science approach is concerned with every detail of the causes (**etiology**) and the steps involved in the progression (**pathogenesis**) of the disease. What is the causative factor? How does it get in? Where does it go? How is it metabolized and excreted? What tissues are affected? What happens to it in water? In air? What exactly does it do at first? What happens then?

The clinician is concerned with the impact on the individual. What measurable changes occur in the exposed human that might be used to detect the presence and determine the extent of disease? What are the overt physiological symptoms? What will arrest the disease? What will relieve the symptoms?

The third approach, the community, population, or epidemiological approach examines the *relative* frequency of disease within a defined population and within subgroups of that population. What kinds of people are getting sick? Is the disease more prevalent among the young? The old? Factory workers? Does the disease exhibit a pattern that indicates that it is communicable?

The three approaches are usually employed in concert. In one exemplary pattern, epidemiology might discover that those who work with a particular chemical have relatively high rates of cancer. Laboratory scientists might then expose experimental animals to a suspected causative agent to confirm or refute the connection experimentally. If and when a connection is confirmed, clinicians would begin to look more carefully for the symptoms of disease among people exposed to the agent. The order of the three approaches is variable; any one approach might initially lead to the suspicion of a connection between specific agents and disease.

In 1974, a physician in Louisville, Kentucky, John Creech, observed that an unusual number of vinyl chloride workers had died of a rare liver cancer (hepatic angiosarcoma). Subsequent (epidemiologic) checks of death certificates confirmed the significance of this relationship. Almost simultaneously, scientists in Italy confirmed that vinyl chloride caused cancer in animals. Laboratory scientists and clinicians throughout the world then went to work investigating just *how* vinyl chloride "caused" liver cancer and how it might be detected, diagnosed, and treated.

What Do Epidemiologists Do?

Epidemiologists study the patterns of disease (magnitude over time, spatial distribution, etc.) within defined groups of people (a county, a state, a metropolitan area, etc.) and the relationships of these patterns to *other* patterns within that group (e.g., occupational patterns, residential patterns, who drinks water coming from what sources, etc.). Epidemiologists try to match up patterns of disease with other patterns, in an effort to identify possible cause-and-effect relationships. More often, epidemiologists try to *confirm* or *refute* match-ups already under suspicion. For example, after the initial observation that "an unusually large number of vinyl chloride workers died of liver cancer," epidemiologists went to work to assess just how much greater is the risk of liver cancer among vinyl chloride workers with varying degrees of historical exposure. Another way of defining **epidemiology** is to say that it is the study of patterns of disease within defined populations and the factors that are responsible for, or that influence, those patterns.

One of the key words in the preceding definition is *defined*. Perhaps the most easily misunderstood feature of the epidemiological approach to studying disease is that epidemiology depends on *rates* of disease. The importance of the word *defined* (as a modifier of group or population) lies in the need for a denominator to give dimension to expressions of magnitude. For example, 300 cancer deaths in a year would be high in a group of 6,000 people. The same number might be normal in a group of 100,000 people and low in a group of 1 million. The numbers of people with a certain disease have meaning only in terms of the number of people who *might* have developed the disease in some standard or control population.

Time is another important dimension. Epidemiologists can work with "morbidity" expressed in terms of time; that is, the percent of people who *have* the disease at one particular point in time (**prevalence**), or the number who are diagnosed within a given *period* of time (**incidence**). If **mortality** (death) is used, mortality must also be qualified in terms of some defined period of time.

Back to our earlier example: if someone came up to you and said he or she had found three cases of liver cancer, you might reply, "So what? A lot of people die of liver cancer each year—especially in Africa." If someone came up to you and reported the discovery of three cases in two years of a "rare" form of liver cancer in a single group of 1,200 American vinyl chloride workers, you might be more impressed. You might be moved to ask the key question, "How prevalent or how common *is* liver cancer among people in general?" If someone reported three cases of a certain type of liver cancer among 1,200 vinyl chloride workers in a single plant and noted that only 25 or 30 cases of this type of liver cancer were reported worldwide that year, you could be fairly sure that an occupational disease had been discovered. Although the vinyl chloride-hepatic angiosarcoma relationship was discovered in just such a way, usually differences in relative rates are not nearly so impressive. Epidemiologists usually work with *small* relative differences in rates of disease between the group of people exposed to some agent and those *not* exposed.

In epidemiological investigations, precise mathematical analyses are required, and extreme care must be given to the methods by which disease is observed, measured, or cataloged in well-defined groups. Great caution must be exercised to ensure that "apples are always being compared to apples." Chemical workers may have significantly greater *or less* risk of developing certain diseases than people in general. But these rates might be identical to groups of nonchemical workers with similar distributions of age, sex, race, socioeconomic status, and so on. Let's consider the concept of controls in a bit more detail.

Control Groups

As pointed out by Lave and Seskin (1979), if an association is found between "exposure to air pollution in cities" and "lung disease"—say, lung cancer—four explanations are possible:* (1) the observation is a false, chance occurrence resulting from the way the sampling was done; (2) air pollution causes or contributes to lung disease; (3) lung disease causes or contributes to air pollution; and (4) some *third* factor is responsible for *both* lung disease and air pollution. In order to conclude that air pollution is a cause or contributing factor in lung disease, the other three explanations must be ruled out. Generally, the first type of possibility is ruled out by repeating the study a number of times, and the third possibility is usually ignored. It is the fourth possibility that gives epidemiologists the most trouble, and this is where controls come in. The selection of a control group is intended to minimize the possibility that *other* factors might line up on one side or the other side of the comparison being made.

In the example just discussed, an association between exposure to air pollution in cities and lung cancer would result if old people, males, and smokers had high lung cancer rates no matter *where* they lived, and if cities tended to attract high proportions of old people, males, and smokers.

Age offers a particularly good case in point—that great care must be taken to compare apples with apples in cancer epidemiology research. Since cancer is largely a disease of the relatively old, investigators must be sure that differences in cancer rates between two populations are *not* a result of the fact that one population has proportionately more old people in it. This restriction does not mean that comparisons cannot be made between populations having different age profiles; it does mean that if such comparisons *are* made, the data must be "age-

---

*Assuming that no *bias* influenced the sampling of city and country dwellers, and smokers and nonsmokers.

adjusted." Typically this adjustment is made by comparing the age-specific rates of the two populations in some way. If a particular population is being compared to a large standard population—say, that of the whole United States—then the age-specific rates for the standard population can be used to calculate an expected number of cancers for the number of people in each age bracket of the population being evaluated. This expected number of cancer cases can then be compared to the actually observed number, with any difference or ratio then subjected to a statistical test of significance. This indirect method or other methods of making mathematical adjustment in populations being compared can also be applied to sex and race and other factors that might influence rates of cancer in "populations."

Epidemiologists work very hard to find control groups matched for as many other factors as possible. The effects of benzpyrene on lung cancer would best be studied (epidemiologically) by comparing the rates of lung cancer in a city having high benzpyrene levels with the rates in a city with low levels—but otherwise "identical."

Obviously, no two cities or groups of any sort are identical, and this inexactness is the "curse" with which all epidemiologists must live. The task then amounts to controlling confounding variables to the extent possible. Among the most common variables controlled in epidemiological studies are age, sex, race, and socioeconomic status.

Retrospective and Prospective Epidemiology

Epidemiology has the advantage of being able to look forward and backward. Suppose, by way of example, that we were concerned that a certain type of skin cancer was possibly caused by exposure to a certain pesticide. One first step might be to identify as many people as possible in whom the cancer was diagnosed within a certain (large enough) period of time. These people would then be matched with an equal number of similar people who have never had the cancer

and do not have it now. We could then look into the histories of the two groups and determine the proportion of those with the cancer exposed to the pesticide versus the proportion of those without the cancer exposed to the pesticide. If a very high proportion of those with the cancer in question was exposed to the pesticide and relatively few of the control group had ever been exposed, we might hypothesize that there *was* a connection. This type of backward-looking study (**retrospective study**) is called a "case control study."

Our second step might be to watch groups of exposed and nonexposed people over time to see how many of each group develop skin cancer. This would be a forward-looking, **prospective study**. Prospective studies start with exposure and look into the future for disease; retrospective studies generally start with newly diagnosed cases of disease today and look back for exposure (Fig. 13.1). Retrospective studies may also look back for both exposure and disease. Perhaps we should describe and contrast prospective and retrospective studies more completely.

Retrospective case control studies are those in which people with the disease in question are compared to similar people who do not have the disease (controls). Epidemiologists look to see if members of the two groups were exposed differently to various environmental or other factors; that is, if more of those with the disease (or those who died of the disease) were exposed to something suspected as a cause of the disease.

In retrospective studies, criteria establishing the study groups must be delineated as precisely as possible and the number of cases of disease should include all (or nearly all) of those who are newly diagnosed in a specified (and long enough) time period. This caution is necessary to avoid missing patients with a very short disease course (because they die rapidly or because they are cured quickly). Controls must be *very* carefully selected in such studies. If the control group is not matched with the disease group for important variables other than exposure to the factor under suspicion, then it is possible that

Study	Past	Present	Future

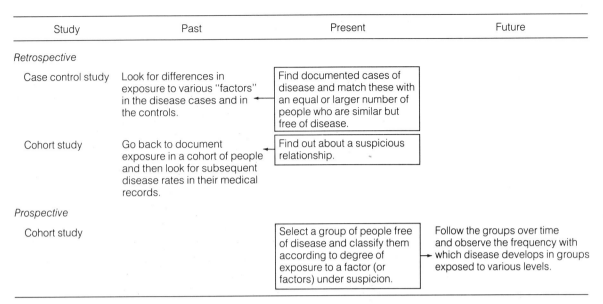

Retrospective

Case control study — Look for differences in exposure to various "factors" in the disease cases and in the controls. ← Find documented cases of disease and match these with an equal or larger number of people who are similar but free of disease.

Cohort study — Go back to document exposure in a cohort of people and then look for subsequent disease rates in their medical records. ← Find out about a suspicious relationship.

Prospective

Cohort study — Select a group of people free of disease and classify them according to degree of exposure to a factor (or factors) under suspicion. → Follow the groups over time and observe the frequency with which disease develops in groups exposed to various levels.

Figure 13.1 The difference between retrospective and prospective epidemiological studies is the way in which the study groups are assembled. In retrospective case control studies, epidemiologists select groups of people with disease and matched groups without disease and then look for exposure to the alleged causative agents in the history of these two groups. In both prospective and retrospective cohort studies, epidemiologists begin by fixing exposure; they then follow high-low or exposed-nonexposed groups for a period of time to see how many of which group will or did develop disease. (Adapted with permission from Mausner and Bahn, 1974, p. 313. Used by permission of W. B. Saunders Co. Reprinted from Kupchella and Hyland, 1986, p. 302, courtesy of Allyn and Bacon, Inc.)

some factor could confound any relationship between the suspected factor and the disease.

Incidence rates (see Chapter 1) cannot be derived in case control studies because the number of people at risk is not known (i.e., no basis exists on which the size of the group from which the identified cases arose can be determined). Once a case control study is completed, however, the relative degree of extra risk for those exposed can be estimated. Case control studies can yield a **relative risk estimate** or **odds ratio**, defined as the ratio of the odds of a diseased person having been exposed divided by the odds of a disease-free person having been exposed. We might learn from such a study that a person who smoked more than two packs of cigarettes per day is roughly 24 times more likely to have died of lung cancer than a "matched" nonsmoker.

The main advantage of case control studies is that they are quick and inexpensive—because the number of subjects to be evaluated is relatively small. The main disadvantages of all retrospective studies are that information about past exposure may not be available or may be inaccurate. Information provided by an informant about the past may be biased, as well. Another serious disadvantage is the difficulty in selecting an appropriate control group. More on this problem later.

Cohort studies are really organized ways of collecting data from inadvertent "experiments" with human subjects. Such studies start with a group of people (usually much larger than a case control study would require) free of disease but with known exposure to some suspicious agent. This group is then followed to see which people in the group develop disease, and/or whether those who have higher exposure to the suspected agent are more likely to develop the disease. The **cohort** (as used in epidemiology, a cohort is a group of people under epidemiological observation) selected for a prospective epidemiological study may be either heterogeneous with respect to previous exposure to the factor under study, or restricted to those having high (or low) exposure only. Cohort studies may be retrospective or prospective as long as the starting point is exposure, not disease.

The size of the cohort to be studied depends on a number of factors, not the least of which is the expected incidence or, reciprocally, the relative rarity of the disease. The study group would obviously have to be very large if it were expected at the outset that only a small percentage would develop disease. Other size-determining factors include availability of subjects, access to medical records, and size of the group that has been exposed to reasonably quantitative levels of a particular agent.

Cohort studies allow investigators to determine the "absolute" as well as the relative risk of developing disease in people exposed to a factor under question. Data derived from cohort studies can be expressed as either *relative risk* or *attributable risk*. **Relative risk** is an expression of how many times more likely one group is to develop disease than another. **Attributable risk** is the absolute difference in incidence rate between the members of the exposed group and the nonexposed group. Attributable risk is literally the number of deaths per unit number of people that can apparently be directly *attributed* to exposure to any factor (e.g., smoking) under consideration.

A major advantage of cohort studies over case control studies is that there are fewer opportunities for bias to creep in. The people under study are classified as to exposure before anything is known about disease. One other major advantage of the cohort approach is that it is more likely to reveal relationships between exposure and disease *other* than the one under suspicion. That is, in addition to confirming or refuting a specific relationship, prospective studies offer a good chance to discover other relationships as well (since a large number of people are followed very closely).

The main disadvantage of the cohort approach is that it involves large numbers of people over a *long* period of time and is therefore very expensive.

The Trouble with Controls and the Trouble with Epidemiology

We mentioned earlier that there is no such thing as a perfect control group. A consequence of this and some other limitations inherent in the epidemiological approach is that the conclusions derived from epidemiological investigation are far from absolute. This much may be obvious to the sophisticated reader who knows that absolute answers really don't come even from much more precise and more completely controlled laboratory investigations. Epidemiologists can be fairly exacting in establishing the degree of correlation between a disease and suspected etiologic agent. But even when correlations are nearly perfect, no cause-and-effect chain can be *absolutely* inferred.

In science, as in courtrooms, association is considered circumstantial evidence, although "guilt" can eventually become established through consistent association. Proof of the sort that comes from elegantly constructed laboratory experiments doesn't happen in epidemiological investigations. Proof usually emerges only gradually. Often it doesn't emerge fast enough. This problem is one of the major reasons why despite large volumes of circumstantial evidence, pollution control, and smoking and health continue to generate controversy.

Cancer Patterns Revisited and Expanded

Epidemiological methods provided the descriptive epidemiological data considered in the "Cancer Patterns" section of Chapter 1. Investigative or analytical epidemiology was the source

Several years ago, late one summer afternoon at the University of Louisville Health Sciences Center, we received a crate of live, but sick chickens suspected of having cancer. We were to make a tentative diagnosis and to prepare samples to be sent to the state veterinary diagnostic laboratory. We planned to keep some of the material for our own studies.

One of us reached into the cage and grabbed a chicken, presumably at random, and we were *not* surprised to find that the chosen one had a large ovarian neoplasm. We prepared a sample for shipment to the state lab; we provided the rest of the chickens with food and water; we turned off the lights and left for the day—planning to begin our studies of the tumors in the remaining chickens the next morning.

Not one of the remaining seven chickens had cancer.

It could have been pure chance that we happened to pick the only tumor-bearing chicken first, but is more likely that it was a result of bias. The sickest or otherwise slowest chickens are simply more likely to "get grabbed." We had probably experienced "sampling bias"—the consequence of which was a false impression of the population being sampled.

One example of how equivalent problems might arise in human studies is by using volunteers to represent a "control" population and failing to take into account the possibility that volunteers might be healthier, more health-conscientious, richer, more likely to be nonsmokers, more highly educated, and so on than nonvolunteers and thus than the population as a whole.

Another example of bias might be using the patient population of a particular hospital as a "control" group in the evaluation of a new anticancer drug and failing to take into account that the cancer patients in that hospital tend to have more advanced cancers than the cancer patient population as a whole.

Bias can also come from data collection (e.g., if different interviewers interview individuals with disease and "perfectly" matched controls, and some interviewers are better at extracting information about chemical exposure histories). Recall bias (in case control studies) can creep in if people with disease tend to be better able to remember their chemical exposure histories than "control" individuals).

---

of the data linking cancer to chemicals, radiation, viruses and to the environment described throughout Part III. Here we will expand a bit on these patterns.

More on Patterns through Time; Are We Having a Cancer Epidemic?

In the last three or four decades, mortality has increased for some kinds of cancer and decreased for others; mortality for most kinds of cancer has remained about the same (Fig. 1.5). Overall, cancer hasn't increased much at all, if age and the size of the U.S. population are properly taken into account. More people are dying of cancer today than in 1900, but there are more people to die and the population has proportionately more old people in it (Fig. 13.2). There is certainly no modern "epidemic" of cancer—except possibly for lung cancer.

This is not to say that cancer has not increased, after age and population size are taken into account. The 40 years between 1930 and 1970 show a 9.5 percent extra increase in cancer incidence—0.24 percent per year (Devesa and Schneiderman, 1977). The "adjusted" rate of increase from 1970 to 1985 has been somewhat higher. Some of the "real" excess is probably a result of improved detection and diagnosis—an improvement in the proportion of cancer deaths being recognized as cancer deaths (it is not im-

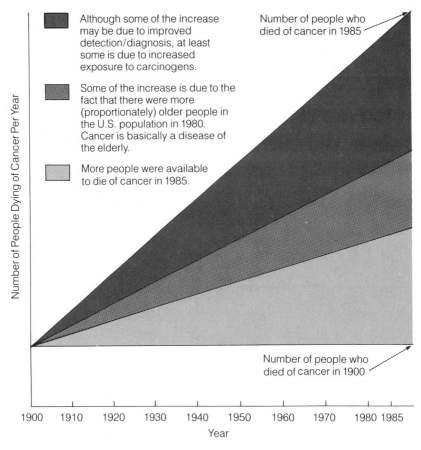

Figure 13.2 Increase in cancer with time. This figure shows cancer mortality in absolute numbers. Some of the increase in cancer that we see today can be accounted for by the fact that more people are alive today to die of cancer. Also, because cancer is a disease of the old, some of the increase is due to increased life expectancy. Although some of the rest of the increase may be due to improved detection and diagnosis, much of the excess increase is most likely a result of an increase in the barrage of carcinogenic insults over time (such as smoking). (Adapted with permission from Süss, Kinzel, and Scribner, 1973, p. 3; reprinted from Kupchella and Hyland, 1986, p. 429, courtesy of Allyn and Bacon, Inc.)

possible to mistake a cancer death for something else). Much of the remainder is a result of the real and significant increase in *lung* cancer.

Over the last half century, there has been a marked change in the incidence rates attributable to different kinds of cancer (Fig. 1.5). The most significant changes in cancer death rates have been (1) a dramatic increase in lung cancer deaths (reflecting an increase in incidence re-

lated to increased cigarette smoking and, possibly, air pollution); (2) an almost equally dramatic decline in stomach cancer deaths (most likely reflecting a decrease in incidence resulting from some unknown dietary change); and (3) a dramatic decline in death from cancer of the uterine cervix (in this case at least partly a result of early detection leading to cure, made possible by the Pap test).

The Lack of Clustering or Other Infectious Disease Patterns in Cancer

Epidemiologists in cancer research centers, state health departments, and elsewhere often get asked to come and investigate what is thought to be an outbreak of cancer in a particular town or neighborhood:

"We have had ten cases of leukemia this year, could it be something in the water?"

"I personally know of four cases of cancer within a block of the city incinerator, could there be a connection?"

Occasionally there is something to such clustering, but far more often they turn out *not* to be clusters at all or to be chance occurrences. Cancer is not uncommon, and sometimes the initial realization of this fact is perceived as something new. As for chance, if cancer is a relatively random occurrence, then it will, from time to time, occur in small bunches—in the same way that if you toss enough coins you will eventually (inevitably) get ten heads in a row.

In an earlier chapter, we reviewed the significance of infectious disease patterns in connection with virus-induced cancer. We discussed the fact that chickens and cats do indeed get virus-induced cancers that occur as outbreaks or local "epidemics." No hard evidence exists for any such epidemics in human beings—with the possible exception of Burkitt's lymphoma (see Chapter 11).

Occupational Cancer Patterns

One of the first published cancer epidemiologists was Percival Pott (see Chapter 8), who described an epidemic of scrotal cancer among chimney sweeps. This cancer was an occupational problem, and occupational cancer epidemiology has continued to run ahead of general cancer epidemiology. Nearly all the (few) *certain*, specific causes of human cancer are carcinogens identified in industrial settings. One reason is that, in occupational settings, human beings tend to get exposed to relatively known and relatively large amounts of rather particular agents—in contrast to the hodgepodge of exposures out in the world at large.

In Chapter 1 we looked at data showing that working with asbestos increases one's risk of lung cancer—particularly if one also happens to be a smoker (Fig. 1.1). In Chapter 8, we considered other "occupational cancers" in the context of chemical carcinogenesis. Table 13.1 summarizes cancer-occupation relationships revealed by, or strongly suspected by epidemiological investigations (see Schottenfeld and Haas, 1978).

We won't go into occupational cancer epidemiology further here, except to point out that improved medical monitoring of workers in industry and improved screening of chemicals as required by the Toxic Substances Control legislation should help identify occupational-cancer patterns sooner than they have been recognized in the past and should help prevent (see Chapter 15) additional occupational cancers in the future.

Smoking and Cancer

Epidemiology has provided overwhelming evidence that smoking is an important cause of cancer (Fig. 13.3). But it took a while, and the story is an instructive one, pointing out some of the problems inherent in epidemiology.

Lung cancer increased most dramatically in men in the last half century; it went from being a relative medical rarity to the most common form of cancer. Smoking also underwent a dramatic increase, but this happened 20 years before the increase in lung cancer and so the connection wasn't made right away. After it was noted that the two patterns matched well, the same general pattern began to appear in women, who took up smoking with a vengeance about forty years after the men. Women have now begun to generate their own lung cancer epidemic about forty years after men began theirs.

Epidemiology has long since confirmed that lung cancer tends to appear in the very same people who took up smoking twenty years before. Wynder and Hoffman (1966), Doll and Hill

Table 13.1   Some of the Agents Linked to Cancer in Occupational Groups

Agent	Organ Affected	Occupation
Arsenic	Skin, lung, liver	Miners, smelter, insecticide makers and sprayers, tanners, chemical workers, oil refiners, vintners
Asbestos	Lung (pleural and peritoneal mesothelioma)	Miners, millers, textile, insulation, and shipyard workers
Benzene	Bone marrow (leukemia)	Explosives, benzene, or rubber cement workers, distillers, dye users, painters, shoemakers
Bis(chloromethyl) ether, chloromethyl methyl ether	Lung	Chemical workers
Chromium	Nasal cavity and sinuses, lung, larynx	Chromium producers, processers, and users, acetylene and aniline workers, glass, pottery, and linoleum workers, battery makers
Coal soot, coal tar, other products of coal combustion	Lung, larynx, skin, scrotum, urinary bladder	Asphalt, coal tar, and pitch workers, coke oven workers, miners, still cleaners
Iron oxide	Lung, larynx	Iron miners, metal workers, iron foundry workers
Isopropyl oil	Nasal cavity	Isopropyl oil manufacturing
Leather	Nasal cavity and sinuses, urinary bladder	Leather workers
Nickel	Nasal sinuses, lung	Nickel ore processors, electrolysis workers
Vinyl chloride	Liver, brain	Plastic workers
Wood	Nasal cavity and sinuses	Woodworkers

Source: Kupchella, C. E. 1986. Data from Williams, R. R., Stegens, N. L., and Goldsmith, J. R., 1977. Associations of Cancer Site and Type with Occupation and Industry from the Third National Cancer Survey Interview, *JNCI*, 59:1147–86. Used by permission of Grune and Stratton.

(1964), and others (Hammond and Horn, 1958) have carried out prospective studies *all* of which have produced the same conclusion, namely, cigarette smoking increases one's risk of lung cancer and the more one smokes, the greater the risk (Fig. 13.3).

Some of the epidemiological findings (National Clearinghouse for Smoking and Health, 1974):

After age 35, death rates (all causes) are higher for cigarette smokers than for nonsmokers at every age.

In men between ages 45 and 54, the death rate for smokers is roughly three times that of nonsmokers.

For two-pack-a-day smokers, the risk of lung cancer is 20 times that of nonsmokers.

For smokers who quit, death rates approach those of nonsmokers in 10 to 15 years.

Some tobacco companies still challenge the connection between smoking and lung cancer, citing the fact that *most* heavy smokers do *not* develop lung cancer and using a technicality—that the link is circumstantial. Never mind that the circumstantial evidence is overwhelming, they feel—the fact that it is "only" circumstantial leaves open the possibility that smoking and cancer are linked only through some third factor—some possibly genetically inherited mystery factor that predisposes a person to taking up and becoming addicted to cigarette smoking *and* simultaneously predisposes that person to developing lung cancer.

An epidemiologist colleague once face-

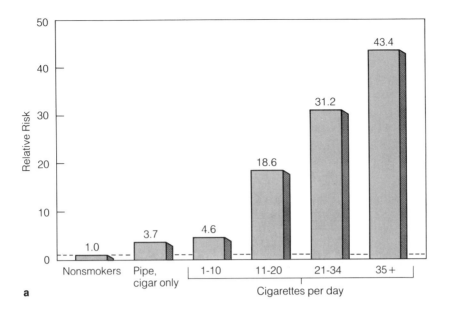

a

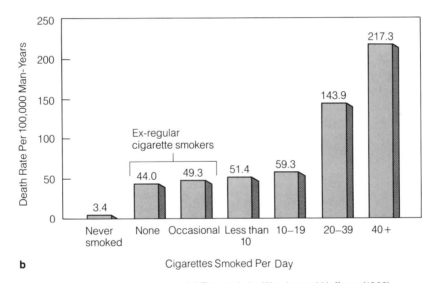

b

Figure 13.3 The epidemiology of smoking and cancer. (**a**) The study by Wynder and Hoffman (1966) looked at the relationship between smoking and *getting* lung cancer; (**b**) the study by Hammond and Horn (1958), a prospective study involving some 187,000 men, examined the relationship between cigarette smoking and dying of lung cancer.

tiously described the kind of experiment that it would take to eliminate this possibility: As babies are born over several years at a particular hospital, an envelope would be drawn from a large number of thoroughly mixed envelopes in a drum. Half of the envelopes in the drum would contain a card bearing the word *smoker*; the other half would have *nonsmoker* cards. A baby for whom a smoker card was drawn would be made to begin smoking at some particular age and continue to do so until death; the nonsmoking babies would be prohibited from smoking for life (they would have to be watched carefully). The numbers of lung cancer deaths would then be determined for both groups. Although this design is less than perfect, it would not allow any "mystery" factor to determine smoking (even if it did determine lung cancer susceptibility). The drum would determine smoking. Having thus disconnected smoking from any other determinant, its relationship to cancer would become clear.

Race and Sex

The biggest differences between men and women with respect to cancer naturally have to do with reproductive organs. Prostatic cancer is the second most common kind of cancer in both white and black men; it is *the* most common form in hispanic men. Breast cancer is the most common form of cancer in females of all three ethnic groups; ovarian cancer, cancer of the uterine cervix and cancer of the uterine corpus rank in the top ten in all three.

Apart from reproductive organs, lung cancer is more common in men than cancer of the colon or rectum; the reverse is true for women (Fig. 1.2). This difference will soon disappear if present trends continue.*

There are several other *ethnic* differences in the patterns of cancer incidence. Blacks have had higher incidences of cancers of the uterine cervix, prostate, lung, and certain digestive organs; whites tend to have more melanoma and cancer of the breast and body of the uterus. Multiple myeloma is in the top ten for both male and female blacks but not for whites (or hispanics). Overall, blacks have more cancer than whites.

Some differences between blacks and whites are in fact genetic; for example, darkskinned people tend to have lower rates of skin cancer because of the increased shielding from carcinogenic radiation their pigmentation affords them. Many differences have been shown to be derived from the fact that ethnic groups tend to line up on particular sides of socioeconomic strata and to other (e.g., cultural) differences that constitute ethnic group-specific environmental exposures.

Socioeconomic Cancer Patterns

Rich women get more breast cancer and less cancer of the uterine cervix. Although the reason(s) for this difference is not known, it is generally hypothesized that some kind of environmental factor lines up the same way as one or more elements of lifestyle. Poor women have many more things in common than the lack of money. They tend to have poorer health care, less adequate diets, earlier marriages, earlier childbirths, more of certain kinds of stress, and on and on. Since breast tissue is a sex hormone "target" tissue, an obvious place to look for risk factors would be in elements of lifestyle that have something to do with hormone changes or sex and reproduction. And indeed, MacMahon, Cole, and Brown (1973) have shown that breast cancer risk lines up with the "age of first birth." Rotkin (1962) and others have shown that cancer

---

*Note that the last few sentences refer to *incidence* rather than *mortality* (see Chapter 1). Lung cancer is already the leading cancer killer in both men and women. In 1982, *lung* cancer mortality in Texas women matched breast cancer mortality. During the 12-year period ending in 1982, breast cancer mortality

stayed about the same while lung cancer death rates doubled— from 11.9 women per 100,000 to 22.6 (*Morbidity and Mortality Weekly Report*, p. 266). Lung cancer is now the leading cause of cancer death in all American women (Fig. 1.2).

of the uterine cervix is associated with early first coitus, promiscuity, and adolescent coitus in particular. It has been hypothesized that the immature cervical epithelium may be particularly susceptible to virus transformation or other unknown carcinogenic agents associated with coitus.

U. S. Geographic Patterns

Some of the most intriguing and dramatic epidemiological cancer data ever published were those presented as maps of U. S. cancer mortality, in the volume *Atlas of Cancer Mortality*, published by the National Cancer Institute (Mason et al., 1975). These maps showed those counties in which cancers of each major type were significantly higher or lower than the average for the United States as a whole. One of these maps is shown here as Figure 13.4 (see also Fig. 9.4). Among the things the maps show are (1) concentrations of lung cancer in the Northeast and along the Gulf Coast; (2) breast cancer concentrated in the Northeast; (3) cervical cancer concentrated in Appalachia; (4) stomach cancer concentrated in the upper Midwest; (5) pancreatic cancer pretty well evenly distributed throughout the country; (6) skin cancer concentrated in the Sunbelt states; and (7) cancer, overall, concentrated in metropolitan counties to the extent that most of the rest of the United States is below average!

Skin cancer in the Sunbelt (Fig. 9.4) comes as no great surprise, but the reasons for *most* of the clustering illustrated in the cited report are unknown. It has been suggested that stomach cancer in Minnesota and neighboring areas is related to diet—more specifically, to dietary habits carried from the countries from which the people of the upper Midwest emigrated. The relevant parts of Austria, Scandinavia, and the Soviet Union also have higher average rates of gastric cancer than the United States.

While the concentration of lung cancers along the Gulf Coast do not line up particularly with smoking patterns, this may reflect the higher incidence of lung cancer in counties with petrochemical and/or shipbuilding industry. The concentration of lung cancer in cities throughout the United States may reflect greater amounts of cigarette smoking in cities or possibly the synergistic interaction between cigarette smoke, air pollutants, and humidity.

Breast cancer and cervical cancer patterns are apparently consistent with the risk factors discussed above for these forms of cancer. Breast cancer is more common among those who marry late and among the well-to-do; cervical cancer is more common in lower socioeconomic groups and those who marry early. People in the Northeast tend to marry later and to have more money than people in Appalachia, but this is a long way from making a definitive statement about cause and effect.

New Jersey stands out like the proverbial "sore thumb." Nearly every one of the counties of New Jersey have significantly higher cancer death rates for virtually every form of cancer than the rest of the United States. Industrial exposures are believed to be responsible for the striking concentration of bladder cancer deaths in males in New Jersey and in most of the rest of the East. The abnormally high rates of cancer of the esophagus, larynx, mouth, and throat *as well as* the bladder in the Northeast, were limited to males—suggesting an occupational connection. That the industrial connection may not be the *whole* story is suggested by the fact that states in the upper end of New England also have high death rates, and these states are neither highly populated nor industrialized. What, then? It has been suggested that the lack of selenium—a mineral known to have some anticancer effects—in northeastern soils may be a factor (Kubota et al., 1967).

The mortality mapping data suggest that it is bad to have lived in a city, and other data indicate that this rule is also true in other countries. Lave and Seskin (1970), who evaluated a number of studies done in England comparing rural and urban air, claim that there is significant evidence of an association between air pollution and lung cancer and note that the incidence of

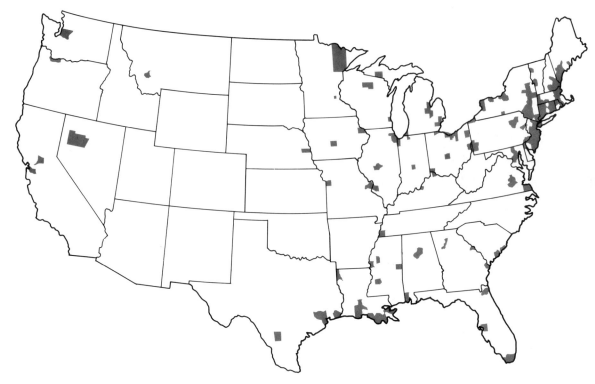

Figure 13.4 Historic patterns of cancer death in the United States. This map shows those U.S. counties in which there were statistically significantly high, age-adjusted, rates of cancer mortality, for all sites combined, for white males during the period 1950 to 1969. (Adapted from Mason et al., 1975; reprinted from Kupchella and Hyland, 1986, p. 437, courtesy of Allyn and Bacon, Inc.)

some sixteen different kinds of cancer was higher in cities than in rural areas. The National Research Council once estimated that if air pollution were reduced in and around U. S. cities by one-half, the lung cancer rate might be reduced by as much as 20 percent. Air pollution is obviously not the only likely city "factor." Many things about cities are different.

The *Atlas of Cancer Mortality* revealed no obvious patterns of distribution for cancers of the pancreas, brain, salivary gland, nose, or sinuses.

In keeping with the relationship between epidemiological and other scientific approaches to disease described at the beginning of this chapter, these maps amount to epidemiological observations awaiting further scientific expla-

nations. They amount to starting points for hypotheses about specific environmental or other connections that can be tested by laboratory scientists, clinical researchers, and other epidemiologists.

Geographic Patterns in the World

Striking differences show up in cancer mortality patterns worldwide (Fig. 13.5; see also Table E.1, p. 196). Comparisons made in recent years have shown, for example, that

Liver cancer is 70 to 100 times more common in certain African countries than in the United States and other western nations.

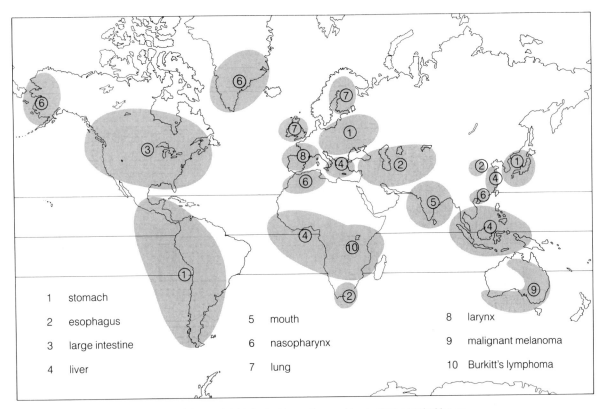

Figure 13.5 Cancer hotspots around the world. (Adapted from *Cancer News*, 1983; used with permission of the American Cancer Society; reprinted from Kupchella and Hyland, 1986, p. 437, courtesy of Allyn and Bacon, Inc.)

1	stomach				
2	esophagus	5	mouth	8	larynx
3	large intestine	6	nasopharynx	9	malignant melanoma
4	liver	7	lung	10	Burkitt's lymphoma

Lung cancer in women is more than fifty times less common in certain Central American countries than in Scotland or Hong Kong.

Breast cancer in Denmark and England is five times more common than in Japan or the Philippines.

Esophageal cancer is 300 times more common in parts of Iran than in Nigeria (Table E.1).

Skin cancer is 200 times more common in Queensland, Australia, than in Bombay, India (Table E.1).

These differences are nearly all presumptively attributed to environmental differences (see Epilog to Part III). Again, differences from country to country together with the fact that immi-

grants, and particularly their descendants, adopt the patterns of cancer mortality of the country to which they migrate are the bases of the idea that 90 percent of cancer is environmental.

Nevertheless, genetics is still important. Indeed, genetics is certainly part of the basis for some geographic differences. High rates of skin cancer in Queensland, for example, is at least partly a result of the fact that Queensland has many genetically fashioned, fair-skinned descendants of Celtic immigrants.

Diet and Other Factors

It is relevant to the preceding discussion that there are Mexican, Chinese, French, African,

Italian, Indian, and German restaurants, among others. Just about every ethnic group has its own cuisine, which is one probable explanation for some international differences in cancer. Many differences we have pointed out may well be linked—with further study—to specific dietary factors. Doll (1976) has pointed out that the relationship between per capita gross national product and a nation's colon cancer incidence may be related to high-meat, low-cereal diets. We don't know why this association exists but one possibility is that the relative lack of fiber in the high-meat, low-cereal diet slows down GI motility, possibly allowing more time for carcinogens to be formed in bowel contents and to act on the GI lining cells. The diet connection is one of the main topics in the chapter on prevention, coming up.

Survival Patterns

Some kinds of cancer are more likely to be survived than others (Table 1.3). Some cancers are inherently more deadly than others. And certain cancers tend to be diagnosed earlier (Fig. 1.3). Five-year survival rates for blacks are lower for practically every form of cancer; presumably this difference is related to certain cultural characteristics and to the socioeconomic and health care status of blacks as a group. Their cancers tend to be diagnosed later, and subsequent care is less good than for whites.

It is important to note here—in anticipation of Chapter 17—that survival does not necessarily *always* reflect quality of treatment. The reason for this has to do with the definition of the words *survival* and *cured*. Survival is measured in years following diagnosis. By convention, survival for five years without evidence of recurring cancer serves as a working definition of **cured**. Cure rates are thus based on five-year survivals. The fact that it takes five years to see what the cure rates will be for therapy administered today, sets up two sources of "slippage" between survival rates and quality of or improvements in treatment. One source is early detection. If a cancer

is detected *earlier* in its natural history, more people will survive five years simply because it takes longer for deaths to occur from earlier points of detection. Also, if survival is generalized from the gross difference between incidence and mortality, a sudden increase in incidence rates with little or no change in mortality rates *could* easily be mistaken for an improvement in survival.

Cancer Registries, Surveys, and Record Keeping

The value of cancer record keeping should be clear by now; many things can be learned from good data and the only way to identify carcinogens and risk factors for humans is to see, systematically, *what* people, exposed to *what*, gets *which* cancers, at *what* rate. Unfortunately, we have not always had good records.

One of the earliest statistical analyses of cancer *mortality* was published by a statistician with the Prudential Life Insurance Company, F. L. Hoffman, in 1915: *The Mortality from Cancer Throughout the World*. A number of states began to register cancer cases after the turn of the century, and J. W. Schereschewsky of the Public Health Service published in 1925 an analysis of cancer mortality trends in the United States: *The Course of Cancer Mortality in the Ten Original Registration States for the 21 Year Period, 1900–1920* (see Shimkin, 1977).

A national, state-by-state, death registration system has been in place in the United States only since 1933. Cancer deaths are included in this system, which permits the American Cancer Society to publish a very thorough summary of cancer mortality statistics each year. But this still leaves the problem of documenting the prevalence and incidence (see Chapter 1) of cancers—because obviously not all cancer causes death.

Cancer incidence-prevalence record keeping was virtually unheard of before World War I, and only in the last 25 years have cancer record-keeping operations moved beyond part-time clerks with a few battered file cabinets. Many individual American hospitals began cancer registries in the 1950s after the American College of Surgeons began to require them as a condition of approval for a hospital's cancer program (see Chapter 19). Over 800 hospitals are on the "approved" list today. Today there are also more than 60 **population-based** (covering a defined population) cancer registries in operation throughout the world, staffed by statisticians and epidemiologists.

The **Connecticut Tumor Registry** was begun in 1941 as the first of the population-based registries that have remained in continual operation to the present day. Data on incidence, survival, and mortality in this registry have become an invaluable resource. The oldest national population-based registry is the Danish Registry, established in 1942 in Copenhagen.

Cancer incidence has been relatively regularly estimated for the United States in national surveys conducted in 1937, 1947–1948, and 1969–1971. Current, continual data has been available through the Surveillance, Epidemiology and End Results (SEER) program of the National Cancer Institute. The SEER program, which has been in operation since 1973, compiles data from ten different population-based registries throughout the country and includes Hawaii and Puerto Rico. This program counts all cancers except nonmelanoma skin cancers and *in situ* cervical cancer. International incidence rates are now regularly compiled by the International Agency for Research on Cancer (IARC) headquartered in Lyon, France.

The roots of systematic evaluation of end results in cancer *treatment* go back to A. Winiwarter in Austria and M. Greenwood in Britain. In 1885 Winiwarter published one of the first statistical reviews of treatment effect, and in 1926 Greenwood published some of the first complete descriptions of the "natural history" of cancer; that is, the survival of *un*treated patients. To this day, Greenwood's work is used as a baseline in expressing the effectiveness of various modes of treatment (see Shimkin, 1977).

Cancer registries in which patients are followed until death are able to generate survival statistics, which are obviously also of great value. Survival data make it possible to document progress being made against various cancers; survival data that take into account age, histologic type, stage at diagnosis, and treatment are absolutely essential in evaluating the effectiveness of new treatment.

Summary

Epidemiology is the study of disease at the population level. Epidemiology seeks to match up patterns of disease with other characteristics of populations in order to identify probable cause-and-effect relationships. Epidemiology can look backward or forward; it can start with disease and look backward for exposure to suspect disease-causing agents, or it can start with exposure and "wait" for disease. It can also look into the historical record for both exposure and disease. Difficulty in eliminating biases, difficulty in defining control groups, difficulty in obtaining good records, and other factors conspire to make epidemiology a science of association and probable cause; rarely does it provide proof. Still, largely because we cannot ethically experiment with human beings, most of what we know about causes of cancer in human beings specifically, we have learned through epidemiological investigation. The resounding fact that jumps out of the cancer epidemiological data is that cancer is largely an environmental disease. If this is true, then cancer must be at least partly preventable. Prevention is the subject of Chapter 15.

References and Further Reading

American Cancer Society. 1983. The Geography of Cancer. *Cancer News*. April. (Translated from *Vivre*, the magazine of the French National League against Cancer, by Andrea Colls-Halpern.)

Andervont, H. B., and Dunn, T. B. 1963. Occurrence of Tumors in Wild House Mice. *Journal of the National Cancer Institute*. 28:1153–63.

Armstrong, B., and Doll, R. 1975. Environmental Factors and Cancer Incidence and Mortality in Different Countries, with Special Reference to Dietary Practices. *Int. J. Cancer*. 15:617–31.

Braun, A. C. 1975. Plant Tumors. In F. F. Becker, ed., *Cancer: A Comprehensive Treatise*. New York: Plenum Press.

Creech, J. L., and Johnson, M. N. 1974. Angiosarcoma of the Liver, in the Manufacture of Polyvinyl Chloride. *J. Occup. Med.*, 16:150–51.

Cutler, S. J., and Young, J. L., eds. 1975. *Third National Cancer Survey: Incidence Data*. NCI Monograph No. 41. Washington, D.C.: National Cancer Institute.

Dawe, C. J. 1973. Comparative Neoplasia. In J. F. Holland and E. Frei, eds., *Cancer Medicine*. Philadelphia: Lea & Febiger.

Devesa, S. S., and Schneiderman, M. A. 1977. Increase in the Number of Cancer Deaths in the United States. *Am. J. Epidemiology*. 106(1):1–5.

Doll, R. 1976. Epidemiology of Cancer: Current Perspectives. *Am. J. Epidemiology*. 104(4):396–404.

Doll, R., and Hill, A. B. 1956. Lung Cancer and Other Causes of Death in Relation to Smoking. *Brit. Med. J.* 2:1071–81.

Doll, R., and Hill, A. B. 1964. Mortality in Relation to Smoking: Ten Years Observations of British Doctors. *Brit. Med. J.* 1:1399–410.

Doll, R., and Peto, R. 1981. The Causes of Cancer: Quantitative Estimates of Avoidable Risk of Cancer in the U.S. Today. *Journal of the National Cancer Institute*. 66:1191–308.

Dorn, H. F., and Cutler, S. J. 1958. *Morbidity from Cancer in the United States*. PHS Monograph No. 56. Washington, D.C.: U.S. Public Health Service.

Ernster, V. L., Sacks, S. T., and Petrakis, N. L. 1983. The Tools of Cancer Epidemiology. In S. B. Kahn et al., eds., *Concepts in Cancer Medicine*. New York: Grune & Stratton.

Hammond, E. C., and Horn, D. 1958. Smoking and Death Rates—Report of Forty-Four Months of Follow-Up of 187,783 Men. *JAMA*. 166:1159–72; 1249–308.

Hoffman, F. L. 1915. *The Mortality from Cancer Around the World*. Newark: Prudential Press.

Kelsey, J. L., and Hildreth, N. G. 1983. *Breast and Gynecologic Cancer Epidemiology*. Boca Raton, Fla.: CRC Press.

Kubota, J., et al. 1967. Selenium in Crops in the United States in Relation to Selenium-Responsive Diseases of Animals. *J. Agr. Food Chem*. 15:448–53.

Kupchella, C. E., and Hyland, M. C. 1986. *Environmental Science*. Boston: Allyn & Bacon.

Kupchella, C. E. 1986. Environmental Factors in Cancer Etiology. *Seminars in Oncology Nursing*. 2:161–69.

Lave, L., and Seskin, E. P. 1970. Air Pollution and Human Health. *Science*. 169(3947):723–33.

Lave, L., and Seskin, E. P. 1979. Epidemiology Casuality and Public Policy. *American Scientist*. 67:178–86.

Levin, D. L., et al. 1974. *Cancer Rates and Risks*. 2nd ed. DHEW Publication No. 75-691. Washington, D.C.: Department of Health, Education, and Welfare.

Lilienfeld, A. M., and Lilienfeld, D. E. 1980. *Foundations of Epidemiology*. 2nd ed. New York: Oxford University Press.

Lombard, L. S., and Witte, E. J. 1959. Frequency and Types of Tumors in Mammals and Birds of the Philadelphia Zoological Garden. *Cancer Research*. 19:127–41.

MacMahon, B., Cole, P. and Brown, J. 1973. Etiology of Human Breast Cancer: A Review. *Journal of the National Cancer Institute*. 50:21–42.

Mason, T., et al. 1975. *Atlas of Cancer Mortality for U.S. Counties, 1950–1969*. NIH Publication No. 75-780. Washington, D.C.: Department of Health, Education, and Welfare, Public Health Service.

Mausner, J. S., and Bahn, A. K. 1974. *Epidemiology: An Introductory Text*. Philadelphia: Saunders.

Moodie, R. L. 1923. *Antiquity of Disease*. Chicago: University of Chicago Press.

Myers, M. H., and Hankey, B. F. 1980. *Cancer Patient Survival Experience*. NIH Publication No. 80-2148. Bethesda, Md.: Department of Health, Education, and Welfare.

National Clearinghouse for Smoking and Health. 1974. *Facts: Smoking and Health*. DHEW Publication CDC No. 74-8717. Bethesda, Md.: Department of Health, Education, and Welfare.

Pollack, E. S., and Horm, J. W. 1980. Trends in Cancer Incidence and Mortality in the United States, 1979–1976. *Journal of the National Cancer Institute*. 60: 1091–103.

Rotkin, I. 1962. Relation of Adolescent Coitus to Cervical Cancer Risk. *JAMA*. 179:486–91.

Scarpelli, D. G. 1975. Neoplasia in Poikilotherms. In F. F. Becker, ed., *Cancer: A Comprehensive Treatise*. Vol. 4. New York: Plenum Press.,

Schereschewsky, J. W. 1925. *The Course of Cancer Mortality in the Ten Original Registration States for the 21 Year Period, 1900–1920*. Washington, D.C.: U.S. Public Health Service.

Schottenfeld, D., and Fraumeni, J. F. eds. 1982. *Cancer Epidemiology and Prevention*. Philadelphia: Saunders.

Schottenfeld, D., and Haas, J. F. 1978. The Workplace as a Cause of Cancer. *Clinical Bulletin*. 8(2):54–60 and 8(3)107–119 (two parts).

Segi, M., et al. 1979. *Age-Adjusted Death Rates for Cancer for Selected Sites in 51 Countries in 1975*. Nagoya, Japan: Segi Institute of Cancer Epidemiology.

Shimkin, M. G. 1977. *Contrary to Nature*. DHEW Publication No. 76-720. Washington, D.C.: Department of Health, Education, and Welfare.

Süss, R., Kinzel, V., and Scribner, J. D. 1973. *Cancer: Experiments and Concepts*. New York: Springer-Verlag.

Symington, T., and Carter, R., eds. 1976. *Scientific Foundation of Oncology*. Chicago: Heinemann Medical Books/Yearbook Medical Publishers.

Wynder, E. L., and Hoffman, D. 1966. Current Concepts of Environmental Cancer Research. *Medical Clinics of North America*. 50:631–50.

The relationship between cancer and the immune system has many intriguing aspects. Let's pose them as questions: (1) If cancer cells are not normal, why does the immune system not attack all cancer cells and destroy them? (2) If cancer is a consequence of impaired immune defense, what exactly goes wrong? (3) Could the immune system be stimulated to attack cancer cells? (4) How? (5) Can antibodies made elsewhere—in another organism or in flasks—be used to destroy cancer cells? (6) Can such antibodies be used to carry toxic chemicals to cancer cells and kill them indirectly? (7) Can antibodies be used to carry radioactive tags to cancer cells and thus aid cancer detection? We will deal with these questions throughout the remainder of the book in the contexts of detection, diagnosis, and treatment. Here our purpose is to describe the immune system and to outline the general relationships between cancer and immunity.

14

The Immune System and Cancer

The Immune System

The immune system as one of several lines of defense against invading microorganisms and foreign substances was introduced in Chapter 3. There, the immune system was identified as the line of defense that singles out and attacks each type of foreign substance in a unique way tailored specifically to that foreign substance. Microorganisms and other foreign substances able to elicit an immune response are said to be **immunogenic** or **antigenic**. The specific molecules that do the eliciting are called **antigens** (see chemical description below).

The antigen-sensitive, specific responder cells of the immune defense system are the lymphocytes. These bone marrow-derived white cells are divisible into two functional types: B-cells and T-cells. **T-cells** undergo part of their final development in the thymus gland. The T in T-cells comes from the expression "thymus derived." T-cells are the principal components of *cell-mediated immunity*; they deal with invaders directly (Fig. 14.1) (see Chapter 3). **B-cells** are

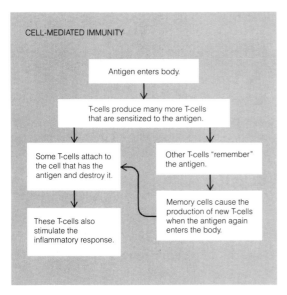

Figure 14.1 The sequence of development of T-cells

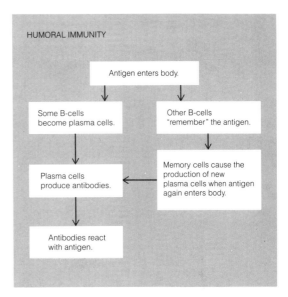

Figure 14.2 The sequence of development of B-cells

believed to develop and mature in the bone marrow; they are called B-cells not because of the bone marrow connection, but because they were first studied in birds (but B does not stand for bird, either), where these cells mature in an organ called the bursa. Antigens cause *bursa-equivalent cells*, or B-cells, to give rise to **plasma cells**, which produce antibodies (Fig. 14.2). B-cells are the basis of humoral immunity (see Chapter 3); they attack antigens from a distance via antibodies released into the blood.

B-Cells and Antibodies

According to the clonal selection hypothesis, there are many, many different kinds of B-cells in every human body, each with a different antibody on its surface. There are at least a few B-cells whose surface antibodies would enable them to react to virtually any soluble antigen that might come along. When a B-cell meets an antigen with which its surface antibodies can combine, it is stimulated and begins to divide—it is called back into the cell cycle. Some of the

resultant progeny cells become **memory B-cells**—cells like the originally stimulated B-cell, only more of them—which establish an *enhanced* ability to deal with that particular antigen the next time it is encountered. The rest of the progeny differentiate into antibody-producing cells called plasma cells, each one of which sends thousands of antibody molecules into the bloodstream per second. If this antibody barrage helps to eliminate the invading organism, as it usually does, the antibodies gradually disappear (plasma cells live only a few days)—but the memory B-cells remain.

B-cells apparently need the help of T-cells and macrophages in order to be "turned on" to a particular antigen. Although the details of the interaction are not yet crystal clear, it appears that the full activation of B-cells requires interaction with macrophage-activated helper T-cells (see below).

Antibodies are proteins capable of combining with particular antigens. The word **antigen** is short for *antibody generator*, and in effect antigen stimulates the production of particular antibodies that can then attack that antigen.

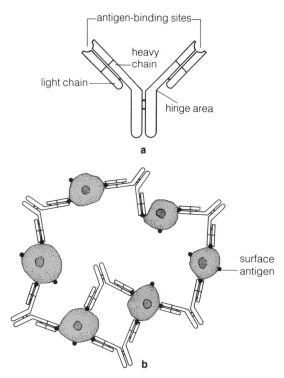

Figure 14.3 (**a**) The general structure of an IgG antibody; (**b**) antibodies shown clumping foreign cells.

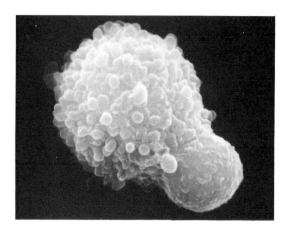

Figure 14.4 A lymphocyte (smaller cell on the right) attacks a cancer cell; the death of a cancer cell induced by a lymphocyte is indicated by the blebs or deep folds that appear on the surface of the cancer cell. (This scanning electron micrograph was made by Andrejs Liepins of the Sloan-Kettering Institute for Cancer Research and was provided courtesy of Lloyd J. Old, M.D., Vice President of the Sloan-Kettering Institute. It appeared originally in *Scientific American*; see Old, 1977. Used by permission.)

Chemically, antigens may be proteins or polysaccharides or combinations of one or both of these with lipids and/or nucleic acids.

There are five different classes of antibodies (also called **immunoglobulins**), identified by the designations IgM, IgG, IgA, IgE, and IgD. Each immunoglobulin molecule is composed of one or more basic units consisting of two heavy and two light polypeptide chains (Fig. 14.3). Each basic type or class of immunoglobulin has a characteristic constant region (amino acid sequence) and a variable region that gives the antibody its reaction specificity. The basic four-chain immunoglobulin has two antigen binding sites per molecule, and this is the basis of the ability of antibodies to serve as bridges between antigen-bearing cells or particles, thereby clumping them.

What do antibodies do? For one thing, they can react with, and neutralize, antigens that are toxins. For another, antibodies can cause cells and other particles that bear complementary antigens to clump, thereby making it easier for macrophages, neutrophils, and other scavenger cells to phagocytize them and making it more difficult for invading viruses to attach to host cells (see Chapter 10). Some phagocytic cells and killer cells (see below) can only attack cells previously coated with antibody. Antibody-antigen reactions also serve to activate the **complement system** (a group of interactive plasma-proteins activated by antibody/antigen reactions and that amplify the immune response, e.g., help bring about the lysis of cells on which the antibody/antigen reaction takes place).

The most amazing thing about antibodies, though, is that they are tailor-made to deal with specific antigens.

T-Cells

For our purposes, there are basically four types of T-cells (see Table 14.1): (1) **killer T-cells** are able to kill other cells (Fig. 14.4); (2) **helper T-cells** help other T-cells, macrophages, and B-cells respond to antigens; (3) **supressor T-cells** actually inhibit the reactions of both T- and B-

Table 14.1 Types of Immune Cells

Cell	Origin	Function
B-cell	Bursa equivalent (bone marrow)	Differentiates into antibody-secreting cell
Plasma cell	Bursa equivalent	Secretes antibody
Cytotoxic or killer T-cell	Thymus	Destroys virally infected and allogeneic cells
Helper T-cell	Thymus	Cooperates in activating B-cells and cytotoxic T-cells
Suppressor T-cell	Thymus	Regulates strength and type of immune response by inhibiting other T- and B-cells
Memory T-cell	Thymus	"Remembers" exposure to particular antigens
Macrophages	Bone marrow	Presents antigen in an immunogenic way to T-cells and B-cells

Adapted from Sondel, 1983. Reprinted by permission of Grune and Stratton and the author.

cells and apparently serve in some regulatory capacity; and (4) **memory T-cells** "remember" exposures to particular antigens in the past. The relationships between these entities is partially illustrated in Figure 14.5. The narrative description of the relationship between macrophages, T-cells, and B-cells goes as follows:

Soluble antigens interact directly with those B-cells already having surface receptors (antibodies) that complement the structure of the antigen like an enzyme complements its substrate. After the antigen and receptor combine, the antigen is internalized by the B-cell and then displayed on the B-cell's surface. Meanwhile, macrophages, having also ingested some of the antigenic material, also display antigen fragments on their surfaces. The macrophages present the displayed antigen to yet-unactivated killer (cytotoxic) T-cells and helper T-cells. In a sense, the macrophages select, for subsequent activation and proliferation, those T-cells whose receptors match the antigen that started the activation cascade. As part of their presentation to the T-cells, macrophages release a hormone called *interleukin-1*. **Interleukin-1** or **IL-1** helps activate T-cells (and may also help induce fever). As they are being activated by macrophages, killer T-cells and helper T-cells release **interleukin-2** and sprout receptors for interleukin-2 which serve to accelerate or intensify their own activation and that of other T-cells.

It is noteworthy that without either an IL-2 or IL-2 receptor, there is no T-cell response; a number of acquired immunodeficiency diseases are the consequence of the failure of one or the other of these to be induced (Waldman, 1986). The interaction of IL-2 with IL-2 receptors determines the *magnitude* and the *duration* of the T-cell mediated immune response—after the interaction of T-cells and antigens gives *specificity* to that response. We might also note here that the activation of T-cells by IL-2 (essentially a T-cell growth factor) involves the same sort of hormone–receptor–second messenger interaction discussed in Chapter 7. T-cell activation appears to be mediated by increased intracellular calcium and the activation of protein kinase C (Waldman, 1986). This also appears to be the mechanism of B-cell and macrophage activation.

Once it is fully activated, a killer T-cell goes about the business of killing cells bearing the antigen that led to its activation; some become memory killer T-cells, enabling the body to mount a quicker, more resounding killer T-cell response should the antigen in question ever be encountered again. Some mature helper T-cells become memory helper T-cells; some release IL-2, which helps activate killer T-cells (helper cells

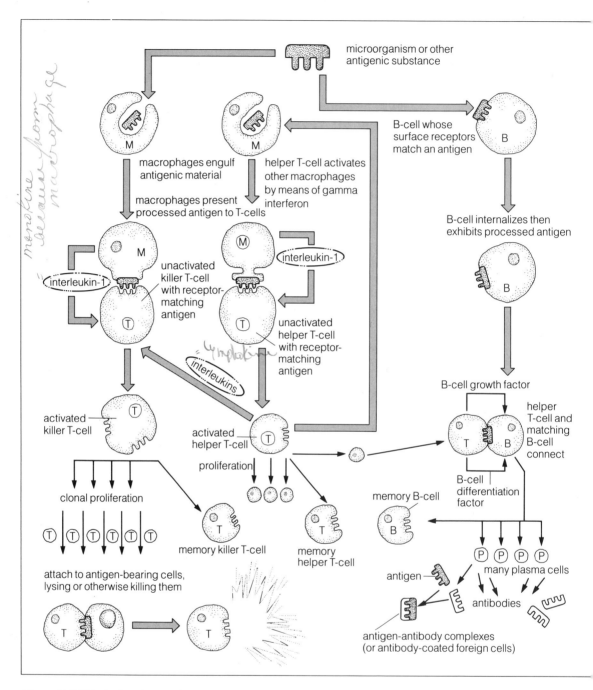

Figure 14.5 This, believe it or not, is a simplified diagram showing the major relationships between and among lymphocytes and lymphokines of the immune system. A description of these relationships is given in the text.

also release gamma interferon and this also helps activate macrophages); other helper cells stimulate the proliferation of B-cells. The interaction between activated helper cells and activated B-cells (see Fig. 14.5) causes the helper T-cells to release **B-cell growth factor** and then **B-cell differentiation factor**. The growth factor causes B-cells to proliferate (some becoming memory B-cells); the differentiation factor causes most of the activated B-cells to become antibody-spewing plasma cells.

Interleukins and Lymphokines

Protecting the body is obviously a complicated business requiring the coordinated interaction of many different kinds of cells in close chemical communication. The **interleukins** are one class of chemical signal molecules through which the cellular elements of the immune system communicate. In addition to interleukin-1 and 2 mentioned above, interleukins-3 and 4A have also been described. **Interleukin-3 (IL3)** is a T-lymphocyte–derived chemical substance that is believed to play a role in the regulation of hematopoiesis by the immune system (Clark-Lewis et al., 1986). IL-1 is one of a class of macrophage-derived immune-cell stimulants called **monokines**. Interleukins produced by lymphocytes belong to a large class of lymphocyte-derived chemical products called **lymphokines**.

T-cells employ lymphokines to communicate with one another, to communicate with other cells of the immune system, and as weapons against target cells. Some lymphokines are directly toxic; some are able to hold macrophages in the vicinity of an invasion; and still others are able to activate other unexcited T-cells or to stimulate macrophages to be more aggressive and efficient in their attack on foreign cells. Some additional specific examples: **Macrophage chemotactic factor**, a lymphokine released by activated T-cells, attracts macrophages to the site

of the battle. Another lymphokine, **migration inhibitory factor** keeps macrophages from leaving the battlefield until the battle is over. **Transfer factor** converts unactivated T-cells into activated T-cells. B-cell growth factor and B-cell differentiation factor are also lymphokines. **Interferon-gamma** is a lymphokine by which T-cells activate macrophages.

Lymphokines, Monokines, and Cancer

With the advent of recombinant gene technology, it has become possible to produce large quantities of lymphokines and other similar substances found normally only in extremely small quantities. The ability to make multiple copies of the genes that specify the structure of these substances and then use them to generate large quantities of gene product has made it possible to study the effects of giving IL-2, for example, first to experimental animals and then to human cancer patients. Clinical trials employing Il-2 were under way at the time we went to press. These involved taking T-cells from patients and growing them in culture with IL-2. The resultant lymphokine-activated killer cells are then put back into the patient together with more IL-2. (Other studies had shown that neither IL-2 nor activated T-cells alone were effective.)

The results of the very first clinical trial with IL-2 was reported in late 1985 (Rosenberg et al.). In this study, 11 of 25 patients with advanced cancer, all of whom failed to respond to other treatment, showed partial shrinkage of tumor; there was also one complete remission. Among the side effects of IL-2 discovered in this trial were fluid retention, malaise, fever/chills, nausea, diarrhea, and anemia (Marx, 1985a).

Even if the side effects are diminished somehow and IL-2 continues to be shown to be effective, we are apparently a long way from the common use of IL-2 in treating cancer. The treatment schemes used in early clinical trials were very expensive and technologically cumbersome; they are not at all practical as a routine treatment.

Other possibilities for IL-2 exploit the fact that the cells of adult T-cell leukemias all bear IL-2 receptors, whereas normal T-cells do not (unless induced). Monoclonal antibodies (called **anti-Tac** because they are antibodies to activated T-cells) to the IL-2 receptors have been used to treat patients, and some have gone into complete (albeit short-lived) remission. Studies are now under way in which toxins are affixed to the IL-2 receptor antibodies. Still another possibility is the use of IL-2 to reverse the immune-suppressive effects of cancer treatment (see Chapter 17).

The relationship between IL-2 and IL-2 receptors is also being exploited in diseases other than cancer. For example, anti-Tac might be useful in eliminating the T-cells that go astray in autoimmune diseases such as diabetes. It may also be used to suppress activated T-cells following organ transplants—thereby obviating rejection.

TNF/Cachectin

Cachectin is a hormone produced by activated macrophages (and NK cells, see below); it is responsible for, among other things, the shock that sometimes accompanies bacterial infections (at the time this was written, cachectin was being studied as a possible mediator of toxic shock syndrome). Cachectin and **tumor necrosis factor (TNF)**, a substance found to cause malignant tumors to regress, are one and the same thing. TNF causes hemorrhagic necrosis (localized cell death/hemorrhage). We will refer to the substance as TNF from this point on. The story of how TNF was discovered and the prospects it holds in cancer treatment are interesting and certainly relevant to our consideration of immunity and cancer. Let's start at the beginning.

The spontaneous regression of tumors has long been fascinating to cancer researchers. Although the phenomenon has often been explained as miraculous, scientists have continued to be interested in the mechanisms of why and how. Cancer researchers have particularly been interested in how spontaneous remissions might be made to happen more often. In the late 1800s, William B. Coley in the United States and physician/scientists in other countries experimented with the idea that *hyping*, or priming, the immune system by giving cancer patients bacterial infections might induce the immune system to "take on" the malignancy as well. Coley, in particular, experimented with killed bacterial preparations that came to be known as **Coley's toxins**. The results of his early studies and others were mixed, and the idea of treating humans with toxins fell out of fashion after Coley's death; it was largely forgotten for most of this century. Studies of the effects of microbial products on tumors using experimental animals continued, however, and eventually generated some promise in the form of *filtrates of* **gram-negative** *bacterial cultures* (bacteria whose cell walls are lipid-rich and, as a consequence, react to a special stain in a particular way)—the active ingredient turned out to be a lipopolysaccharide (LPS). Other bacterial preparations that have shown some promise are *Bacillus Calmette-Guerin (BCG)*, and *Corynebacterium parvum* (or *C. parvum*), both of which showed some therapeutic effect on animal tumors. Problems with toxicity and other difficulties with LPS, BCG, and C. parvum have conspired to make the transition to human tumors disappointing, however.

LPS, BCG, and C. parvum were thought to somehow, sometimes induce the hemorrhagic necrosis of tumors indirectly through some kind of effect on the host; it was during an investigation of the antitumor effect of serum from mice treated with BCG and LPS that TNF was discovered and reported in 1975 by Lloyd Old and co-workers (see Old, 1985). Cloning of the TNF gene (and expression of the cloned gene) was reported in several laboratories in 1985 (see Old, 1985).

Just how TNF causes the hemorrhagic necrosis of tumors is unknown. It may be directly toxic to tumor cells, and there is some evidence that it interferes with tumor capillaries. TNF is known to cause some kinds of cells to stop dividing and others to divide faster, and it has no effect on the proliferation of still other cells. The effects of TNF on cell division are not limited to tumor cells (see Sugarman et al., 1985).

One of the strategies suggested by the isolation of TNF is blocking its effects, thereby blocking cachexia (see Chapter 12). The basis of this idea is the fact that TNF administered to experimental animals produces fever, diarrhea, weight loss, and lethal shock. And it has also been found that endotoxin-resistant mice have macrophages only weakly able to generate TNF in response to endotoxin. Beutler, Milsark, and Cerami (1985) found that passive immunization against TNF protects mice from lethal effects of endotoxins. The latter finding provides strong evidence that TNF somehow mediates these effects and provides basis for hope that cachexia might one day be blocked by blocking TNF.

The normal role of TNF is not yet known. Work with cachectin suggests a role in mobilization of energy reserves—perhaps tumors inappropriately stimulate the production of TNF, or they produce TNF themselves, resulting in cachexia. Investigations of TNF's effects on infectious microbes have not yet supported the notion that it is directly antimicrobial.

The prospects of using TNF as a cancer therapeutic agent are very real. TNF has had some dramatic effects on subcutaneous, transplanted human and animal tumors. Some animal tumors are apparently completely refractory to TNF, however. Among the possibilities being tried are combinations of TNF and interferon and combinations of TNF with other cytotoxic agents. Clinical trials are already under way and hopes are running high.

The Immune System Is Everywhere

B-cells and T-cells take up residence in the spleen, in lymph nodes, and in various other lymphoid tissues scattered throughout the body. Some B-cells and T-cells are always on the move, circulating throughout the body as monitors of the presence of foreign substances, constantly on the lookout for (that is, responsive to) antigens that they do not recognize as "self." The notion of "self" raises an interesting question: How does the immune system know? Although the exact mechanism is not clear, apparently, during neonatal development the immune system somehow surveys all potential antigenic material present at the time and declares these to be "self" and then programs itself such that it will not normally attack proteins that make up the body it is assigned to protect.

Natural Killer (NK) Cells

One other component of the immune system is the **natural killer cell**, or **NK-cell**; we will call them NK-cells here. NK-cells have neither T-cell markers nor B-cell markers, and they exhibit nonspecific killer activity. NK-cells are a subtype of lymphoid cells found in most mammals and birds. They have been described as intermediate in target cell recognition, between the highly specific T-cells and "generalist" macrophages. The NK cell-killing mechanism is believed to involve the release of granules containing proteins called **polyperforins** which somehow destroy the integrity of the target cell membrane. The same mechanism is believed to operate in cytotoxic T-cells. The mechanisms by which NK-cells are stimulated to attack a variety of abnormal cells including cancer cells and cells infected by viruses are unknown (see Herberman and Ortaldo, 1981). Indeed, NK-cells seem to specialize in defense against viruses and cancer. Among the considerable evidence that NK-cells are important defenders against cancer are the facts that, generally speaking, high levels of NK-cells have been associated with (1) resistance to experimental tumor induction and tumor transplantation, (2) enhanced tumor clearance, and (3) diminished metastases (Brodt, 1983). NK-cells have recently been shown to be suppressed in both lung cancer patients and in heavy smokers with no cancer (Phillips et al., 1985).

The Cancer Connections

The immune defense system has an awesome ability to help us survive in a sea of infectious organisms. The normally remarkable efficiency of the immune system raises the question: "Why doesn't it protect us from cancer?"

Perhaps it actually does. Some scientists believe that our bodies reject skin grafts and transplanted kidneys because a system was developed during evolution for snuffing out virus-infected/altered cells and possibly other kinds of normal cells gone wrong. They argue that, otherwise, evolution didn't need to provide us with a foreign-tissue rejection system. It could very well be that in its prime, the immune system snuffs out incipient cancers as a regular part of its job. Maybe only after it gets old—only after the body is past the time of having and rearing offspring and is "biologically dead" anyway—does it then become less effective and allow cancer cells to grow. The facts that the immune system does decline with age, and that most cancers emerge in those old enough for the decline to have begun, lends some credence to this hypothesis. And the fact that the risk of developing cancer goes up in immuno-suppressed patients—those who are being treated following kidney transplants, for example—offers even stronger evidence. Human beings with immune-system deficiencies caused by drugs or disease have 100 times the normal risk of developing certain kinds of cancer (Sondel, 1983; Krueger and Tallent, 1985).

Stress, the Immune System, and Cancer

There is some evidence that psychological factors, including stress, may play some role in predisposing human beings to cancer.

Stress can suppress the immune response. A number of studies of stressed human beings—for example, husbands in mourning over the deaths of their wives, or medical students taking final exams—have shown that stress suppresses cell-mediated immunity (see Marx, 1985a).

Bereavement and depression have both been found to diminish white-cell responsiveness to immune stimulants. Pettingale (1985) summarizes a number of recent studies in human beings, showing, for example, that sleep deprivation influences phagocytosis and depresses lymphocyte responsiveness. Many animal studies have also shown that stress reduces the immune response. It has even been shown that the immune response can be conditioned—upward or downward. Stimuli (which themselves have no known influence on the immune system), if associated for a while with immune-enhancing or immune-suppressing drugs, have been shown to themselves be able to enhance or suppress the immune response when later given alone (see Dixon, 1986).

How is it that the psyche and the immune system might be connected? There are several possibilities. Perhaps the best-known connection is via the adrenal glands. These glands, which are under the control of the pituitary, which itself is under the control of the part of the brain called the hypothalamus, produce cortisone, adrenalin, and other hormones that help the body deal with stress. Cortisone is a well-known suppressor of the immune system. Another possibility is *endorphins*. Endorphins are a class of neuropeptides that diminish pain and induce euphoria. Endorphins have been shown to react with lymphocytes and to impair lymphocyte response *in vitro*.

Biologically, it is not clear *why* stress should suppress the immune system; perhaps this suppression minimizes immunity-related damage to healthy tissue following trauma. This might be beneficial over a short term.

The Antigenicity of Cancer Cells

If cancer cells did not bear unusual antigens—things that the immune system could recognize—this section would not have been written. But cancer cells do have antigens that their norma counterparts do not have. It should be noted here that while **tumor-specific antigens** are antigens that appear *only* on tumor cells, **tumor-associated antigens** are antigens found on normal cells as well as on tumor cells—but on tumor cells they occur at higher levels and/or at the "wrong" time, e.g., antigens normally associated primarily with fetal cells sometimes appear on tumor cells. As indicated in Chapter 4, while tumor-specific antigens are demonstrable in many animal tumor and cell-culture models, the evidence for the existence of tumor-specific antigens in human tumors is rather weak. A wealth of evidence indicates that tumor-associated antigens exist in both animal models and in human cancer, however (see McKhann, 1982, and Old, 1977). Tumor-associated antigens borne by and shed by human cancer cells serve to mark the presence of cancer and can be used in diagnosing cancer (see Chapter 16). A problem seems to be that many human cancers are only weakly antigenic.

It has been shown many times that if a transplantable tumor is allowed to grow for a while in an animal and then removed, other transplants of the same tumor line cannot be established in the same animal (Fig. 14.6). There is an interesting difference between chemically and virally induced cancers in this regard. Most chemically-induced tumors bear unique antigens. If tissue from a particular chemically induced tumor is used to immunize another animal, immunity is conferred only against that particular tumor. Immunological cross reactivity even between different tumors induced by the same chemical, even in the same animal, is rare. This specificity is most likely related to the fact that a chemical carcinogen can elicit any number of mutations, each expressed as a unique antigenic character at the cell surface. Tumors induced by the same viruses, on the other hand, are cross reactive—undoubtedly due to the constancy of the virus-specific antigens expressed on the transformed cell surfaces. In any case, these and other direct elements of evidence indicate that not only are some neoplasms antigenic, but also immune responses are in fact

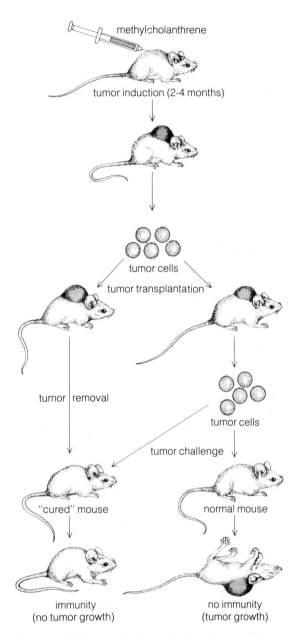

Figure 14.6 Mice can be immunized against specific neoplasms. Immunity to carcinogen-induced tumors can be shown in mice as follows: if cells from a chemically induced tumor are transplanted into another mouse of the same inbred strain, and the resultant tumor removed surgically, the mouse that received the transplant will resist subsequent transplants of the same tumor. (Reprinted by permission of *Scientific American* © 1977. All rights reserved.)

mounted against them. The fact that the initial neoplasm would normally go on to kill the host if it were not removed (Fig. 14.5) suggests that cancer somehow gets ahead of the immune system and can stay ahead.

In animals, successful vaccines against cancers caused by viruses have been developed. A neurolymphoma, Marek's disease, in chickens is caused by a virus. Chickens can be protected from Marek's disease by inoculating them with a similar but not pathogenic (for chickens) virus found in turkeys. A vaccine is also now available for infectious feline (cat) leukemia. The search for viruses as causes of human cancers has borne some fruit (see Chapter 10), and those human cancers caused by viruses are the most likely prospects for anticancer vaccines in the future.

Evidence for immune responses against cancer in humans includes the following: (1) spontaneous remissions—documented cases in which widespread cancers disappeared without treatment or in which metastases disappeared following surgical removal of a primary mass; (2) circulating complexes of antigens and antibody are found in cancer patients; (3) lymphocyte infiltration is seen in human cancer at the edges of neoplasms; (4) proliferation of T-cells and B-cells in lymph nodes draining areas that have cancers; and (5) the increase in cancer incidence in immunosuppressed people. It must be noted, however, that immunosuppressed people are at greater risk only of some kinds of cancer, not all; and "nude" mice, which have no cell-mediated immunity, get no more cancers than normal mice.

But even if the immune system is usually active against cancer, something goes dreadfully wrong in a third of all Americans. What goes wrong in these cases? Again, the only explanation appears to be that cancer is somehow able to evade the immune system.

Escape Mechanisms

It may well be that for many, if not most human cancers, the problem will continue to be that the cancers are not antigenic or not sufficiently antigenic. But even those that *are* antigenic escape the immune system. There are a number of plausible escape mechanisms (see McKhann, 1982):

1. *Antigen modulation.* Cancer cells that have tumor-specific antigens (TSAs) may have them only for a short time and then lose them somehow—by being covered up, by being changed, or by being shed.

2. *Selection.* The cancer cells in a neoplasm are not all the same at any one time. The immune system may in fact destroy all cancer cells that are strongly antigenic, allowing nonantigenic or only weakly antigenic cancer cells to become dominant.

3. *Secretion of excess antigen.* Neoplasms may shed so much antigen into the bloodstream that the elements of the immune system are neutralized, blocked, and/or exhausted before they even reach the site of the cancer.

4. *Indirect immunosuppression.* Neoplasms shed substances other than antigens known to be able to suppress T-cell and B-cell function. It has been known for some time that patients with cancer are often immunosuppressed.

5. *Suppressor T-cell stimulation.* Since the normal function of suppressor T-cells is to hold other T-cells and B-cells in check, another possibility is that neoplasms somehow stimulate suppressor cells. Experiments with mice have in fact shown that after a period of tumor growth, cells previously able to attack cancer cells lose this capacity, and this loss coincides with the appearance of suppressor T-cells (see McKhann, 1982).

6. *Tolerance.* If a large amount of normally antigenic material is administered to an individual, this may not only result in no detectable immune response, but the individual may not respond to a small amount of the same antigen later. This situation is called **immunological tolerance**. The antigen load imposed on a cancer-bearing individual may ultimately cause the im-

mune system to tolerate that antigen in a similar manner.

7. *Protective antibody coating.* It is conceivable that if a tumor-associated or tumor-specific antigen stimulates the production of a non-complement-fixing, noncytotoxic antibody, the antibody could interact with cancer cells and mask their antigens in such a way as to prevent other cytotoxic reactions.

8. *Outrunning the immune system.* A tumor may simply grow faster than the immune system's ability to deal with it. For example, the location of a tumor and the nature of its antigenicity could be such that the production of specific antibody and reactive cells may never catch up to the tumor.

Prospects for Using the Immune System Against Cancer

Throughout the world, cancer researchers are at work on ways in which the immune system might be exploited in the fight against cancer. Their strategies can be subdivided into a number of broad categories, some of which are diagnostic and most of which are therapeutic. Consider the following possibilities (see also Chapter 17):

1. Give patients substances able to stimulate the immune system in a general way; for example, BCG, C. parvum, interleukins, or interferon—alone or in combination with other anticancer agents.

2. Immunize the host with some of the antigen from his or her own tumor cells or cells from a similar neoplasm removed from another person. Cells removed from the patient can be used if the cells are killed or rendered incapable of division first. The cells can also be treated to enhance their ability to elicit an immune reaction.

3. Inject immune enhancers directly into the neoplasm (as in Item 1, except that the adjuvant is put directly into the neoplasm or next to it).

4. Give an antibody. Using monoclonal antibody production techniques (see below), produce antibodies against antigens present on a patient's tumor cells but not on the patient's normal cells. Give the patient the antibody. One of the problems with this kind of "passive immunity" is that antibody molecules made elsewhere are often themselves attacked by the body's immune system. Up to now, part of the problem has been that we have had to for technical reasons use monoclonal antibodies of mouse origin. Now it is possible to make *chimeric* antibodies—part human and part mouse, and these are expected to be less likely to elicit an immune reaction against the monoclonal.

5. Make antibodies more potent by affixing toxic chemicals, chemotherapeutic agents, or radioisotopes to them. The National Cancer Institute is now supporting clinical trials of *drug-antibody conjugates.* In one such trial, people with inoperable lung cancer are being given an anticancer drug bonded to the monoclonal antibody of an antigen associated with lung-cancer cells. Clinical trials with monoclonal antibodies alone have been carried out with mixed results.

6. Isolate lymphocytes from a cancer patient and expose them to tumor-associated or tumor-specific antigen from that patient's neoplasm. Put the "activated" lymphocytes back into the patient.

7. Stimulate T-cells in such a way that they recognize tumor-specific, or tumor-associated antigen as foreign—for example, by giving the patient the lymphokine "transfer factor" isolated from T-cells that had been exposed to the tumor antigen in a patient cured of the same kind of tumor or in volunteers.

8. Find ways to block the cachexic effects of the tumor necrosis factor while enhancing its tumor-necrosis–inducing effects; then give patients more of the factor.

9. Use antibodies to demonstrate the presence of neoplasms as an aid in early detection or staging. Affix a radiolabel to an antibody and

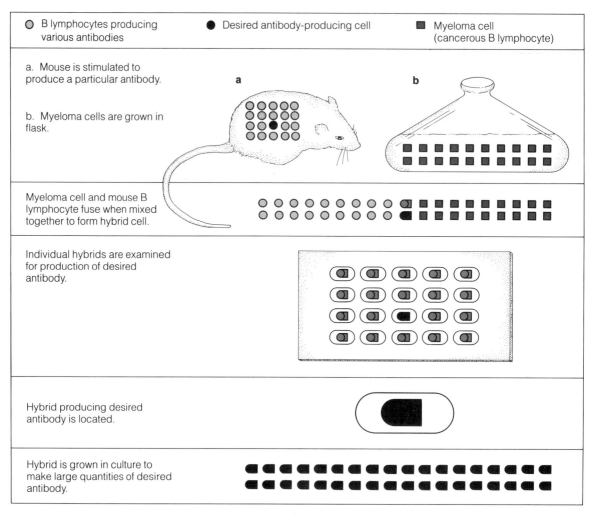

Figure 14.7 General procedure for making monoclonal antibodies

Legend items in figure:
- ○ B lymphocytes producing various antibodies
- ● Desired antibody-producing cell
- ■ Myeloma cell (cancerous B lymphocyte)

a. Mouse is stimulated to produce a particular antibody.

b. Myeloma cells are grown in flask.

Myeloma cell and mouse B lymphocyte fuse when mixed together to form hybrid cell.

Individual hybrids are examined for production of desired antibody.

Hybrid producing desired antibody is located.

Hybrid is grown in culture to make large quantities of desired antibody.

---

then allow the antibody to react with cells bearing the antigen. Use a scanner to detect any concentrations of antibody-tagged antigens in the body thereby indicating tumor sites.

Interferon and monoclonal antibodies promise to accelerate the evaluation of immunological possibilities in the war against cancer. Interferon (see Chapters 10 and 17) is a family of antiviral agents generally able to activate macrophages, T-cells, and NK-cells and to enhance the inflammatory response. Genetic engineering tech-

niques have made it possible to produce large quantities of interferons, making it possible to evaluate the use of interferon in treating cancer (see Grady, 1982).

Monoclonal antibodies (a full description of monoclonal antibody production techniques is given in Chapter 16) are antibodies with a degree of specificity and homogeneity heretofore unobtainable (see Fig. 14.7). The ability to prepare exquisitely specific and pure antibody to an antigen will make it much more efficient to look for elusive tumor-specific antigens—to see which or even tumor-associated antigens can help patients having tumors bearing such antigens. If tumors outrun the immune system, monoclonal antibodies may be the means by which to help patients catch up. As already mentioned, monoclonal antibodies can also be used to carry radioactive tags to cells bearing tumor antigens, thus marking the presence of primary cancers and metastases; they can also be used to carry lethal doses of radiation or cytotoxic chemicals to cancer cells.

Summary

For the time being, although some progress has been made, the application of immunology to the treatment and diagnosis of human cancer has been painfully slow. Measured against the promise of immunology and the early enthusiasm it engendered, progress has seemed even slower. After much work, a little of the promise has been realized and some of it may never be realized. Some of the promise remains, however. The prospect of vaccines for some forms of cancer remains one of the most important prospects for cancer prevention.

References and Further Reading

Beutler, B., Milsark, I. W., and Cerami, A. C. 1985. Passive Immunization Against Cachectin/Tumor Necrosis Factor Protects Mice from Lethal Effect of Endotoxin. *Science.* 229:869–71.

Beutler, B., et al. 1986. Control of Cachectin (Tumor Necrosis Factor) Synthesis: Mechanisms of Endotoxin Resistance. *Science.* 232:977–80.

Brodt, P. 1983. Tumor Immunology—Three Decades in Review. *Ann. Rev. Microbiol.* 37:446–76.

Clark-Lewis, I., et al. 1986. Automated Chemical Synthesis of a Protein Growth Factor for Hemopoietic Cells, Interleukin-3. *Science.* 231:134–39.

Dianzani, R., and Rossi, G. B., eds. 1985. *The Interferon System.* New York: Raven Press.

Dixon, B. 1986. Dangerous Thoughts. *Science 86.* April, pp. 63–66.

Dixon, F., and Kunkel, H., eds. 1982. *Advances in Immunology.* Orlando, Fla.: Academic Press.

Goding, J. 1984. *Monoclonal Antibodies: Principles and Practice.* Orlando, Fla.: Academic Press.

Grady, D. 1982. What Ever Happened to Interferon? *Discover.* 3:83–85.

Hancock, B. W., ed. 1984. *Immunological Aspects of Cancer.* Hingham, Mass.: Kluwer Academic Publishers (Kluwer-Nijhoff).

Herberman, R., and Ortaldo, J. 1981. Natural Killer Cells: Their Role in Defenses Against Disease. *Science.* 214:24–30.

Hurrell, J. G., ed. 1982. *Monoclonal Hybridoma Antibodies: Techniques and Applications.* Boca Raton, Fla.: CRC Press.

Kluger, M. J., Oppenheim, J. J., and Powanda, M. C., eds. 1985. *The Physiologic, Metabolic, and Immunologic Actions of Interleukin-1.* New York: Alan R. Liss.

Krueger, T. C., and Tallent, M. B. 1985. Neoplasias in Immunosuppressed Renal Transplant Patients: A 20 Year Experience. *Southern Medical Journal.* 78:501–06.

Lotzová, E. 1986. *Immunobiology of Natural Killer Cells.* Boca Raton, Fla.: CRC Press.

Luderer, A., and Weetall, H., eds. 1982. *Clinical Cellular Immunology: Molecular and Therapeutic Reviews.* Clifton, N.J.: Humana Press.

Marrack, P., and Kappler, J. 1986. The T Cell and Its Receptor. *Scientific American.* 254(2):36–45.

Marx, J. 1975. Antibody Structure: Now in Three Dimensions. *Science.* 185:1075–76.

Marx, J. 1976. Immunology: Role of Immune Response Genes. *Science.* 191:277–278.

Marx, J. 1985a. The Immune System Belongs in the Body. *Science.* 227:1190–92.

Marx, J. L. 1985b. Burst of Publicity Follows Cancer Report. *Science.* 230:1367–68.

McKhann, C. 1982. Tumor Immunology Past, Present, and Future. In J. Fortner and J. Rhoads, eds., *Accomplishments in Cancer Research 1981.* Philadelphia: Lippincott.

Milgrom, F., Abeyounis, C., and Kano, K. *Principles of Immunological Diagnosis in Medicine.* Philadelphia: Lea & Febiger.

Milstein, C. 1986. From Antibody Structure to Immunological Diversification of Immune Response. *Science*. 231:1261–68.

Mizel, S., ed. 1982. *Lymphokines in Antibody and Cytotoxic Responses*. Orlando, Fla.: Academic Press.

Myrvik, Q., and Weiser, R. 1984. *Fundamentals of Immunology*. 2nd ed. Philadelphia: Lea & Febiger.

Old, L. J. 1977. Cancer Immunology. *Scientific American*. 236(5)62–79.

Paul, W., ed. 1984. *Fundamental Immunology*. New York: Raven Press.

Pettingale, K. W. 1985. A Review of Psychobiological Interactions in Cancer Patients. In M. Watson and T. Morris, eds., *Psychological Aspects of Cancer*. New York: Pergamon Press.

Phillips, B., Marshall, M. E., Brown, S., and Thompson, J. S. 1985. Effects of Smoking on Human Natural Killer Cell Activity. *Cancer*. 56:2789–92.

Pick, E., ed. 1983. *Lymphokines*. Orlando, Fla.: Academic Press.

Prehn, L. 1981. Role of Immunity in Cancer Remains a Puzzle. *Bioscience*. 31(6):449–52.

Ray, P. K., ed. 1985. Advances in Immunity and Cancer Therapy, Vol. 1. New York: Springer-Verlag.

Reif, A. E., ed. 1984. *Immunity to Cancer*. Orlando, Fla.: Academic Press.

Riley, V. 1981. Psychoneuroendocrine Influences on Immunocompetence and Neoplasia. *Science*. 212:1100–09.

Rosenberg, S. A., et al. 1985. Observations on the Systematic Administration of Autologous Lymphokine-Activated Killer Cells and Recombinant Interleukin-2 to Patients with Metastatic Cancer. *N. Engl. J. Med.* 313:1485–92.

Rosenberg, S. A., Spiess, P., and Lafreniere, R. 1986. A New Approach to the Adoptive Immunotherapy of Cancer with Tumor-Infiltrating Lymphocytes. *Science*. 233:1318–21.

Schwartz, L., ed. 1980, 1982, 1983. *Compendium of Immunology*. Vols. 1, 2, 3. New York: Van Nostrand.

Sibley, C. 1984. How Do B Lymphocytes Control Antibody Production? *Bioscience*. 34(1):30–35.

Siegelman, M., et al. 1986. Cell Surface Molecule Associated with Lymphocyte Homing Is a Ubiquitinated Branched-Chain Glycoprotein. *Science*. 231:823–29.

Sondel, P. 1983. The Immunology of Cancer. In S. Kahn et al., eds., *Concepts in Cancer Medicine*. New York: Grune & Stratton.

Springer, G. 1984. T and Tn General Carcinoma Autoantigens. *Science*. 224:1198–206.

Stinnett, J. D., ed. 1983. *Nutrition and the Immune Response*. Boca Raton, Fla.: CRC Press.

St. John, T., et al. 1986. Expression Cloning of a Lymphocyte Homing Receptor cDNA: Ubiquitin Is the Reactive Species. *Science*. 231:845–50.

Sugarman, B. J., et al. 1985. Recombinant Human Tumor Necrosis Factor-(alpha): Effects on Proliferation of Normal and Transformed Cells in Vitro. *Science*. 230:943–45.

Waldman, T. A. 1986. The Structure, Function, and Expression of Interleukin-2 Receptors on Normal and Malignant Lymphocytes. *Science*. 232:727–32.

PART FIVE
DEALING WITH CANCER AND THE THREAT OF CANCER

This is the last part of the book. Although Part V contains five chapters, there are really three topics here: prevention, detection, and treatment. Chapter 15 covers prevention. In essence, it translates what we know about the *causes* of cancer into specific strategies that should reduce the risk of getting cancer. Chapter 16 emphasizes the *next* best thing to prevention—which of course is early detection—in an overall description of the ways in which cancer is detected, diagnosed, and assessed. Chapter 16 describes

the ways in which medicine gathers data about particular neoplasms so that treatment can be planned and carried out accordingly. Chapter 17 summarizes the ways in which surgery, radiation therapy, chemotherapy, and immunotherapy are used to fight cancer. Chapter 18 outlines the key features of each major type of human cancer. Chapter 19 deals with the problem of coping with a diagnosis of cancer and the aftermath of both successful and unsuccessful treatment.

15

Preventing Cancer

The very best thing you can do about cancer is avoid getting it. If you prevent cancer, you don't need doctors, hospitals, diagnostic procedures, staging, treatment, rehabilitation, or medical bills. Prevention is especially important because present-day cures are only 35 percent effective on the average, and they themselves are life threatening. There is no question that the best personal anticancer strategy is prevention.

Prevention is also, potentially, the most effective thing doctors and other health professionals can do about cancer. Despite the fact that some significant gains have been made in the treatment of acute lymphocytic leukemia, Hodgkin's disease, testicular cancer, and other kinds of cancer, the fact is the medical profession has *too little* to offer cancer patients in the way of effective treatment. Despite the dictum "Treat the sick and leave the well alone," and despite the fact that preventive medicine still does not fit very well into the grand scheme of medical care, prevention presently offers much more than treatment in terms of potential for doing something about cancer.

Is Prevention Possible?

We know that cancer is a family of diseases with mostly external, environmental causes. Depending on the attributor, anywhere from 80 to 90 percent of all cancer is attributed to the environment—in the most general meaning of the term *environment*. Because we know about specific environmental agents in relatively few instances, because it may turn out that some of the unknown environmental "factors" are hopelessly complicated combinations of things that may never be identified, and because some environmental factors are simply unavoidable— such as sunlight and background radiation— "environmental" does not necessarily mean "avoidable." Still, some experts believe that maybe as much as 90 percent of all cancer will ultimately prove to be preventable (Berg, 1977).

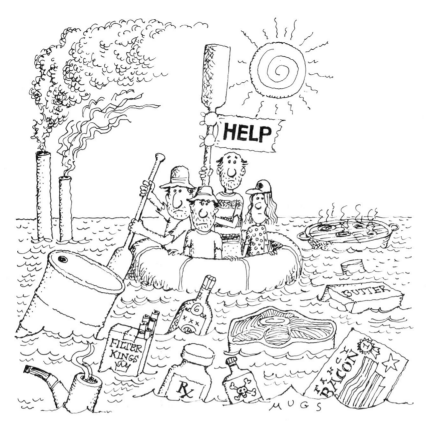

Figure 15.1 Adrift in a sea of carcinogens

Others estimate that at least 60 percent will ultimately prove to be preventable (see Reif, 1981).

Consider the following:

Counting skin cancer, about half of all cancer is linked to sunlight or tobacco.

Lung cancer is almost entirely (85 to 90 percent) related to smoking.

Breast cancer is related to reproductive history and diet; cancer of the colon is also related to diet.

Breast cancer, lung cancer, and colon cancer account for half of all cancer.

Recently (1982), the National Research Council (NRC) predicted that we will one day very soon

be able to prescribe a diet that will reduce cancer incidence in the United States by 30 percent.

A summary of cancer-associated environmental factors is given in Table E.4 (p. 200). An estimate by Newell and Boutwell of the proportion of "preventable" cancers related to the environment is given in Table 15.1. Other estimates will be given throughout this chapter.

Can Cancer Prevention Efforts Make a Difference?

The connection between smoking and lung cancer offers the most striking, doubly incriminat-

What Exactly Does Prevention Mean?

The word *prevention* can be used all across a spectrum that begins with carcinogenesis and ends with cancer death. Cancer can be prevented from happening, it can be prevented from ever producing symptoms, and it can be prevented from causing death. Unqualified, these different meanings of prevention as it applies to cancer are potentially confusing. Qualified, these different types of prevention become primary prevention, secondary prevention, and tertiary prevention. **Primary prevention** refers to strategies that keep cancer from getting started in the first place. Two examples are (1) blocking exposure to carcinogenic agents and (2) removing an organ in which the later development of cancer is practically in-

evitable—as in familial polyposis (see Chapter 5). We consider primary prevention in this chapter.

Secondary prevention means "catching cancer early," before it does any harm—after it produces very early symptoms but before it produces disruption in normal host function. Secondary prevention is, in essence, what happens as a result of effective early detection by vigilance or by screening. Secondary prevention is the subject of the next chapter. **Tertiary prevention** refers to the effective treatment of cancer after its presence becomes obvious through some constellation of signs and symptoms. Tertiary prevention is the featured topic of Chapter 17.

---

ing evidence that specific actions make a big difference. The more cigarettes smoked, the greater the risk of dying of lung cancer (see Fig. 13.3); and the more time that passes after one quits, the nearer the risk comes to normal. What could be plainer? We have already discussed the fact that Mormons run about a third of the cancer risk as the average American (Fig. E.1, p. 199). Mormons do not use tobacco or alcohol, thus avoiding certain carcinogens, and they get less cancer. We discuss other such evidence throughout the chapter.

A Checklist of Prevention Strategies

Because new carcinogens are found continuously, people often say, "*Everything* causes cancer; so why worry about it?" But this notion is both false and dangerous. The facts clearly indicate that people who avoid known carcinogens tend not to get cancers associated with those carcinogens. A more general "great truth" is that the risk of developing cancer can be reduced significantly by taking identified carcinogens into account in living life. In this part of the

chapter we will review what could be called a checklist of cancer prevention strategies. We will convert the associations we covered in the section on carcinogenesis (Chapters 7–10 and in Chapter 13) into a set of do's and don't's that will reduce cancer risk. It cannot be said with any certainty exactly how *much* risk reduction following each of these suggestions provides. The impact of each action will vary, but it is highly likely that each will have some impact. Let's begin with diet.

Diet

Inappropriate diet will probably turn out to be the main villain as we continue to identify specific environmental carcinogens. As pointed out earlier, the National Research Council (NRC) has (1982) suggested that we may one day be able to specify a diet that will reduce cancer incidence by a full third. Other estimates go even higher. While it is clear that there is an association between diet and cancer, the only pronouncements we are able to make now are vague and somewhat general. The NRC compares what we know now about diet and cancer to what we knew about cigarettes and cancer twenty years ago. The council goes on to say, however, that it is time to offer some pretty solid "interim guidelines" regarding cancer and diet.

At the outset, we must remember that food is not "just food." The various categories of cancer-causing substances that may be present in or on food are outlined in Table 15.2. Dietary cancer prevention strategies must take natural components, additives, contaminants, and residues into account, suggesting that cancer prevention via diet will be a team effort involving both government and the individual. The government's responsibility for pesticide residues, contaminants, and the safety of food additives will be addressed later, under the more general heading of public policy. Since naturally occurring substances and nutritional balance are probably more important, these will be considered first. The following is an annotated list of dietary do's and don't's, based on things we already know about cancer and diet:

Eat Well (Quality Not Quantity) A well-balanced diet is always a good idea because it brings many well-documented health benefits. The same holds for the admonition "Don't overeat." Maybe reducing total food intake simply reduces the total amount of dietary carcinogens ingested, but (whatever the reason) it *has* been shown that a reduction in total food intake in animals decreases the incidence of cancer (National Research Council, 1982). Although the evidence is not entirely clear for humans, the relatively few specific diet-cancer associations that have been documented all point to the benefits of a classical good diet. Some specifics follow.

Eat Fruit and Vegetables For many of the reasons related to vitamins and fiber (as well as for health reasons unrelated to cancer), it is a good idea to include fresh fruits and vegetables in one's diet. A North Carolina study revealed (see Winn et al., 1984) that women who had 21 or more servings of fruit and vegetables a week had half as many cancers of the throat, tongue, gum,

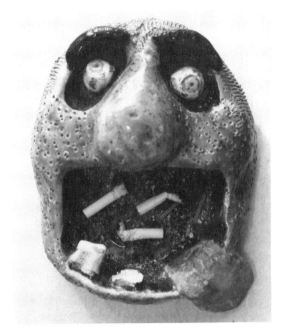

Figure 15.2 Don't smoke

or mouth as women who had 11 or fewer servings of fruit and vegetables per week, other things being "equal."

Eat Foods Rich in Fiber There have been many conflicting findings with respect to the importance of the relationship between fiber and cancer. Where it has been shown that a high-fiber diet has a protective effect, investigators have simply matched cancer incidence with relative amounts of fiber-containing foods without regard to the exact composition of the fiber. The fact that some studies have shown no connection between fiber and cancer, led the NRC (1982) to conclude that "if there is an effect, specific components of fiber, rather than total fiber, are more likely to be responsible." Since high-fiber diets protect against other kinds of digestive problems, such as constipation, irregularity, and diverticulitis, a high-fiber diet is clearly a good idea even if it turns out to have little relationship to cancer. Foods high in fiber include whole-grain bread and cereals, brown rice, nuts,

Table 15.1 Estimated Preventable Cancers

Cancer Associated With	Site	Annual Incidence	Preventable
Cigarette smoking plus alcohol	Lung and larynx	90,000	80,000
	Head and neck, esophagus	13,500	8,500
Industrial exposure	Bladder	9,000	5,000
Diet	Breast	30,000	10,000
	Colon	30,000	10,000
Sex	Cervix	7,500	7,500
Sunlight	Melanoma and other skin	5,000	1,500
Total		185,000	122,500

Source: Modified from National Cancer Institute data by Newell and Boutwell, 1981, p. 79. Used by permission.

pears, apples, beans, cabbage, carrots, and other raw fruits and vegetables (with skins).

Make Sure That You Get All Essential Vitamins Evidence exists that vitamin A, its chemical precursors (beta-carotene and retinoids), and vitamins C and E may block the carcinogenic process. Diets low in vitamin A have been associated with a higher than normal risk of cancers of the prostate, uterine cervix, skin, bladder, and colon (National Cancer Institute, 1984). The results of a study of some 2,107 male workers at the Western Electric Company in Chicago, beginning in 1959 and running some 19 years, suggested that diets rich in beta-carotene reduced the risk of lung cancer in cigarette smokers. In Norway, a study of more than 8,000 men including both smokers and nonsmokers showed that the risk of lung cancer was six times higher in subjects who had diets low in vitamin A (Blonston, 1984). Other studies in the United States and in Israel, Great Britain, France, and Japan have also indicated that beta-carotene affords some protection against lung cancer. Retinoids have been shown to inhibit the development of chemically induced cancers in animals (National Research Council, 1982). Foods rich in vitamin A include greens, asparagus, broccoli,

carrots, squash, tomatoes, sweet potatoes, apricots, peaches, and vitamin A-enriched milk. Vitamin A is toxic above certain levels, and this fact suggests that people not take vitamin A supplements (see later discussion of chemo-prevention).

According to the NRC, case control and correlation studies suggest that foods rich in vitamin C may be associated with a lowered risk of cancers of the stomach and esophagus. **Ascorbic acid** (another name for vitamin C) has also been shown to retard the chemically induced transformation of cells grown in culture and even to cause the reversion of cells already transformed (see Chapter 4).

The fact that vitamin E is an antioxidant and that it, like vitamin C, can inhibit the formation of nitrosamines, suggests that it too may have some anticancer properties. Available data do not allow any firm conclusions at this time, according to the NRC. Nor can any conclusions be drawn yet about the B vitamins.

The anticancer effects of vitamin A and its precursor retinoids may be related to the normal role of vitamin A in epithelial cell differentiation (see below). As for vitamin C and vitamin E, both are chemical antioxidants. They may work to prevent cancer by blocking some of the oxi-

Table 15.2 Categories of Substances in Food That May Increase Cancer Risk

Food Categories	Examples
An added poisonous or deleterious substance	Mercury in fish; aflatoxin in peanuts
A naturally occurring poisonous or deleterious substance	Inherent constituents of food such as solanine in potatoes, oxalic acid in rhubarb
An added poisonous or deleterious substance that is required in the production of food or cannot be avoided by good manufacturing practice	Environmental contaminants such as polychlorinated biphenyls in fish
A food additive	Intentional food ingredients such as saccharin; indirect food additives such as food-packaging migrants
A generally recognized as safe (GRAS) substance	Salt, sugar, vinegar
A prior-sanctioned substance	Nitrites in meat and poultry; caffeine in soft drinks
A pesticide chemical	DDT
A color additive	Red Dyes 2 and 40
An animal drug residue	Nitrofuran residues in cattle; diethylstilbestrol residues in cattle

Source: From *Science*, Vol. 223, March 9, 1984, pp. 1034-1040. Copyright 1984 by the AAAS. Used by permission of the author and the publisher.

dation reactions involved in the conversion of precarcinogens to ultimate carcinogens (Chapter 8). Foods rich in vitamin C include oranges and other citrus fruits, peaches, strawberries, cantaloup, and melons. The NCI indicates that two helpings per day of dark green vegetables and yellow-orange fruits and vegetables will provide the right amount of vitamins A and C.

Vitamins and minerals are often mentioned in the same breath. What about minerals? The NRC review (1982) looked into claims that nine different minerals have some relationship to cancer incidence. There were reasonably significant data for only iron and selenium, however. The NRC states that although "both the epidemiological and laboratory studies suggest that selenium may offer some protection against the risk of cancer . . . firm conclusions cannot be drawn on the basis of the present limited evidence" (p. 168). The NRC review was likewise unable to find enough basis for firm conclusions about the association of cancer with dietary iron, copper, zinc, molybdenum, iodine, arsenic, cadmium, or lead.

Restrict Fat Intake According to the NRC (1982) and the National Cancer Institute (1984), this strategy should include limiting both saturated and unsaturated fat. According to the NRC report, animal studies suggest that only when fat intake is relatively *low* do polyunsaturated fats seem to enhance the development of cancer. The NRC claims that—so far, anyway—the association between fat intake and cancer was the strongest of any of the dietary associations evaluated in terms of both epidemiological (case control and correlation studies) and laboratory (experimental animal) studies. Cancers associated with high fat intake include cancers of the breast, prostate, and colon. Although the mechanisms involved in the linkage of dietary fat intake and cancer are not known, there is reason to suspect that fat may somehow act as a promoter. In colon cancer, this action may take the form of the effects of bile acids in the gut—the amounts of bile acids secreted into the gut are determined by the amount of fat consumed. Lower fat intake can be accomplished by eating lean meat, poultry, and fish; removing fat from meat before cooking; avoiding fried foods; limiting butter, margarine, cream, shortening, and oils; using low-fat milk; and eating fruit for dessert.

It should be noted that the NRC was unable to come to any conclusions relative to protein and carbohydrate consumption, although its review of the data available suggested the *possibility* of a relationship between *high* protein intake and certain cancers.

Be Particular about How Food Is Prepared
Frying foods adds fat to them; eat foods that are baked, boiled, or broiled. Very high temperatures such as those reached in barbecuing or broiling food can cause mutagens to be formed via the **pyrolysis** (heat-induced breakdown) of protein. Mutagens can also be formed in meat cooked at low temperatures, however. Barbecuing foods can also deposit mutagenic and even carcinogenic polycyclic compounds such as benzo(a)pyrene via smoke.

Avoid Smoked and Salt-Cured Foods
Throughout the world where diets include large quantities of smoked and salt-cured foods, there are greater incidences of certain cancers particularly of the stomach and the esophagus. Country ham has two strikes against it—three, counting fat.

Eat Vegetables of the Family Cruciferaceae (Cauliflower, Broccoli, etc.) To botanists, the Cruciferaceae is a plant family whose members have four-petaled flowers suggestive of a cross; the word *crucify* comes from a common Latin root. An association has been found between the members of this family (used as food) and cancer prevention. Although epidemiologic evidence for this association has been found in many different places (National Research Council, 1982), the exact reason or the nutritional benefit is unknown. To be sure, these foods are relatively rich in some likely anticancer vitamins such as A and C, but perhaps the effect is due to the anticarcinogenic properties (i.e., suppression of free radical formation, stimulation of de-

toxification pathways, etc.) of constituent indoles, aromatic isothiocyanates, and phenols, and such other nonnutritive substances as selenium.

Avoid Moldy Foods and Foods Containing Excessive Levels of Pesticides As was discussed earlier, molds such as *Aspergillis flavus* produce a substance called *aflatoxin*, which is one of the most powerful cancer-causing substances known (see Chapter 8). Aflatoxin and other such mold toxins (**mycotoxins**) are believed to be associated with high levels of liver cancer in many countries of the world where generally poor storage facilities and practices promote the growth of mold. Pesticides are invisible, so all foods should be washed thoroughly; we must look to federal and state governments to monitor the pesticide residues on produce (see below).

Do Not Use Certain Artificial Sweeteners Such as Saccharin Casually Although saccharin (and possibly cyclamate) is a relatively weak carcinogen (see Chapter 8) as determined by animal experiments, it must be presumed to be linked to bladder cancer in humans, even though epidemiological studies have not provided a clear indication of an association between any of the nonnutritive sweeteners and cancer (National Research Council, 1982). The Food and Drug Administration has concluded that aspartame is not carcinogenic in animals. Since aspartame has been on the market only since 1981, there are no epidemiological data yet available on its carcinogenicity in humans.

Eat Sparingly of Luncheon Meats and Other Cured Products with Nitrates or Nitrites Added In the body, nitrate can be converted to nitrite (e.g., by bacterial action in saliva), which can in turn react with amines and other dietary components to yield N-nitroso compounds (see Mirvish et al., 1980). Epidemiological studies in more than a half dozen countries have shown an association between increased stomach and esophageal cancer to increased ingestion of nitrate or nitrite (National Research Council, 1982; see also National Academy of Science, 1981). Direct assessments of the carcinogenicity of nitrate and nitrite in animals, however, have been inconclusive (National Research Council, 1982). Even if nitrates and nitrites, themselves, turn out to be "clean," many *N*-nitroso compounds are potent carcinogens, and since nitrates and nitrites can be converted to these, the National Academy of Science (1981) recommended that exposure to nitrate, nitrite, and *N*-nitroso compounds be reduced.

Be Generally Careful about Other Food Additives and Contaminants The NRC points out that some 3,000 chemical substances are added to foods deliberately during processing, and another 12,000 chemicals used in packaging materials, and that these substances sometimes end up in food. Although the Delaney Clause in the Food, Drug, and Cosmetic Act (see below) prohibits the deliberate addition of known carcinogens to food, relatively few deliberate and inadvertent additives have been adequately tested. According to the NRC (1982), "certain nonnutritive constituents of foods, whether naturally occurring or introduced inadvertently (as contaminants) during production, processing, and storage, pose a potential risk of cancer to humans" (p. 15).

Don't Drink Too Much Alcohol Excessive consumption of alcohol has been linked to cancer of the mouth, esophagus, liver, and possibly other organs. Alcohol may be related to cancer in a number of different ways—for example, by enhancing the carcinogenic effects of tobacco (see below) or through a connection between alcohol-induced liver damage and liver cancer. Excessive alcohol consumption is generally defined as more than two ounces of alcohol per day.

Lifestyle

The word *lifestyle* means "the way one lives." Usually it is an all-encompassing term, but we will use it here narrowly, to mean "miscellaneous elements of the way one lives other than diet and occupation." The following lifestyle adjustments help reduce the risk of cancer. Again, the impact of each on risk is highly variable; in most cases, the degree of impact is unknown.

Don't Smoke The relationship between cigarette smoking and lung cancer has been known for several decades (see Fig. 13.3). Cigarette smoking also increases the risk of esophageal, laryngeal, oral, pancreatic, kidney, cervical, and bladder cancer. In the late 1960s, it was reported that tobacco use and cigarette smoking in particular was responsible for in excess of 33 percent of all deaths in men aged 35–59 and 44 percent of those 44–49 (U.S. Public Health Service, 1967). Smoking is also a positively synergistic risk factor (that is, in combination with various other substances, the cancer-causing effect is greater than the sum of the effects of each alone) for cancers associated with other cancer-causing agents such as asbestos, uranium ore, and other radioactive substances.

A congressional study released in 1985 found that disease and lost productivity related to smoking cost the United States $65 billion a year—more than $2 for every pack of cigarettes smoked. The National Research Council (1982) states, "It has become absolutely clear that cigarettes are the cause of approximately one-quarter of all the fatal cancers in the United States" (p. 1). Cigarette smoking has been called the single most important cause of disease and death in the United States (Schuman, 1984).

Don't Live with or Otherwise Associate with Smokers There have been many studies that have shown a relationship between cancer risk and exposure to household tobacco smoke; a number of studies in several countries have shown that nonsmoking females married to smokers have a higher risk to lung cancer than nonsmoking females married to nonsmokers. The American Cancer Society, for instance, reported in a recent study that a nonsmoking woman was 10 to 30 percent more likely to

It's no secret that tobacco farmers make money. In Kentucky (where tobacco brings farmers about $1 billion per year) and in other tobacco-producing states, tobacco is a big cash crop. Revenue from tobacco can spell the difference between profit and loss and thus survival on many a farm. Tobacco farmers need to make a living, and this argument has preserved the tobacco price support system that has been in place since long before we became sure that tobacco smoking was the single most important preventable cause of cancer in America.

There are even some unspeakable (if not unprintable) economic arguments in favor of allowing people to smoke all they want. Smoking not only kills people via lung cancer, it also is related to increased mortality via emphysema, heart disease, and other forms of ill health. Cairns (1978) points out that while preventing tobacco from taking lives prematurely via these diseases can be translated into a socioeconomic benefit in terms of increased years of productivity and directly related, decreased health care costs, it would also show up as a social cost in terms of increased Social Security payments and subsequent health care costs. He cites a study done in England (Department of Health and Social Security, 1972) in which it was calculated that the *savings* on health care and Social Security benefits, as a result of cigarettes keeping down the number of old people, would pay for all government-sponsored medical research in England many times over. Then of course there is tax revenue. In the United States, tobacco products are heavily taxed, providing state and federal governments with nearly $9 billion annually (in 1983—see *Louisville Courier Journal*, November 11, 1984). In the English study, tobacco tax revenue was about equal to the cost of running and staffing all the hospitals in England. Little wonder governments are not generally eager to snuff out tobacco.

---

develop lung cancer if exposed to the smoke of others than was a woman who was not so exposed (see also Sandler, Everson, and Wilcox, 1985).

Don't Smoke Pipes or Cigars, Either Cigar and pipe smokers run greater risk of cancer of the mouth, tongue, and throat and maybe lung cancer (see Fig. 13.3).

Don't Chew Snuff or "Scrap" Chewing tobacco causes cancer of the mouth. A National Institutes of Health Consensus Development Conference in January 1986 (see NIH Consensus Development Conference Statement, 1986) concluded that: "The human evidence that use of snuff causes cancer of the mouth is strong. . . . [The data are insufficient] to come to any conclusions regarding the relationship . . . to cancers at other sites."

Don't Smoke Marijuana Tars derived from marijuana smoke have been shown to induce cancers in animals.

If You Drink, This Amounts to One More Reason Not to Smoke Heavy consumption of alcohol along with heavy smoking increases the risk to cancer of the mouth and esophagus.

Consider City Life Carefully The risk of developing many cancers is significantly greater for city dwellers than for people who live in rural areas. There are probably many reasons for this increase, including carcinogens and cocarcinogens in polluted air and carcinogens in drinking water; fast pace-induced stress may also be a factor.

Stay Out of the Sun and Use Sun Screens When You Don't Sunlight and skin cancer, including malignant melanoma, are unquestionably related (see Fig. 9.4). The riskiest time is between 11 A.M. and 2 P.M., and at greatest risk are fair-skinned (e.g., Celtic) people because of their relative lack of the pigment **melanin**, which blocks out harmful rays. Fair-skinned people should, whenever they are out in the sun, (1) wear long-sleeved shirts and long pants, (2) wear hats, (3) use sun screen lotions; a rating of 15 will block nearly *all* the sun's harmful rays (National Cancer Institute, 1984).

Minimize Your Exposure to Radiation in General Avoid all unnecessary ionizing radiation of any kind. In Chapter 9, we noted that some effects of radiation were proportional to dose, and some effects were proportional to the *square* of the dose. But for all practical purposes, the relationship between radiation dose and cancer is linear—the more radiation, the more of an effect. Although the effects of very low levels of radiation are subject to continuing controversy, we must assume that there is no threshold until we find out otherwise. A good working conclusion is that every bit of radiation will make a difference in terms of cancer risk. The nature of the risk is such that while the benefit of necessary medical X-rays *outweighs* the increased cancer risk, "consumers" should consider each X-ray carefully and ask about its necessity.

Don't Take Unnecessary Drugs In Chapter 8, we listed some drugs known to be associated with cancer risk, and other, yet-undiscovered drugs may be associated with cancer. Many potential problems can arise with unnecessary and otherwise inappropriate prescription drugs and "recreational" drugs, and there are *many* reasons to avoid unnecessary drugs of any kind. Women who took estrogen in the past in much higher doses than are given today to relieve symptoms of menopause have a greater risk of developing uterine cancer. We pointed out in Chapter 8, that the hormone estrogen has been linked to cancer of the uterus. Although the linkage between estrogen in oral contraceptives and breast cancer is still controversial. A Center for Disease Control study reported in 1983 found no connection (*Morbidity and Mortality Weekly Report*, June 29, 1983), but another report about the same time (Pike et al., 1983) found that women who took high-progestogen oral contraceptives before age 25 have an increased risk of developing breast cancer before age 37. A study released in 1985 showed that the risk of uterine cancer among women who use estrogen during menopause remains significantly higher for several years after they stop taking estrogen (Page and Asire, 1985). Birth control pills may actually reduce the risk to ovarian cancer (National Cancer Institute, 1984). In Chapter 18 we discuss the use of drugs in cancer treatment; later on in this chapter we discuss the prospects for cancer prevention drugs.

Don't Get Fat, and Don't Stay Fat Develop the right balance between physical activity and food consumption. Obesity has been associated with cancer of the breast (especially postmenopausal) and cancer of the endometrium. Androstenedione, which is a steroid hormone originating in the adrenal gland, is converted to estrogen in the fat of postmenopausal women. This extra-ovarian estrogen would be higher in obese women and may account for the association between obesity and hormone-dependent cancers.

Avoid Chronic "Severe" Stress This goes without saying, actually because chronic severe stress is bad for *many* reasons. Relative to cancer, stress is a presumptive immune system suppressor, which could conceivably allow cancer to develop. A well-known relationship exists between negative stress or excessive stress and suppression of the immune system and animal experiments with transplanted, or chemically induced, cancers have shown that stress makes cancer more likely.

Occupation

Watch Where You Work   We covered the association between occupation and cancer in several earlier chapters. Occupation is *clearly* a risk factor for cancer. If you have a choice, stay away from occupations and industries (e.g., foundries, coke ovens, rubber working, metal mining, chemical) associated with cancer risk. If you cannot or choose not to take this course, then become informed about all the things you may be exposed to in your occupation. Be on the lookout for asbestos, benzene, chromium, nickel, vinyl chloride, carbon tetrachloride, and other chemicals listed earlier. Use all the caution you can bring to bear relative to work with presumptive or suspect carcinogens and, of course, *documented* carcinogens. Wear protective clothing, and follow all the safety rules.

Some Other Cancer Prevention Strategies

Chemoprevention

Our "pill for every problem" penchant raises the possibility of chemoprevention of cancer. Suppose something could be identified that could block some key step in the development of cancer? Wouldn't that be nice? We would not have to forgo any pleasurable activity—at least, not in the interest of cancer prevention—if we had "after the act" pills. This is not such a wild idea, actually!

Theoretically, given what we know about carcinogenesis (see Chapters 7–9), carcinogenesis could be blocked by at least three, maybe four, chemical strategies. One strategy would be to block the pathway or pathways by which a "precarcinogen" is converted into an "ultimate" carcinogen. Another plan would be to accelerate metabolic pathways that do not produce carcinogens along the way. A third would be to block the binding of carcinogens to DNA. A fourth might be to suppress oncogenes or to neutralize oncogene products.

The general pattern of activation of many "ultimate" carcinogens is a chemical oxidation (see Chapter 8). It has already been shown in animals that antioxidants such as butylated hydroxyanisole (BHA) and butylated hydroxytoluene (BHT) can reduce the carcinogenicity of many carcinogens by one or more of the mechanisms discussed earlier (see Ruddon, 1981; National Research Council, 1982). Ruddon also points out that these chemicals are used to "preserve freshness" in many foods—at levels shown to protect against carcinogenesis in mice. Other "chemicals" that *may* offer some protection against cancer include selenium, vitamin C, vitamin E, and vitamin A (see Table 15.3).

Retinoids are particularly interesting because they apparently act at the promotion but not the initiation phase of carcinogenesis. They can even reverse the malignant phenotype of already completely transformed cells, apparently by stimulating differentiation (Meyskens and Fuller, 1980; Sporn, 1978; Maugh, 1974; Bertram, 1980). Unfortunately, the retinoids are toxic (**hypervitaminosis A** is a disease caused by too much vitamin A), and in this respect are associated with the same general problem found with chemotherapeutic drugs (see Chapter 17).

Even if we do not give up on the idea of behavioral modification, the chemoprevention approach would still be attractive because of the simple fact that it will not be possible to remove every carcinogen from the environment no matter how we try. This limitation suggests a double-barreled strategy: removing all the carcinogens we can, and chemically neutralizing the rest!

Vaccines

Vaccines effective in preventing cancers have already been used for some time—in animals other than humans, such as virus-caused leukemias in cats and chickens (see Chapter 10). Certain viruses have now been linked to human cancers—and isolated. The next step will be to develop vaccines.

Table 15.3   Some Possible Chemopreventatives

Anticancer Agent	Example(s) of Systems Studied
Vitamin A and derivatives	Inhibits chemically induced carcinomas in a variety of laboratory animals and at a variety of anatomical sites. Dietary deficiency of vitamin A enhances susceptibility to chemical carcinogenesis. Human population groups ingesting low levels of vitamin A are at increased risk for developing lung and bladder cancers.
Vitamin C	Blocks nitrosamine formation
Vitamin E	Helps reduce level of mutagens in human intestine
Riboflavin	Inhibits chemically induced liver cancers
2-bromo-alpha-erogcryptine together with retinylacetate	Inhibits carcinogen-induced mammary cancer
ε-aminocaproic acid	Inhibits carcinogen-induced colorectal tumors
Indomethacin	Inhibits carcinogen-induced colon tumors
Butylated hydroxyanisole	Inhibits carcinogen-induced lung, forestomach, mammary tumors
Butylated hydroxytoluene	Inhibits carcinogen-induced lung, forestomach, mammary, liver tumors

Source: Oppenheimer, 1983, p. 71. Used by permission of American Laboratory.

No Preventive Gain from Avoiding People with Cancer

Cancer is not contagious. True, certain infective microorganisms have been implicated as causes of a few, relatively rare forms of cancer, but the organisms involved are very difficult to transmit. And cancer itself is *not* contagious.

Cancer Prevention by Intercepting Precancerous Conditions

We discussed precancerous conditions in Chapter 5. Any account of cancer prevention would be incomplete without some mention of maneuvers designed to identify and do something about precancerous conditions so that cancers never develop. Some examples: for people with family histories of colon cancer, colonoscopy should be done at regular intervals beginning at age 20 or so and if polyps are found, they should be removed. Similarly, those at risk of uterine

cervical cancer should have regular Pap tests and appropriate treatment for any dysplasias found.

Problems Putting Prevention into Practice

If cancer is preventable and if prevention strategies work, why are cancers not being prevented? Good question! This is, in fact, the most important question we will deal with in this chapter.

Three major kinds of barriers block cancer prevention: (1) technical, (2) personal, and (3) public policy. The technical barriers come from our inability to identify all specific causes or to avoid all identified, specific causes at the same time. Personal barriers have to do with ignorance and behavioral science; people may not know what to do, and they often fail to act according to what they know. Public policy barriers have to do with government policies governing the release of cancer-causing substances into the environment. Let's consider the technical problems first.

Cancer Prevention as a Technical Problem

In Chapter 8, we discussed the difficulty of conclusively identifying specific causes of cancer. All these difficulties have relevance here because the first step in avoiding an environmental cause of cancer is to identify the cause. You can't avoid something, usually, unless you know what it is! The cancer prevention problem is partly technical—we simply don't have tests that can yield 100 percent conclusive determinations as to carcinogenicity in human beings. The tests that we do have, such as microbial prescreening followed by a rodent bioassay, are time consuming and costly. Part of the technical difficulty is related to cost. Some cancers related to the "environment" may be caused by complicated combinations of complex sequences of exposures that will be very difficult if not impossible to figure out.

Also, even when a specific thing is *clearly* carcinogenic, it may "technically" be impossible to avoid. Sunlight is carcinogenic yet exposure to some sunlight is inevitable; exposure to some background radiation is likewise inevitable.

But by far the most perplexing prevention problem, hands down, is that even clearly *avoidable*, clearly carcinogenic substances are not avoided—because of combinations of ignorance, stupidity, industrial-commercial irresponsibility, and ineffective government regulation.

Cancer Prevention as a Behavioral Science Problem

By emphasizing personal motivation in this section, the author does *not* mean to downplay the importance of public and professional education relative to cancer prevention. It's just that motivation is clearly a bigger problem than ignorance. More can be done than is being done in

cancer education, to be sure, but good, well-funded organizations and agencies such as the American Cancer Society and the National Cancer Institute are in place, doing a good job of educating professionals and the public.

In case the connection hasn't occurred to the reader yet, many causes of cancer are sources of pleasure. After sex, alcohol, sunlight, smoking, and rich, good-tasting food, music is perhaps the only general source of pleasure that is not carcinogenic—but then, we all know the kinds of things go on in and around many places where there is music! This connection predicts that cancer prevention will continue to be an uphill battle. It could be argued that personal motivation is the *single biggest hurdle* in the way of diminishing the cancer problem.

Some years ago, I happened to be in Washington, D.C., at the National Cancer Institute for a meeting. The meeting was called by the Division of Cancer Control, that part of the NCI charged with making sure that what we already know about cancer is put into practice. A high official of that division smoked cigarettes during the entire meeting, sitting directly under a No Smoking sign. It struck me at the time that the cigarette habit must be one of the most powerful forces loose on earth. A surgeon friend (who later did quit smoking) smoked even though nearly all the surgery he did amounted to removing cancers of the mouths and throats of smokers. A pathologist I know who spends a good part of every day looking at cancer cells collected from smokers, smokes a pipe almost continuously. *I* smoke one.

Look at it this way. We already know very well that tobacco smoke is loaded with carcinogens and that cigarette smoking in particular causes cancer and all kinds of other health problems (Fig. 13.3). And we know that it pays to quit. Still, the most we have been able to get out of our government (until recently—see Box) is a requirement for a wimpish warning on cigarette packs and continuation of the tobacco price-support system. The most we have been able to get out of the tobacco companies is a call by one for an open debate on the evidence about cigarette smoking and advice to "young people" not to smoke because smoking is for "grown-ups." Saddest of all is that the most we have been able to do individually is illustrated in Figure 15.3.

An initial decline in per capita cigarette consumption followed the Surgeon General's landmark report (U.S. Public Health Service, 1964) but it lasted only one year; consumption was higher in each of the next three years (Fig. 15.3). The labeling act was passed in 1968, and after that the trend spiraled downward through 1983.

A number of influences are collectively responsible for the overall downward trend. After the Surgeon General's original report, a cigarette health warning labeling act was passed in 1968, various state laws restricted the sale of cigarettes to minors, a number of antismoking campaigns were sponsored by various private and governmental agencies, the Federal Trade Commission required that tar and nicotine content be posted, advertising was restricted (no cigarette ads on television), and the insurance companies came up with premium penalties for life, homeowners, and even automobile insurance sold to smokers.

Figure 15.3, as an indication of a trend, is also encouraging—if not by its slope, by its apparent ultimate destination. Warner (1981) attributes the decline to an antismoking public attitude, which in turn reflects a painfully slow but successful conversion of knowledge into behavioral change. Still, there is reason to be disap-

pointed in the slope of the decrease in cigarette consumption. After more than 30,000 studies documenting the health effects of smoking, the fact is that a third of our population 21 years and older, and a fifth of all teenagers continue to smoke (Schuman, 1984).

Perhaps we should quit spending money finding carcinogens until we find better ways to motivate one another to avoid the carcinogens we already know something about. Perhaps all cancer research money should go to behavioral research, at least for a while, until the behavioral scientists catch up to the chemists and the tumor biologists.

Education is not really the whole answer, at least not for those who already have the habit. As indicated above, even people who know "fool" well what the risk is still smoke—and in public, yet. When being "completely" educated makes no difference, what then?

Help from the Helpers?

The health professions offer little help to the individual in terms of education or in putting knowledge into practice—apparently because the health care system as presently constituted has little or no provision for helping people prevent disease. The following is probably the utterance least likely ever to be heard in a doctor's office:

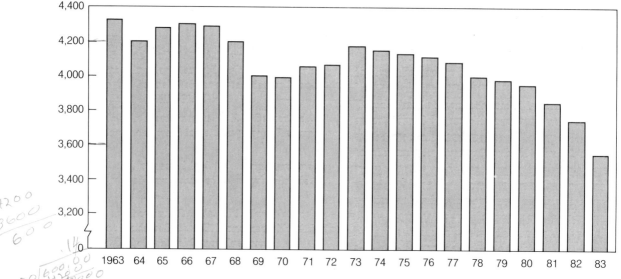

Figure 15.3 Per capita cigarette consumption since the Surgeon General's Report. (*Source:* U.S. Department of Agriculture)

Doc, I feel fine. I took off work today, and I sat in your office—for three hours—with some forty people, all with obviously fatal contagious diseases, just so I could ask some advice about cancer prevention. What can I do to avoid cancer . . . you know . . . to keep from getting cancer 20 or 25 years from now? Whaddaya say, Doc?

Many barriers block good preventive medicine. Some are patient related, like the one implied in the preceding paragraph—that prevention is not considered an acceptable reason to visit the doctor. Also, habits are hard to break, and much-delayed gratification does not reinforce. Some barriers to preventive medicine are physician related; for example, prevention has low priority, because sick people have to be helped first. There are also the problems of low financial incentive and delayed gratification. Still other barriers to good preventive medicine are related to the health care system—prevention has a low priority in this system, and there are simply too few financial incentives.

Among the things health care professionals *could* do fall into three broad categories: (1) convincing people that they are indeed in danger (education), (2) putting cancer prevention strategies into terms of specific behavior changes, and (3) helping people actually change behavior.

The typical communication between a physician and a patient works fairly well in situations where a specific action leads to a specific outcome. But this mode is totally inadequate for prevention outcomes. If a physician tells (and "tells" is a key word here, because the communication typically is one-way) a patient that he or she needs an injection, the patient will usually submit to the injection whether or not he or she really knows why it is being given. This same approach to prevention would amount to saying, "Smoking is bad, and you better quit." Without further elaboration and explanation, this statement rarely has any effect whatsoever—because in this case the patient is required to do more than be passively submissive. But it takes time to point out the details of cigarette smoke on the lungs, to explain "how in the world" there could be a connection between smoking and bladder cancer, to outline what happens to risk when a smoker also works with

Table 15.4 Some Primary Prevention Strategies for Health Professionals

Factor	Possible Intervention	Preventable Cancers
Tobacco smoking	Counseling to motivate cessation	Lung, oropharyngeal, laryngeal, esophageal, bladder, pancreas
	Strategies to achieve cessation	
	Strategies to maintain cessation	
	Support strategies for at-risk children, adolescents	
Diet high in total and saturated fat	Counseling to balance diet	Colorectal, prostate, ovary, endometrial, breast
	Strategies for at-risk families	
Large bowel polyps	Identification by sigmoidoscopy and stool guaiac	Colorectal
	Polypectomy	
Cervical dysplasia	Identification by properly performed Pap test	Cervical
	Appropriate treatment	
Ultraviolet light	Counseling on use of sun screens and on times to avoid sun exposure	Skin, melanoma
Alcohol	Counseling/referral to community resources	Oropharyngeal
Asbestos	Counseling to identify hazard, e.g., school building insulation	Lung, pleural
	Counseling to wear respirator	

Source: From Jon K. Sternburg, "Identification and Management of Risk Factors for Cancer," in *Concepts in Cancer Medicine*, eds. Kahn, et al., 1983, p. 242. Reprinted by permission of Grune and Stratton, Inc. and the author.

asbestos, or to clear up misconceptions such as one pack a day isn't bad or that smoking filter cigarettes is all right. It takes time to explain the connection between specific symptoms (to which a patient can relate) to damage caused by cigarette smoke. It takes time to answer questions. But doctors (and nurses) don't have much time, and most of them are not really able to talk to patients in lay terms. Sternburg (1983) suggests that physicians should work outside of their practices and take the cause of prevention into the schools and into the greater community via public meetings, television, radio, and so on.

Even at that, the task really only begins with the patient's conviction that there is danger and the identification of specific behavioral changes that will reduce risk. Beyond the kinds of intervention suggested in Table 15.4 (note that this includes some diagnostic maneuvers to identify risk factors), health care professionals have a certain obligation to motivate people to launch behavioral modification and to help them develop a plan. Those who would help must even become a source of sustained motivation by serving as external monitors of progress. Obviously, in order to be believable, health professionals must serve as good examples. A physician with nicotine-stained fingers and cigarette burns in his or her white smock is hardly going to be very credible.

Perhaps because of the combined tyranny of our entrenched health care system and the problems of personal motivation, cancer prevention will not come of age until it can be made to fit the system. As perverted though this may seem, it may well come down to being able to take a pill to prevent cancer and maybe to be vaccinated against it.

Cancer Prevention as a Problem of Public Policy

Government can do a number of things to help prevent cancer. Our government is already doing many things, but it needs to do more. With respect to environmental carcinogens turned loose by industry, the individual is relatively powerless. The federal government has primary responsibility for this fraction of environmental cancer, no matter how small the fraction, under the constitutional mandate to provide for the general welfare. How can an individual protect him- or herself from carcinogen-contaminated groundwater, surface water, air, or soil? How can states keep citizens from being exposed to carcinogens that blow or flow, or that are trucked or piped across state lines? Who or what, if not the federal government, can protect us from carcinogenic chemicals in food processed in one state and sold in another?

The environmental movement that began in the late 1960s evolved into a deep-seated interest in a clean environment by the general public, and this in turn has become a well-entrenched national commitment in the form of many new and tough environmental laws in the past two decades. But many important unsolved problems in enforcing the laws still remain. Ambiguities will keep the courts busy resolving conflicts between the government and various special-interest groups for many years to come. Nevertheless, the impressive array of environmental protection laws now on the books promises to serve us well in the future. Recent laws or laws that have undergone significant amendment in the past decade and a half and that provide for protection from carcinogenic risk include (1) the Food, Drug and Cosmetic Act, (2) the Resource Conservation and Recovery Act, (3) the Water Pollution Control Act, (4) the Clean Air Act, (5) the Occupational Safety and Health Act, (6) the Safe Drinking Water Act, (7) the In-

secticide, Fungicide and Rodenticide Act, (8) the Toxic Substances Control Act, and (9) the Consumer Product Safety Act (see Fig. 15.4).

The scope of this book will not allow (the editor says the book will be too long) expanded coverage and analysis of all these laws, but let's take a look at one of the most important before we analyze the overall picture.

Food Additives and the Delaney Amendment

Food additives—that is, chemicals added to food to enhance color, or to preserve it—fall under a clause of the 1958 Pure Food, Drug, and Cosmetic Act. A clause in this law, usually referred to as the Delaney Amendment (because it was sponsored by James J. Delaney of New York) specifically bans the use of any food additive found to "cause" (key word) cancer when eaten by humans or by animals or when subjected to any other test "appropriate" (another key word) for evaluating the safety of food additives. The Delaney Clause has been used in recent years in the banning of such things as cyclamates and saccharin, saffrole (root beer flavoring), diethylstilbestrol (DES, an estrogen-like dietary substance fed to livestock to accelerate meat production), and Red Dye No. 2. All these things were shown to produce excess numbers of cancers in experimental animals.

The Delaney Amendment is controversial because it admits *no* threshold level; it is based on the assumption that there is no low level of any carcinogenic substance that is harmless when in food or drink. Sometimes this assumption produces results that the general public finds difficult to understand. The study on which the banning of saccharin was originally based, for instance, involved feeding about 100 rats a diet of 5 percent pure saccharin from the time they were born until they died. Fourteen of these rats developed bladder cancer, compared with only two such animals in a group of 100 animals given no saccharin. Although a human being would have to drink several hundred 12-ounce diet sodas a day for life to accumulate an

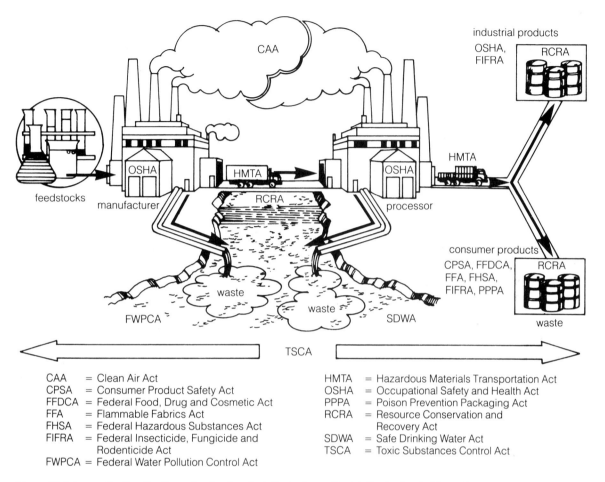

CAA	= Clean Air Act	HMTA	= Hazardous Materials Transportation Act
CPSA	= Consumer Product Safety Act	OSHA	= Occupational Safety and Health Act
FFDCA	= Federal Food, Drug and Cosmetic Act	PPPA	= Poison Prevention Packaging Act
FFA	= Flammable Fabrics Act	RCRA	= Resource Conservation and
FHSA	= Federal Hazardous Substances Act		Recovery Act
FIFRA	= Federal Insecticide, Fungicide and	SDWA	= Safe Drinking Water Act
	Rodenticide Act	TSCA	= Toxic Substances Control Act
FWPCA	= Federal Water Pollution Control Act		

Figure 15.4 Laws affecting the life cycle of a chemical. Each piece of legislation is directed toward a different aspect of the problem from generation to consumption to disposal. There is obviously some overlap. (Adapted from *EPA Journal*, July-August 1979, Washington, D.C. Reprinted from Charles E. Kupchella and Margaret C. Hyland, *Environmental Science: Living Within the System of Nature*. Copyright © 1986 by Allyn and Bacon, Inc. Used by permission.)

equivalent dose, strict application of the Delaney Amendment called for the removal of saccharin from the consumer market (although this was later revised when Congress exempted saccharin from the Food, Drug, and Cosmetic Act. The banning of saccharin offers a particularly poignant example of the complexity of our society and the difficulty of regulating carcinogens in the environment. It has been pointed out that if obesity and cancer are indeed related and if the saccharin ban resulted in a return to natural

sweeteners such as sugar, and if this produced an increase in weight in some people, predisposing them to certain "fat"-related cancers, banning saccharin could result in more cancers than would have been produced if saccharin were left on the market—presuming, of course, that saccharin indeed would cause tumors in human beings.

Interpreted rigidly then, the Food, Drug, and Cosmetic Act allows little room for the consideration of circumstance. Some people argue that this rigidity presents problems in cases where weakly cancer-causing substances are present in extremely small amounts (levels undetectable when the law was written), or if and when there is an overriding benefit to the presence of the substance. The law has no provision for considering benefits. Since no scientific evidence suggests that there *is* a carcinogenic threshold—that is, a dose of any carcinogenic substance that will *not* produce tumors if given to enough people in a large population—it seems prudent that the Delaney Amendment stand at least in the absence of any clear benefit from a particular additive.

Regulating Carcinogenic Hazards: Where to from Here?

It should be clear from the foregoing that regulating carcinogenic hazards is far from "cut and dried." Many laws are written by different Congresses under different circumstances. The laws overlap in their scope, yet each has a different underlying philosophy, a different mandated approach, and many different, unrelated agencies are involved.

The Office of Technology Assessment (OTA) of the U.S. Congress points out the differing approaches. It categorizes both the Delaney Clause and the Resources Recovery Act as "zero risk" laws because the responsible agencies (see Figure 15.4) are charged with completely eliminating risk, without regard to other factors. The Clean Air Act, the Clean Water Act, and the Occupational Safety and Health Act are called "technology-based" laws because they actually specify the "control" devices to be used by the regulated industries. The Toxic Substances Control Act (TSCA), the Consumer Product Safety Act, and the Insecticide, Fungicide, and Rodenticide Act are called "balancing" laws because they specifically direct the regulatory agencies involved to consider factors other than health risk in establishing regulations.

Little wonder that there continues to be a vigorous debate over these laws. Environmentalists call for more vigorous enforcement, in many instances environmental groups have taken the EPA to court to get the EPA to meet its responsibility under the law. At the same time, industry has tended to conjure up public visions of economic ruin if reform does not provide relief from oppressive federal regulation. The government gets caught in the middle and has vacillated, even during the same administration.

In 1984, the Reagan administration issued a document establishing as policy the principle that substances that cause cancer in animals must be presumed to be suspect human carcinogens. Another document published under the same administration a year and a half earlier had discounted the value of nonhuman animal tests—and was vigorously protested by the scientific community (Marshall, 1982).

The fact is, none of the laws governing carcinogenic hazards are perfect. The patchwork of regulations is cumbersome at best, and reform is both inevitable and needed. We should expect to see increasing attention given to the concept of "acceptable risk" as time goes by (see Gori, 1980).

Following its assessment of the way in which the government dealt with environmental cancer risk up through the early 1980s, the OTA proposed a number of what are called "options" for improvement. Their options (which were really alternative recommendations) fell into the following categories: (1) improving our ability to gather information about cancer incidence and mortality, (2) improving the ways in which we evaluate potential carcinogens, and (3) amendments to the Toxic Substances Control Act. These recommendations are still very much worth considering.

In the category of gathering better information about cancer, the OTA makes the following recommendations:

1. Expand the NCI's SEER program (see Chapter 17) to achieve representative coverage of the entire United States.

2. Establish a national cancer registry.

3. Support epidemiological investigations designed to answer specific cancer environment questions; for example, about the workplace and diet.

4. Consider specific recommendations derived from the work of various commissions and study groups, perhaps via a center for health data collection activities.

The OTA's recommendations for improving carcinogen testing were

1. Find something to replace the long-term carcinogenicity bioassay using small mammals.

2. Find better short-term tests for assessing potential carcinogens.

3. Increase support for the National Toxicology Program.

Recommendations concerning the TSCA included

1. Increase the EPA's resources and thus its ability to assess, more expeditiously, the risk associated with chemicals *before* they are introduced.

2. Require industry to submit at least some minimal amount of toxicity data on each new chemical (amend TSCA).

3. Shift to industry the burden of proof that additional testing of a new chemical is not needed (amend TSCA).

4. Consider establishing an oversight panel to make technical decisions for all government agencies involved in the regulatory process.

The fact that enforcement is still far from complete and the fact that carcinogens will never be completely controlled means that the individual is still the most important master of his or her own personal destiny with respect to exposure to carcinogens. The press and popular opinion continue to label industry, and industrial chemicals turned loose in the environment, as the main causes of cancer. But diet and other elements of lifestyle involving personal choice are collectively much more important than pollution when it comes to cancer risk. This fact will not be accepted very readily because of the responsibility it places on the individual. Faceless corporate villains are easy to blame and easier to rail at; it is always difficult to see ourselves as our own worst enemies.

The Greatest Needs in the Future of Cancer Prevention

The greatest research needs and other kinds of needs in the category of cancer prevention include (1) motivational research, (2) the development of preventive medicine as an important part of health care, (3) better ways of identifying carcinogens, (4) research into those aspects of the nature of oncogenes that might suggest prevention strategies, and (5) more systematic ways of monitoring cancer incidence.

Behavioral scientists must find ways to help people shed bad habits and adopt good habits. Health professionals, particularly doctors and nurses, must be taught how to teach prevention to their clients (*patients* is not really the right word here). Medical schools, in particular, must give preventive medicine a loftier place in the curriculum than it now has. Perhaps a no-smoking clause should be added to the pledge that doctors and nurses take when they enter their professions.

Summary

The *essence* of this chapter could be summarized in several ways, all of which lend themselves to a tabular presentation. Table 15.5 gives the major alterable risk factors for cancer and summarizes some specific actions that should lead to cancer prevention. Cancer can, in fact, be prevented. More research is needed to allow us to frame still more prevention strategies by identifying yet

Table 15.5 Cancer Risk Factors and Actions That Can Be Taken to Avoid Them

Known Risk Factor	Risk	Action
Alcohol	Heavy drinking, especially with smoking; increased risk of mouth, throat, liver, and esophagus cancer	If you drink alcohol, do so only in moderation. (One or two drinks per day is considered moderate.)
Cigarettes, cigars, pipes	Increased risk of lung cancer. For cigarette smokers, 10 times that of nonsmokers	Don't smoke. Low-tar, low-nicotine cigarettes do not eliminate risk of getting cancer.
Chewing tobacco, snuff	Increased risk of mouth cancer	Don't use smokeless tobacco products.
Estrogens (for menopause)	Long-term, high-dose use; increased risk of cancer of the uterus	Take estrogens only as long as necessary.
Occupation	Exposure to one or a combination of certain known cancer-causing industrial agents (nickel, chromate, uranium, asbestos, petroleum, vinyl chloride) in many cases with smoking; increased risk of several cancers	Know and follow health and safety rules of your workplace. If provided, wear protective clothing; use safety equipment (masks, respirators, etc.). Don't smoke.
X-rays	Overexposure (for example, a large number of X-rays over a long period of time); increased risk of many types of cancers	Avoid X-rays that aren't medically needed. Be sure X-ray shields are used to protect other parts of your body when possible.
Sunlight	Long exposure and no sun screen protection; increased risk of skin cancer	Don't stay in the sun for more than brief periods of time without protection (hats, long sleeves, long pants, sun screen lotions).
Diet	Many cancers have been associated with diet either through the consumption of carcinogens and/or through the lack of chemopreventive agents (see text).	Eat a balanced diet, low in fat and high in fiber. Don't allow yourself to become overweight.

Source: U.S. Department of Health and Human Services, 1984.

unknown, specific carcinogens. We need to improve the laws designed to keep carcinogens out of our environment, and we need to enforce them. We need to do a better job of educating ourselves about good and bad health habits. We need to find out much more about how to overcome poor health habits, and we need to adopt good health habits.

References and Further Reading

Beebe, G. 1982. Ionizing Radiation and Health. *American Scientist*. 70:35–44.

Berg, J. 1977. World-wide Variations in Cancer Incidence as Clues to Cancer Origins. In H. Hiatt, J. Watson, and J. Winsten, eds., *Origins of Human Cancer*. Cold Spring Harbor, N.Y.: Cold Spring Harbor Laboratory.

Bertram, J. 1980. Structure-Activity Relationships Among Various Retinoids and Their Ability to Inhibit Neoplastic Transformation and to Increase Cell Adhesion in the C3H/10T1/2 CL8 Cell Line. *Cancer Research*. 40:3141.

Blakeslee, A. 1982. 1982 Cancer Research Update. *Cancer News*. Autumn. Pp. 14–17.

Blonston, G. 1984. Prevention. *Science 84*. September. Pp. 36–39.

Cairns, J. 1978. *Cancer Science and Society*. San Francisco: Freeman.

Creasey, W. A. 1985. *Diet and Cancer*. Philadelphia: Lea & Febiger.

Department of Health and Social Security (England). 1972. Smoking and Health: A Study of the Effects of a Reduction in Cigarette Smoking on Mortality and Morbidity Rates on Health Care and Social Security Expenditure and on Productive Potential. London: H. M. Stationery Office.

Doll, R., and Peto, R. 1981. The Causes of Cancer: Quantitative Estimates of Avoidable Risks of Cancer in the United States Today. *Journal of the National Cancer Institute*. 66:1191–1308.

Dominguez, G., ed. 1977, 1983. *Guidebook: Toxic Substances Control Act*. Vols. 1, 2. Boca Raton, Fla.: CRC Press.

Fay, J. R., et al. 1985. Inhibitors of Chemical Carcinogenesis. Report by SRI International (Menlo Park, Calif.) for the National Cancer Institute, Bethesda, Md.

Gori, G. 1980. The Regulation of Carcinogenic Hazards. *Science*. 208:256–61.

Hirschman, R., and Leventhal, H. 1983. The Behavioral Science of Cancer Prevention. In S. Kahn, et al., eds., *Concepts in Cancer Medicine*. New York: Grune & Stratton.

Holman, C. J., Armstrong, B. K., and Heenan, P. J. 1986. Relationship of Cutaneous Malignant Melanoma to Individual Sunlight-Exposure Habits. *JNCI*. 76(3): 403–14.

Josten, D. M. 1984. *Cancer Prevention: It's Up To You*. Madison, Wisc.: Cancer Prevention Program, University of Wisconsin.

Kahn, S., et al. 1983. *Concepts in Cancer Medicine*. New York: Grune & Stratton.

Kessler, D. 1984. Food Safety: Revising the Statute. *Science*. 223:1034–40.

Marshall, E. 1982. EPA's High-Risk Carcinogen Policy. *Science*. 218:975–78.

Maugh, T. 1974. Vitamin A: Potential Protection from Carcinogens. *Science* 186:1198.

Maugh, T. 1982. Cancer Is Not Inevitable. *Science*. 217:36–37.

Meyskens, F., and Fuller, B. 1980. Characterization of the Effects of Different Retinoids on the Growth and Differentiation of a Human Melanoma Cell Line and Selected Subclones. *Cancer Research*. 40:2194.

Mirvish, S., et al. 1972. Ascorbate-nitrite Reaction: Possible Means of Blocking the Formation of Carcinogenic-N-nitroso Compounds. *Science*. 177:65.

Mirvish, S. S., Karlowski, K., Birt, D. F., and Sams, J. P. 1980. Dietary and Other Factors Affecting Nitrosomethylurea (NMU) Formation in the Rat Stomach. Pp 271–77 in E. A. Walker, L. Griciute, M. Castegnaro, et al., eds., *N-Nitroso Compounds: Analysis, Formation and Occurrence*. IARC Scientific Publication No. 31. Lyon, France: International Agency for Research on Cancer.

National Academy of Science. 1981. The Health Effects of Nitrate, Nitrite, and N-nitroso Compounds. Part 1 of a 2-part study by the Committee on Nitrite and Alternative Curing Agents in Food. Washington, D.C.: National Academy Press.

National Cancer Institute publications on cancer prevention (Write to Cancer Communications, National Cancer Institute, Building 31, Room 10A18, Bethesda, MD 20205. Also see the government documents section of your nearest federal depository library):

> *Asbestos Exposure: What It Means, What to Do*. NCI Publication No. 84-1594. 11 pages.
>
> *Cancer: What to Know, What to Do About It*. NCI Publication No. 84-211. 23 pages.
>
> *Clearing the Air: A Guide to Quitting Smoking*. NCI Publication No. 83-1647. 32 pages.
>
> *Everything Doesn't Cause Cancer but How Can We Tell Which Chemicals Cause Cancer and Which Ones Don't?* NCI Publication No. 84-2039.
>
> *Good News, Better News, Best News . . . Cancer Prevention*. NCI Publication No. 84-2671.
>
> *Why Do You Smoke?* NCI Publication No. 83-1822.
>
> *Questions and Answers about DES Exposure During Pregnancy and Before Birth*. NCI Publication No. 81-1118.

National Cancer Institute. 1984. *Cancer Prevention*. Pamphlet. Washington, D.C.: U.S. Department of Health and Human Services.

National Research Council. 1982. *Diet, Nutrition, and Cancer*. Washington, D.C.: National Academy Press.

Newell, G., and Boutwell, W. 1981. Potential for Cancer Prevention. *Cancer Bulletin*. 33(2):78–79.

NIH Consensus Development Conference Statement, 1986. Health Implications of Smokeless Tobacco Use. *JAMA*. 255(8):1045–48.

Oppenheimer, S. 1983. Prevention of Cancer. *American Laboratory.* 15(2) February: pp. 66–72.

Page, H. S., and Asire, A. J. 1985. *Cancer Rates and Risks.* 3rd ed. NIH Publication No. 85-691. Bethesda, Md.: National Institutes of Health.

Pike, M., et al. 1983. Breast Cancer in Young Women and Use of Oral Contraceptives: Possible Modifying Effect of Formulation and Age at Use. *Lancet.* 11: 1414–15.

Reif, A. 1981. The Causes of Cancer. *American Scientist.* 69:437–47.

Roberts, L. 1986. Sex and Cancer. *Science 86.* July/August, pp. 30–33.

Ruddon, R. 1981. *Cancer Biology.* New York: Oxford University Press.

Sandler, D. P., Everson, R. B., and Wilcox, A. J. 1985. Passive Smoking in Adulthood and Cancer Risk. *Am. J. Epidemiology.* 121:37–48.

Schottenfeld, D., and Fraumeni, J., eds. 1982. *Cancer Epidemiology and Prevention.* Philadelphia: Saunders.

Schuman, L. 1984. Progress and Responsibilities of Educators in Smoking Control. The Harvey Lecture, Presented at the Annual Meeting of the American Association for Cancer Education, Minneapolis.

Shamberger, R. J. 1984. *Nutrition and Cancer.* New York: Plenum Press.

Shaw, C., ed. 1981. *Prevention of Occupational Cancer.* Boca Raton, Fla.: CRC Press.

The Sourcebook on Cancer, Diet, and Nutrition. 1985. Chicago: Marquis Who's Who, Inc.

Sporn, M. 1978. Chemoprevention of Cancer. *Nature.* 272:402.

Sternburg, J. 1983. Identification and Management of Risks Factors for Cancer. In S. Kahn, et al., eds., *Concepts in Cancer Medicine.* New York: Grune & Stratton.

Tomatis, L. 1985. The Contribution of Epidemiological and Experimental Data to the Control of Environmental Carcinogens. *Cancer Letters.* 26:5–16.

U.S. Public Health Service. 1964. *Smoking and Health—Report of the Advisory Committee to the Surgeon General of the Public Health Service.* PHS Publication No. 1103. Washington, D.C.: U.S. Government Printing Office.

U.S. Public Health Service. 1967. *Health Consequences of Smoking, A Public Health Service Review.* PHS Publication No. 1696. Washington, D.C.: U.S. Government Printing Office.

U.S. Public Health Service. 1974. Teen-Age Smoking: National Patterns of Cigarette Smoking, Ages 12 Through 18 in 1972 and 1974. DHEW Publication No. (NIH) 76-931. Bethesda, Md.: National Institutes of Health.

U.S. Public Health Service. 1979. *Smoking and Health— A Report of the Surgeon General.* DHEW Publication No. (PHS) 79-50066. Washington, D.C.: U.S. Government Printing Office.

Warner, K. 1981. Cigarette Smoking in the 1970's: The Impact of the Antismoking Campaign on Consumption. *Science.* 211:729–80.

Winn, D. M., et al. 1984. Diet in the Etiology of Oral and Pharyngeal Cancer Among Women from the Southern United States. *Cancer Res.* 44:1216–22.

Wortzman, M., Besbris, H., and Cohen, A. 1980. Effect of Dietary Selenium on the Interaction Between 2-acetylaminofluorene and Rat Liver DNA in Vivo. *Cancer Research.* 40:2670.

f cancer could be prevented in everyone, this and the following chapters would be unnecessary. But we do not know how to prevent all cancers, and we probably never will. For those of us in whom prevention fails and cancer begins to develop, the next best thing is to detect the cancer at the earliest possible moment. A malignant neoplasm is more and more likely to become incurable with the passage of time.

We do not yet have a single test that marks the presence of cancer. If we had one, this chapter would be a short section in the next chapter on treatment. Because we don't have a single test, we need a whole chapter to consider the many things that go into detecting and diagnosing cancer. Most commonly, the diagnosis of cancer involves some sequence of symptomatic complaints by a patient, followed by a physician's suspicions and a battery of diagnostic tests. As long as the results of successive tests continue to suggest the possibility of cancer, the cascade continues to move toward a biopsy. The final diagnosis can only be made after examining cells under a microscope.

Before we consider the elements in the diagnostic pathway, we need to define a few key terms. The word **detection** means the act of discovering or finding out. The phrase "cancer has been detected" technically means that a pathologist has looked at some cells and, given other clinical information, has declared them to be cancer cells; the phrase is sometimes used in a softer way to indicate that something highly suspicious has been found and that a confirming look at some tissue is warranted. **Diagnosis** is a richer word encompassing discovery but going beyond to describe the exact nature of what has been discovered. The phrase "The diagnosis is cancer" may also mean that a pathologist has looked at some cells and has declared them to be cancer cells. Most of the time, a specific kind of cancer is specified in a diagnosis. Sometimes the phrase **definitive diagnosis** is used to specify a complete description (including type, grade, and stage) of a cancer that has been detected.

16

The Detection and Diagnosis of Cancer

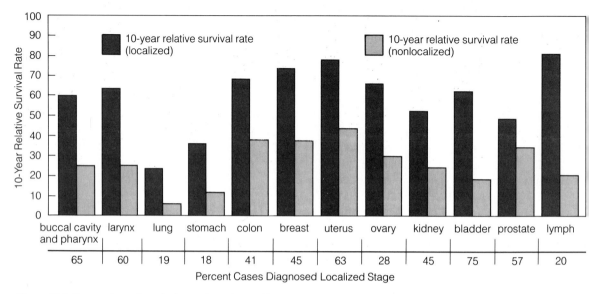

Figure 16.1 Comparison of survival rates in patients with localized and nonlocalized cancer. (*Source:* Miller, 1976, Fig. 1, based on data from the 4th End Results Study of the Biometry Section of the National Cancer Institute. Reprinted by permission of J. B. Lippincott Company and the author.)

The Value of Early Detection

Despite the fact that for certain cancers there has been no demonstration that early detection makes a difference (e.g., cancer of the esophagus and pancreas, and leukemia), early detection of cancer overall makes a great deal of positive difference in prognosis. Generally speaking, the earlier a cancer is found the more likely it is to be localized, which means better prognosis. A striking illustration is presented in Figure 16.1. In this figure, twelve kinds of cancer representing 80 percent of all cancer and accounting for 70 percent of all cancer deaths are shown in terms of the survival rates for patients with localized cancer and patients with nonlocalized cancer. As noted by Miller (1976), for most of these cancers, the 10-year relative survival rates are 50 percent higher for those with localized disease. Overall, more than a third of all cancer deaths could be averted by existing technologies for early detection. By some estimates, future improvements in detection technology will one day make 90 percent of all cancers curable.

Factors That Separate the Beginning of Cancer from Treatment

The point has already been made in this book many times that in the natural history of all malignant neoplasms, invasion and metastasis follow malignant transformation by finite, but highly variable, periods of time. Local invasion, regional extension, and distant metastasis may each occur very early, when the neoplasm is very small, or they may occur after a long period. Early detection can make a difference only if it can reveal neoplasms before they have spread very far.

The significance of, and the problems in the way of, early detection are derived from the degree to which the "windows" of detectability

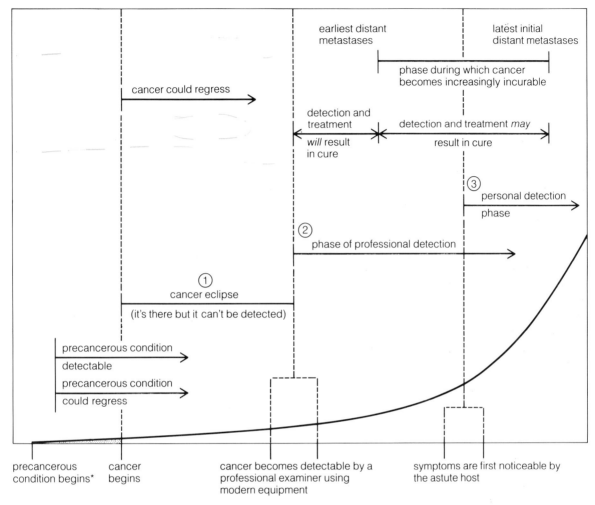

earliest distant metastases

latest initial distant metastases

phase during which cancer becomes increasingly incurable

detection and treatment *will* result in cure

detection and treatment *may* result in cure

cancer could regress

③ personal detection phase

② phase of professional detection

① cancer eclipse

(it's there but it can't be detected)

precancerous condition detectable

precancerous condition could regress

precancerous condition begins*

cancer begins

cancer becomes detectable by a professional examiner using modern equipment

symptoms are first noticeable by the astute host

*If there is one.

Figure 16.2 When early detection makes a difference. Shown here are the generalized phases in the natural history of a malignant neoplasm. The problem is that durations of the phases shown here are rarely known.

and curability do or do not overlap, respectively (Fig. 16.2). The beginning of cancer is separated from treatment by a developmental process called *tumorigenesis*, which has several phases (with indistinct boundaries) relative to detection (see Antonovsky and Hartman, 1979, and Bar-Moar and Davies, 1960). The first phase is the phase of *un*detectability—when the neoplasm is too small to be picked up by any known detection method and the neoplasm produces no detectable general pathology. The second phase is that in which the neoplasm or its effects can be detected, but only by a skilled professional using modern equipment. A third phase begins when the growth of the neoplasm produces symptoms noticeable to the "average" layperson and ends when the layperson reports the symptom to a physician or other health professional. This third phase could be divided in two parts, the point of division being the realization by the layperson that something is really wrong and that he or she should see a doctor. A fourth stage begins when the first health practitioner hears about the symptoms and ends when the patient is referred to, and is first seen by, a cancer specialist. A fifth stage begins with the first visit to a cancer specialist and ends with a confirming diagnosis. Each of these phases can be thought of as a source of delay in getting treatment. Although some part of each phase represents *unavoidable* delay, at least some of the delay in every phase is theoretically avoidable. For example, the first phase can be shortened by improved methods of detection and by more highly developed skill by examiners, in effect extending the range of the second phase. A theoretical absolute limit to this approach is set by the uncertainty as to whether or not what may be detectable as a very, very early cancer will, if left alone, go on to become a life-threatening cancer.

Another way in which treatment delay might be shortened is by having skilled examiners with modern equipment examine more people, in effect moving more detection into the "professional" phase. This approach has some physical and economic limits we will discuss later, in the section on screening. Educating laypeople and improving the efficiency of health care and referral systems can also make a difference in early detection.

Detection Strategies

The detection of a neoplasm is generally not possible until it has reached a size of 10 billion cells and has a mass of about one gram (roughly the size of a sugar cube). Only if the neoplasm secretes a powerful hormone or hormone-like substance can it be detected much earlier (see Chap-

ter 13). If located where they have little physical impact on adjacent structures and otherwise cause little or no physiological disruption, masses many times larger than a sugar cube can be overlooked even by professional examiners using modern equipment. In order to reach the size of one gram, a neoplasm must go through about 30 doublings. Estimated time required for solid tumors to double once ranges from 7 to 120 days (Kahn, 1983). Each increase in cell number increases the likelihood that neoplasms will have spread beyond natural barriers by invasion or metastasis and thus decreases the likelihood that the neoplasm will be completely curable by surgery alone.

Malignant neoplasms of the skin and mouth present one kind of detection and diagnostic problem. Malignant neoplasms of the distal colon, vagina, uterine cervix, throat, esophagus, and stomach that physicians can get at relatively easily, but with *some* difficulty, present another kind of problem. Cancers of the internal organs obviously present special diagnostic problems, and the steps separating the initial symptoms and definite diagnosis may amount to quite a long story. The diagnosis of all these cancers can be enhanced by astute vigilance on the part of patients and physicians.

The Role of Vigilance

Vigilance begins with the seven warning signals described in Chapter 1. The value of these warning signals cannot be overemphasized. They do not always mean that a cancer is present, but they should always be checked out.

According to Cady et al. (1978), (1) changes in bowel or bladder habits may be associated with cancers of the colon, rectum, prostate, or bladder; (2) skin sores that do not heal strongly suggest basal cell or epidermoid cancers (see Chapter 5); (3) unusual bleeding or discharges from such orifices as the vagina, nipple, mouth, or nose, anus, or urethra may indicate erosions (ulcers) secondary to malignant neoplasms of the uterus, breast, respiratory tract, rectum, colon, or the genitourinary system, respectively; (4) lumps or thickenings of the testes, breasts, or other tissue can be caused by growing masses of cells (among other things); (5) indigestion or difficulty swallowing may be caused by obstruction of the digestive tract; (6) changes in moles may mean malignant melanoma; and (7) chronic cough and hoarseness may be early signs of laryngeal cancer or late signs of lung cancer.

There are, of course, more than seven warning signs. As indicated by the range of host effects of cancer described in Chapter 12, a wide variety of symptoms may be harbingers of cancer. It makes good sense to check out anything strange or unusual that happens, especially if the sign lasts more than a few weeks. Self-examination on a regular basis can be very valuable because it can reveal problems well before they announce themselves more obtrusively. Most breast cancers are first detected by women examining their own breasts.

American Cancer Society guidelines for the types and frequencies of self-inspections and inspections that require the services of a health practitioner are given in Table 16.1

Why Delay?

After the typical human being notices some symptom or constellation of symptoms possibly related to cancer, he or she waits a while before reporting the observation to a physician. At first the person waits to see if the symptom is "real" and to see if it won't go away. But even after a few weeks, even after it becomes clear that the symptoms may be there to stay, a highly variable period of *additional* time usually goes by before the person reports the problem. Reasons for this delay are many and varied, and stem from such things as fear of doctors and hospitals; fear of authoritative people dressed in white; fear of big buildings, cities, or pain; and fear of feeling foolish if the problem turns out to be nothing. Other factors include "machismo," misplaced mod-

esty, guilt or shame, emotional disorders, religious conviction, poverty, ignorance, and being "too busy to sit in a waiting room all day with a bunch of really sick people."

The appearance of symptoms can be thought of as increased odds that a cancer is present, making close inspection by a physician worthwhile. The observation and reporting of early symptoms remain the most effective route to detecting cancer early. Mass screening of asymptomatic people simply reveals too few cancers to make it a worthwhile, effective way of looking for early cancer. Screening of asymptomatic people at high risk for the development of a particular cancer is another story, however.

High-Risk Groups and Screening

The term *secondary prevention* was introduced in the last chapter, where it was defined as the detection and eradication of cancer before it disrupts normal body function. For all practical purposes, secondary prevention is synonymous with early detection. The screening of asymptomatic individuals for cancer thus falls into the category of secondary prevention. Screening is most effective when it concentrates on high-risk populations and when directed toward cancers having certain "ideal" characteristics.

In terms of screening effectiveness, the "ideal" cancer would meet the following tests:

1. The cancer is detectable for a long period *before* it produces any serious disruption in normal body function. Love (1983) calls this the "detectable preclinical phase," or DPCP.

2. The cancer progresses from curable to incurable at or near the *end* of the DPCP.

3. The cancer is relatively "easy" to detect, meaning that detection is inexpensive.

4. The defect or change being detected is *always* really cancer and will *always* progress to fatal cancer if left untreated.

5. Effective treatment is available.

Table 16.1   The American Cancer Society's Guidelines for the Early Detection of Cancer in People without Symptoms.

Age 20–40	Age 40 and Over
Cancer-Related Checkup Every 3 Years	*Cancer-Related Checkup Every Year*
Should include the procedures listed below plus health counseling (such as tips on quitting cigarettes) and examinations for cancers of the thyroid, testes, prostate, mouth, ovaries, skin, and lymph nodes. Some people are at higher risk for certain cancers and may need to have tests more frequently.	Should include the procedures listed below plus health counseling (such as tips on quitting cigarettes) and examinations for cancers of the thyroid, testes, prostate, mouth, ovaries, skin, and lymph nodes. Some people are at higher risk for certain cancers and may need to have tests more frequently.
Breast	*Breast*
—Exam by doctor every 3 years	—Exam by doctor every year
—Self-exam every month	—Self-exam every month
—One baseline breast X-ray between ages 35–40. *Higher risk for breast cancer:* Personal or family history of breast cancer, never had children, first child after 30	—Breast X-ray every year after 50 (between ages 40–50, ask your doctor) *Higher risk for breast cancer:* Personal or family history of breast cancer, never had children, first child after 30
Uterus	*Uterus*
—Pelvic exam every 3 years *Cervix* —Pap test—after 2 initial negative tests 1 year apart—at least every 3 years, includes women under 20 if sexually active. *Higher risk for cervical cancer:* Early age at first intercourse, multiple sex partners	—Pelvic exam every year *Cervix* —Pap test—after 2 initial negative tests 1 year apart—at least every 3 years *Higher risk for cervical cancer:* Early age at first intercourse, multiple sex partners *Endometrium* —Endometrial tissue sample at menopause if at risk *Higher risk for endometrial cancer:* Infertility, obesity, failure of ovulation, abnormal uterine bleeding, estrogen therapy
	Colon & Rectum
	—Digital rectal exam every year —Guaiac slide test every year after 50 —Procto exam—after 2 initial negative tests 1 year apart—every 3 to 5 years after 50 *Higher risk for colorectal cancer:* Personal or family history of colon or rectal cancer, personal or family history of polyps in the colon or rectum, ulcerative colitis

Reprinted courtesy of the American Cancer Society, Inc.

Controversy over the value of screening asymptomatic people continues to rage precisely because nearly all cancers fall short of these ideals in highly variable ways—and, for many if not most kinds of cancer, the applicability of Items 2 and 4 is unknown. The DPCP may be so short as to be practically nonexistent for some cancers; some may become uncurable even before they are detectable (see Fig. 16.2). As discussed in Chapter 5, some things look like cancer that are *not* cancer, which raises the possibility of false positive results. In still other cases, detectable precancerous conditions may not always progress to invasive cancer. Cervical dysplasia and cervical carcinoma *in situ* may or may not lead to invasive cancer, and even if they do, the elapsed time may range from 3 to 30 years (Love, 1983). When precancerous conditions are detectable but not treated, well-developed systems are needed by which to follow up or keep track of patients.

The value of screening also depends on how good the tests are. Ideally, screening tests should be able to identify everybody who has disease when the test is applied. Short of this ideal, we speak of the **sensitivity** of a screening test, which is the number of true positives found, divided by the number of people tested who actually had cancer (Table 16.2). Tests whose sensitivity falls short of the ideal result in "false negatives." Such tests can send people home with cancer who believe they are well.

The ideal screening test should also not give any false positive results—should not falsely indicate that a cancer-free person has cancer. Short of this ideal, we speak of the **specificity** of a test, the number of people found to be free of cancer by the test, divided by the number who were in fact free of cancer. The problem with false positive tests is that people who are in fact well are then subjected to further inconvenient, expensive, and possibly risky testing.

Added to the inherent limitations of screening tests is the problem of variable application and human factors. For example, Love (1983) reports that estimates of the sensitivity of the Pap test range from 60 to 99 percent. He cites

Table 16.2 Sensitivity and Specificity; Possible Combinations of Test Results and "The Truth"

	Status of Cancer	
Test Result	*Is Present*	*Is Not Present*
Positive	True Positive	False Positive
Negative	False Negative	True Negative

Derivation of the Terms *Sensitivity* and *Specificity*:

$$\text{Sensitivity} = \frac{\text{True Positives}}{\text{True Positives} + \text{False Negatives}}$$

$$\text{Specificity} = \frac{\text{True Negatives}}{\text{True Negatives} + \text{False Positives}}$$

the vagaries of sampling, variable technique, variable features of specific lesions, and subjective interpretation, as all taking some toll of sensitivity.

Although at first glance it would seem easy to document the value of screening for cancer, such is not the case. Even when studies are done, and even when they apparently show that screening is valuable, such results can stem from several kinds of study bias—they can falsely indicate that screening is better than not screening. Love (1983) lists the sources of bias:

1. *Unrepresentative samples.* Screening groups are sometimes inadvertently selected that are composed of high-risk individuals. Large numbers of cancers are thus found, not because the screening was effective, but because the subjects had unusually high numbers of cancer.

2. *Overdiagnosis.* Screening sometimes finds "cancers" that are not really cancers. Naturally, these are more successfully treated than real cancers and people are counted as having been "saved" by screening who were not really saved at all.

3. *Lead-time bias.* If cures are measured in terms of five-year survival, and if screening detects cancer early, improved "survival" may re-

sult from the fact that the beginning of the five-year count is started early—even though the patients die at the same time they would have, had they not been screened.

These and other forms of bias continue to raise questions about the real value of screening. Another reason for questioning the value of screening is cost, which we'll discuss next.

Populations at high risk for developing certain cancers were described in Chapters 11, 13, and 15. The question we explore here, briefly, is "Why is it better to focus on high-risk individuals in the search for occult cancers?" The answer to this question has to do with economics→economics in the broadest sense, having to do with the allocation of resources, not just money.

In the following discussion, cost means *mostly* money—the cost of doctors, nurses, bookkeeping, time off work, travel; but it also refers to costs in terms of the risk of radiation and drug reactions, grief, anxiety, and assorted stresses. From the perspective of society as a whole, the value of screening can be expressed as the difference between (1) all the costs of finding a cancer early and treating it successfully, and (2) the cost of that cancer being found later and treated *un*successfully. The cost of finding a cancer early is calculated by multiplying (1) the cost of screening one asymptomatic person by (2) the number of people screened and then (3) dividing by the number of cancers found. The result is then the cost per cancer found. Added to this cost, in order to come up with the *total* cost of finding and treating an early cancer, would be the cost of successful treatment. This total is then weighed against the cost to society of dealing with that cancer later, and—more likely than in the former case—unsuccessfully. This cost would include the cost of prolonged treatment, lost earnings, other less objective costs such as grief and suffering, and the cost to society of the premature shortening of a productive life.

Keeping all this calculation from being a simple arithmetic problem are the facts that (1)

no standard value can be set on a year of human life, (2) we have really no way to know just how many cancers found early by screening would have been found early *enough* anyway, and (3) screening can lead to false positive diagnoses and to inappropriate treatment. Still, it should be clear that the greater the difference between (1) the cost of finding a cancer and (2) the cost of not finding it until it is too late, the more justifiable the screening. The cost of finding a cancer goes down when lots of cancers are found, and on this fact is based the strategy of concentrating on high-risk groups and on common cancers in screening. This cost can also be reduced by screening for cancers that are relatively inexpensive (in terms of dollars and health care resources) to find, such as cancers of the skin, mouth, colon, or breast.

After Something Suspicious Is Found

The documentation of an initial array of suspicious symptoms is really only the beginning in cancer diagnosis. Every collection of symptoms has more than one possible cause. To arrive at a diagnosis of cancer, all other possibilities must be ruled out.

The suspicious physician begins a systematic and often time-consuming investigation by asking the patient certain key questions. This "taking of a history" is designed to reveal more detail and to uncover possibly significant events, symptoms, and facts that a patient may have forgotten to mention. This in turn may be followed by a battery of blood tests and the use of some special visualization techniques such as X-rays, CAT scans, ultrasound, and direct observation, with special lighted tubes, of the bronchi, the esophagus, the stomach, the colon, the vagina, and the uterine cervix. Some of the latter techniques may also help the physician obtain some suspicious tissue for examination under the microscope. Let's review the entire diagnostic sequence in detail.

Medical History Taking

First of all, a good medical history may reveal relevant symptoms that the patient may have overlooked and not reported to a physician. The history is also a useful way to identify high-risk individuals. Histories of smoking, alcohol consumption, and other lifestyle elements may all have relevance to the likelihood of cancer.

Earlier cancers may in fact recur many years after being declared as cured. Earlier cancers may also indicate increased risk for another similar cancer or for some other form of cancer. Patients who continue to smoke after being cured of an earlier oral cancer have a 40 percent chance of a local recurrence, while those who quit smoking have only a 5 percent chance (Cady et al., 1978). Patients cured of cancer in any paired organ (breast, kidney, etc.) generally have a "far higher" than normal risk of cancer in the other paired organ (Cady et al., 1978). Cancer treatment, even though successful, may raise the risk of subsequent cancers caused by carcinogenic radiation and chemotherapeutic agents. The combination of radiation and chemotherapy in Hodgkin's disease patients has been shown to increase the risk of leukemia in survivors, for example. Other risk factors that may be discovered by taking a medical history (e.g., family history of breast cancer, colon cancer, or retinoblastoma; history of sexual activity and occupation) were listed in the last chapter.

No matter how someone may have come by an increased risk to cancer, it is important to know that the risk is greater. If the increase is great enough, it may become worthwhile to subject such individuals to costly, time-consuming intensive diagnostic procedures that would otherwise not be justified.

The Physical Exam

The physical examination is so important in medical care that whole courses and entire textbooks are devoted to it in medical education.

Here, we will mention a few aspects of the relationship between the physical exam and cancer detection. For cancer, the physical exam is intended to reveal the symptoms discussed earlier and the physiological changes associated with cancer discussed in Chapter 13. Table 16.3 lists some symptoms that may be found in physical examination that may indicate cancer and that should thus be checked out.

Routine Blood Tests and Analyses

Along with the thorough going-over that constitutes the physical part of the physical exam, certain laboratory tests are usually also done as part of routine "checkups." These tests may include urinalysis, blood counts, and tests for a wide array of markers that are nonspecific indicators of disease. High blood calcium levels, for example, can result from a bone cancer or other malignancy. Changes in many different serum enzymes, long important in diagnosing other diseases, have also been found valuable in cancer diagnosis. Alkaline phosphatase changes, for example, are associated with pancreas inflammation and fracture healing and are also associated with liver metastases and certain bone cancers. Serum amylase is sometimes elevated in pancreatic cancer patients. In addition to *quanti*tative changes, *quali*tative changes may also appear in the nature of serum enzymes associated with particular neoplasms. Many quantitative and qualitative changes are correlated with specific malignancies strongly enough to serve as "markers" of cancer (see below).

Imaging

The general term **medical imaging** applies to all the ways in which some form of energy is used to generate a medically useful visual pattern or image of some structural or functional feature of

Table 16.3 Some Possible Findings on Physical Exam That May Indicate Cancer and That Warrant Further Evaluation

Persistent skin ulcer

Pigmented skin lesion with irregular outline, color, height, or consistency

Small, nodular, roughened areas

Rashes and other skin eruptions, scratching and itching, tiny clots under the skin

Lymph nodes persistently enlarged more than 2 cm without evidence of infection

Hard or firm deep masses palpated from the surface

Salivary gland or thyroid gland masses

Oral ulcers or thickened whitish masses, especially in the mouths of smokers

Ulcerations of the cervix

Masses palpated in the abdomen

Evidence of lung masses (e.g., unilateral wheezing)

Breast masses

Ulceration or mass in the rectum

Testicular mass

Source: Deckers, McDonough, and Shipley, 1978, pp. 14–16.

the human body. Imaging means "looking" inside without actually going inside the body. In some types of imaging, the energy may be passed through the body; in other types, it is reflected. Imaging can confirm the presence or absence of a problem; it is also used to define the extent of disease, to monitor responses to treatment, and to monitor the progression of disease. Imaging techniques range from simple X-rays to nuclear magnetic resonance imaging.

Conventional X-rays

In conventional X-ray films, X-rays (Chapter 9) pass through the body and fall on a fluorescent screen. Light from the screen then blackens a juxtaposed photographic film, yielding a two-dimensional picture of the structures through which the rays passed. X-rays are able to produce pictures, particularly of bone and lung defects. They have the following *dis*advantages: (1)

confusion arises from having to interpret three-dimensional structures from two-dimensional pictures; (2) X-rays are harmful—only 1 percent of the radiation used passes through the body, and the rest is absorbed by body tissues via ionizing interactions (see Chapter 9; see also Jaffee, 1982); and (3) many kinds of defects do not show up on X-rays.

Contrasting materials (that intercept X-rays) are often used to heighten the difference between body compartments. Barium is used to visualize the GI tract, and iodine is used to visualize blood vessels. Soft neoplasms inside soft tissue can be invisible to X-rays unless they visibly distort normal structural relationships.

Digital radiography A variation on the theme of conventional X-ray film is digital radiography. Basically, the kind of television output of X-rays seen in fluoroscopy is converted into a number pattern (a process called *digitizing*). In one kind of digital radiography, called *subtraction*, a baseline image is made and digitized; then a contrasting material is injected into blood vessels, and another image is made. The first image is subtracted from the second, yielding an enhanced image of the blood vessels.

Mammography

Mammograms are X-rays of the breast able to reveal thickenings, calcifications, and cell masses that may be indicative of cancer. The American Medical Association now recommends that all women have a first mammogram made between ages 35 and 40—with the new, low-dose X-ray equipment available. The association recommends that women at higher risk than normal (mother or sister has had breast cancer) get a baseline mammogram even earlier than that (see Table 16.1).

Computerized Axial Tomography (CAT scans)

In the CAT scan, the X-ray source is generated in a tight beam, 10 mm wide or less, aimed at a person's body perpendicular to the long axis. This source is rotated about the body in the perpendicular plane and the X-rays strike detectors on the opposite side of the body. After a complete revolution, the beam has, in effect, passed through only a thin, vertical plane representing a slice of the body. A computer converts the information gathered by detectors and converts it into a two-dimensional cross-sectional image.

In essence, this technology couples X-rays and computers to produce three-dimensional images of lesions. The computer takes information derived from a series of X-rays taken from different angles and integrates it into a composite picture illustrating the shape, size, and exact location of a lesion (see Ledley et al., 1984). The instrument serves both to help detect otherwise undetected neoplasms and to help in planning treatment.

Nuclear Magnetic Resonance (NMR)

NMR, or nuclear magnetic resonance, is based on the principle that the nuclei of certain kinds of atoms in the human body behave like spinning magnets—with north and south poles. When such atoms are placed in a strong magnetic field, they line up in the direction of that field and they wobble at characteristic frequencies. If a second magnetic field is brought into the picture at right angles to the first and made to oscillate (to reverse poles) at a characteristic frequency, nuclei wobbling in resonance with the oscillation will move into a new alignment. As the second field is shut off, the responsive nuclei will return to the alignment dictated by the first field. This move results in a radio signal that can be picked up by a detector. Computerized analysis of such signals coming from a body can be processed to yield a "chemical" picture of the body (see Pykett, 1982). In essence, NMR does chemical analyses electronically; it can reveal how much of a particular chemical is present in a certain location and the nature of the surrounding chemical and physical environment.

NMR is relatively new; only one to two hundred NMR machines were in use by mid 1985.

Positron Emission Tomography (PET)

Positron emission tomography (PET) is a research tool with little or no application to cancer detection as yet; it is included here for the sake of completeness. PET is a form of nuclear medicine in which the injected isotopes are short-lived positron emitters. The isotope is attached to a chemical with specific affinity for some structural or functional chemical feature of the body. As positrons are emitted, they interact with local electrons to produce two gamma rays that move away from one another in opposite directions. Detecting both as they emerge from the body permits a computer to locate the origin providing the same kind of spatial discrimination that a CAT scan provides. The advantage over the CAT scan is that PET makes it possible to visualize chemical *activity* as well as structural features.

The need to have a cyclotron nearby to produce positron emitters with half-lives measured in minutes, plus the high cost of the required detectors, will limit the application of PET in routine cancer detection and diagnosis.

Ultrasound

The ultrasound technique employs ultra high-frequency sound waves that reveal the location, density, size, and shape of internal masses by the nature of the "echos" that bounce back (see Devey and Wells, 1978). This technology is akin to the use of sonar to find sunken ships or submarines. The advantage of ultrasound over the CAT scan is that no ionizing radiation is used. There appear to be no side effects, although some sources of potential problems include chromosomal breaks, cavitation (the development of microbubbles generated from gases dissolved in the tissue), and heating. The disadvantage is that resolution is not nearly as good as that obtained via the CAT scan.

Angiography

If a neoplasm is angiogenic (causes new blood vessels to form) or if it distorts normal blood vessels, these effects can be visualized by injecting a radio-opaque material into the bloodstream and taking an X-ray picture of the vessels. This procedure is called **angiography**, and the result is called an **angiogram**. When the same kind of procedure is applied to lymphatic vessels, the procedure is called **lymphangiography**. Angiography is not without risks. Patients sometimes react badly to the contrast medium, punctured blood vessels present risk of clotting, and X-radiation entails the usual risk.

Nuclear Medicine: Scanning for Radionuclide Deposits

Scanning is based on the high energies of radiation emitted from unstable isotopes as they decay. Isotopes with short half-lives and with particular biological affinities are put into the body and end up in places determined by their chemical affinities and activities. Detectors are then passed over the body to find the radioactive material. Injecting radioactive iodine (^{131}I) and then passing a detector over the thyroid in a systematic pattern can show the pattern in which iodine is taken up by this gland, revealing abnormalities in size and shape and irregularities in the gland. Another example is technetium 99m which is used to visualize (via scanning) the uptake of the isotope by brain neoplasms in which the normal blood-brain barrier has been breached. The brain is a privileged organ in several respects, one of which is the blood-brain barrier. Normally, this barrier prevents some components of blood, otherwise able to diffuse out of the blood into tissue, from entering brain tissue. Technetium is excluded from the normal brain by an intact barrier but tumorigenesis may destroy this barrier, and therein lies the basis of the value of technetium scan. Monoclonal antibodies are now being used to carry radionuclides to neoplasms—the antibody specificity being exploited in marking neoplasms via tumor-associated antigens (see Weinstein et al., 1982).

Scanning is particularly useful in detecting cancer that has spread to bone. Limitations of scanning include (1) the fact that potentially harmful radioactive material is given to the patient and (2) the technical difficulty associated with two-dimensional images.

Thermography

Thermography makes use of the fact that heat is dissipated as electromagnetic energy in the infrared region of the electromagnetic spectrum. It exploits the fact that neoplasms are the sites of wasteful energy metabolism and/or have high rates of blood flow and thus tend to give off more heat than surrounding normal tissue. Subsurface neoplasms—as in breast cancer, for example—indeed do show up as "hot spots" in an infrared photography. In a breast cancer detection trial, however, thermography was found not to offer any advantage over physical examination or mammography. Thermography is the only form of medical imaging in which the energy source generating the image is not provided by some external source.

Other Special Tests and Technologies in Cancer Diagnosis

Immune Response Testing

Because cancer often suppresses the immune response, tests of the immune response have some utility in diagnosing cancer. One such test employs the antigenic compound dinitrochlorobenzene (DNCB). When this or some other antigenic material is applied to the skin of a normal subject, localized inflammation signals a normal immune response. A lack of response suggests a suppressed immune response. Of course, not all cancers suppress the immune response and even those that do, don't all do so to the same degree. The same kind of cancer might also have different effects on the immune systems of different people. This latter fact apparently has some prognostic significance; cancer patients who do have good reactions to antigen challenges tend to do better. Their cancers tend to be detected earlier, and they respond better to treatment. Immune status thus has value both in the diagnostic evaluation of cancer and also in treatment planning.

Endoscopy

Endoscopy is a procedure that allows a physician to look at surfaces that are normally out of sight. By means of a flexible lighted tube called an **endoscope**, which can be inserted into various body openings, physicians can look directly at the inside surfaces of such cavities as the nasopharynx, larynx, bronchus, esophagus, stomach (**gastroscopy**), rectum, colon (**colonoscopy**), bladder, and uterine cervix. In identifying neoplasms, endoscopy is nearly as sensitive as close scrutiny of the outer skin surface.

Laparotomy Sometimes a flexible lighted tube is inserted into a cavity that does not have a normal opening to the outside. This feat is accomplished by first making a small incision (a procedure called a **laparotomy**) through which laparoscopy and/or direct visual examination can be made. Such procedures are done more often to accomplish accurate staging (see Chapter 5) than they are done for diagnosis; there are usually more sensitive and less drastic ways to make a diagnosis.

Tumor "Markers"

Some malignancies shed particular antigens and other chemical compounds that appear in the bloodstream. And some of these compounds are nearly enough uniquely associated with particular neoplasms to serve as useful diagnostic "markers" or signals as to the possible presence of these neoplasms.

A **tumor marker** is a substance produced by cancer cells *or* by the hosts' normal cells in response to the presence of cancer. The marker must differ qualitatively and/or significantly quantitatively from the compounds produced by normal cells. Markers may be present in the blood or other fluid compartments, or they may remain associated with the cancer cells themselves. The "ideal" tumor marker appears with a particular cancer *every time* it appears; it *never* appears in cases where the cancer is not present. The "ideal" marker also appears in amounts that correlate with the size of the cancer, is easy to detect, and costs very little in terms of dollars and patient discomfort.

Markers are used not simply to detect the presence of a cancer. In fact, no tumor marker yet identified is sufficiently specific to warrant its use as a screening test for cancer. Markers are useful, however, in the general asymptomatic population in establishing prognosis, in confirming a diagnosis, in staging cancer, in monitoring recurrence, and in monitoring response to treatment.

Tumor markers fall into four general categories: oncofetal antigens, hormones, enzymes, and "other." Among the more commonly used tumor markers are human chorionic gonadotropin (HCG), prostatic acid phosphatase (PAP), carcinoembryonic antigen (CEA), and alphafetoprotein (AFP). CEA is an example of an oncofetal antigen; human chorionic gonadotropin (HCG) is an example of a hormone marker; prostatic alkaline phosphatase is an example of a marker enzyme; and polyamines and prostaglandins are examples of markers other than antigens, hormones, and enzymes.

Human Chorionic Gonadotropin (HCG) The most specific of the tumor markers is HCG. The presence of this marker is almost a certain indicator of trophoblastic cancer in women and germ cell testicular cancer in men. As with other markers, the principal usefulness of HCG is in assessing the effects of therapy and in signaling the recurrence of disease. HCG is so specific that the cancers it marks are not considered cured until HCG levels return to normal (Kahn, 1983).

Carcinoembryonic Antigen (CEA) When CEA was first discovered, it was recognized as an antigen normally present in fetuses but absent in normal adults. Its appearance in adult blood was thought to possibly be uniquely associated with certain kinds of colon cancer. Further work, however, revealed that CEA in blood was also

associated with lung and pancreatic cancer, and such other diseases as cirrhosis of the liver and ulcerative colitis. Still, the fact that 97 percent of healthy adults have CEA levels below 2.5 ng per ml—while more than 70 percent of those with cancers of the colon or rectum have levels significantly higher—make CEA a useful "marker." In recent years, CEA has become very useful as an indicator of the success of treatment and the recurrence of previously operated bowel cancer (see Fig. 16.3). Failure of CEA levels to fall to normal in a bowel cancer patient who had high CEA levels, suggests that not all the cancer was removed. Steadily rising levels following surgery are often associated with cancer recurrence (Fig. 16.3).

Alphafetoprotein (AFP) A liver protein called *alphafetoprotein*, found in fetuses, appears in the serum of adults who have hepatitis, primary hepatocellular carcinoma, and testicular teratocarcinomas. Again, although AFP is not *specific* for cancer it has some use as a marker, and its importance is enhanced by the fact that liver cancer is difficult to detect. Guidelines for using AFP in diagnosing hepatomas are given by Wepsic (1981).

Prostatic Acid Phosphatase (PAP) A fairly specific indicator for prostatic cancer is prostatic acid phosphatase, when elevated levels are accompanied by bone pain and a nodular prostate gland. A number of isoenzymes of acid phosphatase are found in the blood. (**Isoenzymes** are variations in the molecular forms of enzymes having the same function; isoenzyme patterns vary in different kinds of normal tissue, and changes in the isoenzyme patterns appearing in the blood may indicate destruction of cells in particular kinds of tissue.) Particular isoenzymes are associated with pancreatic cancer and benign prostatic hyperplasia.

Other Markers Claims and counterclaims have been made about other potential markers, such as by-products of melanin in melanoma, cerebrospinal fluid polyamines and central ner-

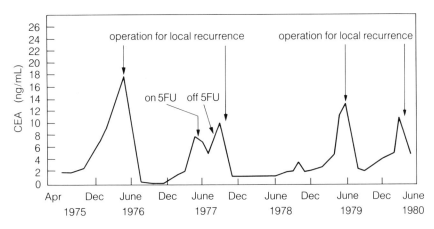

Figure 16.3 CEA and the clinical course of colorectal cancer. This graph shows how a patient's CEA levels reflected four operations and four local recurrences of colorectal cancer over a 5-year period. (*Source:* data from Fabricatorian and Gallagher, 1981; figure adapted from Stein, 1983, p. 11. Used by permission of Abbott Laboratories and Blackwell Scientific Publications Ltd.)

vous system tumors (Marton et al., 1976), and various other proteins, glycoproteins, and complex sugars. **Prostaglandins** (a group of polyunsaturated fatty acids that are short-lived and local-acting, but potent bioregulators found in nearly all body tissues) may become important as markers in the future. Cancers of the thyroid, bronchus, kidney, breast, and endometrium have been reported to be associated with increased prostaglandin synthesis.

Many additional potential tumor markers are under evaluation (see Klug et al., 1984; Magnani et al., 1983; Bast, 1981). The search is driven by a potentially big payoff—as many as 90 percent of all cancers may be cured following very early detection, as opposed to the current 35 percent cure rate.

Although only a few markers are particularly useful at this point, a vigorous search goes on for ways of identifying the chemical fingerprints of different kinds of cancer. The value of early detection and the potential of immunological and biochemical indicators certainly warrant further exploration.

An important property of potential tumor "markers" is their detectability. Not all kinds of

chemical changes are equally detectable. Perhaps a word or two about radioimmunoassays will help make this point.

Radioimmunoassays: Finding Needles in Haystacks

Generally, if large neoplasms cause certain chemical changes in blood, their smaller counterparts cause smaller changes. In such cases, early detection is limited by chemical detection technology. One of the most significant breakthroughs in recent decades in this category has been the development of the radioimmunoassay (RIA).

An RIA couples and then exploits the immunological specificity of a particular chemical and the ease of detecting radioisotopes. It has been used for quite some time in detecting and monitoring (after the response to therapy) hormone-secreting neoplasms. Radioimmunoassays are commonly used to measure elevations in HCG related to trophoblastic tumors; elevations in growth hormone, ACTH, prolactin, and other hormones associated with pituitary tumors; elevated calcitonin levels associated with medullary carcinoma of the thyroid; elevated insulin related to pancreatic tumors; elevated gastrin levels associated with cancers of the stomach; and elevations in various other hormones and "near" hormones (see Chapter 13) related to neoplasms secreting these substances inappropriately (see Yallow, 1981). More recently, RIAs have been used to detect nonhormonal antigens such as CEA and alphafetoprotein.

The RIA represents both (1) a means to search for antigens truly specific for only certain neoplasms and (2) the means to screen for these neoplasms once such relationships are documented.

Monoclonal Antibodies in Cancer Detection

Kohler and Milstein (1975) developed a technique to produce large amounts of antibodies directed toward particular sites on particular antigens (see also Milstein, 1982). The technique involves fusing lymphocytes stimulated by a particular antigenic determinant with mouse myeloma cells. Myeloma cells are cancer cells and are thus "immortal." They also happen to be cells whose chief differentiated character is the production of large quantities of immunoglobins.

The technique for producing monoclonal antibodies was illustrated in Chapter 14. Basically, an antigen is injected into a mouse. Some of the spleen cells begin making antibody to the antigen. Since there may be many different antigenic determinants even on a single antigen, different lymphocytes may make different antibodies to the injected antigen. The spleens of the immunized mice are removed, and isolated spleen cells are fused with mouse myeloma cells. Fusion is accomplished by incubating the cells in the presence of Sendai virus (a virus which even after being killed by ultraviolet light can cause cells to fuse when mixed with them) or polyethylene glycol to make the membranes soft and sticky. Under these circumstances, when a myeloma cell comes into contact with a

spleen lymphocyte, the cell membranes fuse and one cell with two nuclei results. Passage of such cells in culture ultimately results in the fusion of the nuclei and the formation of true hybrid cells called **hybridomas**. Some of these retain (1) the ability to make a particular antibody brought to the union by a spleen lymphocyte, and (2) the ability to "divide and live forever" making large quantities of antibody brought to the union by the myeloma cell. The setup is such that only hybrid cells survive. Plain spleen lymphocytes die off because they can live only a short time in culture. Plain myeloma cells die because the strains used are deficient in nucleic acid synthesis, and the growth medium kills all such cells. The few remaining true hybrids (in which the spleen lymphocyte makes up for the nucleic acid problem) are isolated as single cells (cloned), and clones that make the desired antibody are selected. These may then be grown in large cultures or injected into mice closely related to those in which the lymphocytes were first stimulated. From the cultures or from the mice, large quantities of specific antibodies called **monoclonal antibodies** can be produced. These antibodies have a variety of applications, one of which has relevance to this chapter.

Monoclonal antibodies can be made against cancer cells. More specifically, monoclonal antibodies can be made against particular cancer antigens common to all cancers of a given type. Such monoclonal antibodies can then be used to "find" all cells bearing a particular antigenic determinant. Radioisotopes such as iodine 131 can, and have been (Goldenberg et al., 1980) affixed to monoclonal antibodies against CEA. Since colon cancer tissue has higher concentrations of CEA than normal tissue, more radioactive iodine is taken to the tumor and remains there than anywhere else. The "concentration" of radioactive iodine can then be detected by scanning cameras and thus has obvious utility in detecting otherwise undetectable cancers (see Scheinberg, Strand, and Gansow, 1982). This technique is limited by our ability to identify antigens that are relatively specific for particular kinds of cancer. The availability of monoclonal antibodies has actually facilitated the search for tumor-specific antigens.

But even where tumors have antigens *shared* by other tissues there may be some hope. For example, it has been shown that if monoclonal antibodies can be delivered to the lymphatics before entering the general circulation, they may still effectively mark the presence of lymph node metastases.

Monoclonal antibodies can also be used to classify or subclassify cancers. They can be used to "immunotype" different subpopulations of lymphocytes and thus aid in diagnosing cancer (see Kennel et al., 1984).

Monoclonal antibodies also have treatment applications. We may now reasonably expect one day to be able to produce monoclonal antibodies to antigens from an excised neoplasm and then use the antibodies to fight any remaining cancer. Antibodies may be made even more potent by attaching anticancer drugs, toxic chemicals, or radioisotopes to them, and in fact this has already been tried in human beings. The antibodies can be used to carry poisons directly to cancer cells, acting like guided missiles with destructive payloads (see Vallera et al., 1983). Among the cytotoxic agents that can be taken to tumor cells by monoclonals are radioisotopes, regular chemotherapeutic drugs, plant toxins such as ricin, and even bacterial toxins, such as diptheria toxin (Kennel et al., 1984).

Chromosome Analysis

As discussed in Chapter 11, some evidence exists that chromosome breaks and rearrangements may account for cancer via physical alteration of the relationship between oncogenes and controlling genes. There is already some indication that breaks may tend to occur in certain places—the so-called fragile sites (see Yunis and Soreng, 1984). If this finding holds up and such breaks tend to be associated with cancer with high frequency, chromosomes may one day be routinely examined for breaks associated with particular cancers.

Lumbar Puncture

The lumbar puncture (or spinal tap) is a procedure that enables a diagnostician to examine cerebrospinal fluid (CSF) for cancer cells or tumor markers. The lumbar puncture is accomplished by inserting a needle into the space around the spinal cord and aspirating the fluid. The same mechanical procedure can be used to deliver drugs directly into the CSF.

Bone Marrow Analysis

In this procedure, a needle is used to puncture a flat bone, e.g., the sternum; marrow is then drawn into the needle. The aspirate is spread onto a slide, enabling a pathologist to evaluate the stem cells that give rise to blood cells. This procedure can be useful in diagnosing leukemias (Fig. 16.4), checking responses to treatment (see Chapter 17), or evaluating possible bone metastases.

The Biopsy

All the other diagnostic maneuvers in cancer can be thought of as leading up to the biopsy. Only visual microscopic inspection of biopsy material by a pathologist allows a final answer, yes or no.

Cells of blood cancers such as the leukemias can be obtained by taking a blood sample (Fig. 16.5) or a bone marrow sample from which a smear is made on a glass slide. For solid neoplasms, pieces of tissue can be taken directly from the skin, "core" samples can be taken through a hollow biopsy needle (see Fig. 16.6). Deep internal lesions may require an exploratory operation to obtain tissue.

If the location of a suspicious lesion is such that a biopsy is easily done, then it is done

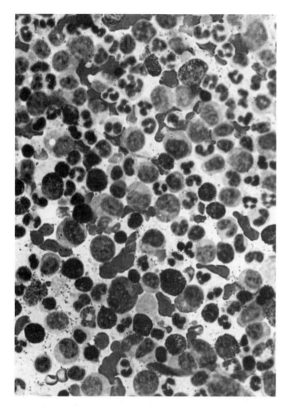

Figure 16.4 Bone marrow aspirate from a patient with chronic myeloid (granulocytic) leukemia. The large cells with the large nuclei are abnormal granulocytic cells. (Photo courtesy of Per H. B. Carstens, M.D., and Alvin W. Martin, M.D., Department of Pathology, University of Louisville School of Medicine.)

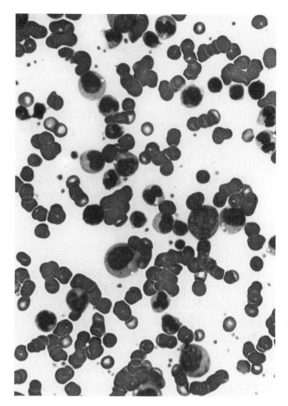

Figure 16.5 Blood smear from the same patient with chronic myeloid leukemia as shown in Figure 16.4. Here, again, the large cells with large nuclei are abnormal granulocytic cells. (Photo courtesy of Per H. B. Carstens, M.D., and Alvin W. Martin, M.D., Department of Pathology, University of Louisville School of Medicine.)

straightaway. If the biopsy is not so easy to do, then other tests are done first—to see if a biopsy is really justified. As long as the diagnostic tests continue to indicate that cancer is a possibility, the tests move through a logical sequence of expense and difficulty, closer and closer to a biopsy.

The word **biopsy** means the removal of some suspicious tissue so that a pathologist can look at it. The responsibility of the person doing the biopsy is to get a representative piece of tissue while inflicting the least amount of harm on the patient.

Biopsy technique depends on the natural history of the neoplasm under consideration

and other factors. The principal techniques are (1) aspiration biopsy, (2) needle biopsy, (3) incisional biopsy, and (4) excisional biopsy.

Aspiration biopsy Drawing cells and tissue fragments through a small needle that has been guided into the tumor mass (Fig. 16.6b). In general, major surgery is not undertaken solely on the basis of aspiration biopsy evidence.

Needle biopsy Obtaining a core of tissue through a specially designed needle introduced into the tumor in a manner not unlike that used by geologists taking core samples of bedrock. The small amount of tissue provided via needle biopsy is enough for diagnosing most types of

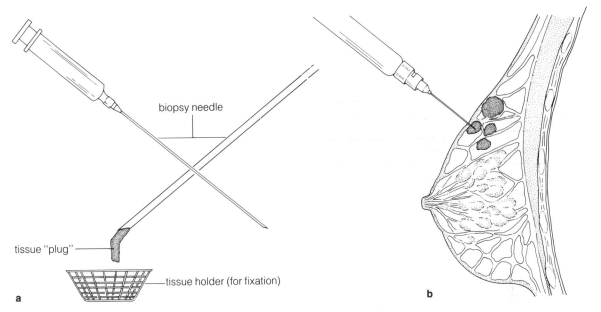

Figure 16.6 (**a**) Solid tissue biopsy; (**b**) needle aspiration biopsy of a breast cyst

neoplasm. However, soft tissue and bony sarcomas sometimes present difficulty in differentiating benign from malignant lesions. With these latter lesions, attempts are often made to get greater amounts of tissue.

Incisional biopsy Removal of a small wedge of tissue from a larger tumor mass. Incisional biopsies are the preferred method of diagnosis for soft tissue and bony sarcomas because of the magnitude of the surgical procedure necessary to get all such lesions.

Excisional biopsy Excision of the entire suspect tumor mass with little or no margin of surrounding normal tissue. Excisional biopsies are the procedure of choice for most tumors when they can be performed without contaminating new tissue planes or otherwise compromising the ultimate surgical procedure.

A list of biopsy techniques is given as Table 16.4. Many factors affect the selection of the technique to be used; for example, accessibility of the lesion, type of neoplasm suspected, impact on patient and hospital resources, reliability, and

the possibility of interference with future management if the lesion does turn out to be malignant.

With good corroborative clinical information and with clear indications of confidence on the part of the pathologist, definite surgery is sometimes done on the basis of scrutinizing a **frozen section** (a thin slice of tissue cut from a quick-frozen specimen). Usually treatment is held off until permanent sections can be prepared. **Permanent sections** are made by first "fixing" the tissue in a fixative such as formalin. If electron microscopic evaluation is to be done—for example, to look for special intracellular markers such as zymogen granules, found only in pancreatic cells—then special fixatives are used. For standard light microscopy, the fixed tissue is embedded in a mounting medium such as paraffin, cut into slices a few micrometers thick, stained with some combination of dyes to reveal particular structural or chemical features, and then covered and sealed under a thin piece of glass. The pathologist then examines the tissue. In order to make a definitive diagnosis, the pathologist must have all of the clin-

Table 16.4 Biopsy Techniques

Technique	Description
Collecting body secretions	Collecting sputum or urine and examining cells therein
Scraping or curettage	Brushing a lesion or a tumor surface with a cotton-tipped applicator or scraping it with a spatula—relatively simple ways to obtain cells for examination
Aspirating fluid	Drawing off fluid that has accumulated in the abdominal cavity or lung with a needle and syringe. Any cells in the fluid can be examined as a smear on a glass slide or made into a block and cut into slices as described in the text.
Needle aspiration biopsy	Sampling accessible masses by inserting an ordinary intravenous needle into them and drawing cells in by applying a slight vacuum
Needle biopsy	Taking core samples from deeper tissue through specially designed long "biopsy" needles. Tissue that can be sampled in this way under local anesthesia include breast, prostate, muscle, liver, lung, bone, and kidney.
Dermal punch	Removing small plugs of tissue from accessible skin or oral lesions via "dermal punches"
Scalpel incision or excision	Using a scalpel to remove a "big" piece of tissue or even an entire lesion for examination; more cumbersome and requires more extensive local anesthesia (internal lesions may even require an "operation") than the foregoing. These are also more definitive than the foregoing.
Biopsy by endoscopy	Using flexible fiberoptic instruments to visualize the esophagus, stomach, genitourinary tract, and the respiratory tract; can be fitted with mechanical devices to collect tissue from suspicious lesions
Full surgical procedures	Surgically removing masses. Generally inaccessible masses of such internal organs as the ovary, thyroid, parotid, brain, liver, lung, pancreas, and kidney require an operation in which the patient is put to sleep.

Source: Wood and Binder, 1978, pp. 19–20.

ical information gathered about the neoplasm (it is important to know where the tissue came from, for example) as well as a good look at the tissue on the slide.

perhaps for easily seen cancers, such as those of the skin or oral cavity. Screening of high-risk individuals does seem to be worthwhile, however. The diagnostic workup leads ultimately to a biopsy.

Summary

Generally speaking, the earlier a cancer is detected, the less likely it is to have spread and the better the prognosis. The value of early detection is actually quite variable for different kinds of cancer. Detection strategies include astute general vigilance on the part of patients and physicians and various physical and chemical methods. Mass screening of asymptomatic individuals is generally not worthwhile except

References and Further Reading

Antonovsky, A., and Hartman, H. 1979. Delay in the Detection of Cancer: A Review of the Literature. In L. Kruse, et al., eds., *Cancer, Pathophysiology, Etiology, and Management*. St. Louis: Mosby.

Bar-Maor, S. A., and Davies, M. 1960. Delay in Diagnosis and Treatment of Cancer of the Digestive Tract. *Harefuah* 59:319–23 (1 Nov.). (Heb).

Bast, R. 1981. Reactivity of a Monoclonal Antibody

with Human Ovarian Carcinoma. *Journal of Clinical Investigation.* 68:1331–37.

Bast, R., et al. 1983. A Radioimmunoassay Using a Monoclonal Antibody to Monitor the Course of Epithelial Ovarian Cancer. *New England J. Med.* 309:883–87.

Boss, B., et al. 1983. *Monoclonal Antibodies and Cancer.* New York: Academic Press.

Bragg, D. G., Rubin, P., and Youker, J. E., eds. 1985. *Oncologic Imaging.* New York: Pergamon Press.

Busch, H., and Yeoman, L. C., eds. 1982. *Methods in Cancer Research.* Vol. 19: *Tumor Markers.* New York: Academic Press.

Cady, B., et al. 1978. History Taking for Cancer Detection. In *Cancer, A Manual for Practitioners.* 5th ed. Boston: American Cancer Society, Massachusetts Division.

Cancer, A Manual for Practitioners. 1978. 5th ed. Boston: American Cancer Society, Massachusetts Division.

Cancer Screening and Diagnosis: An Annotated Bibliography of Public and Patient Education Materials. 1980. Washington, D.C.: National Institutes of Health.

Dao, T., Brodie, A., and Ip, C., eds. 1986. *Tumor Markers and Their Significance in the Management of Breast Cancer.* New York: Alan R. Liss.

Deckers, P., McDonough, E., and Shipley, W. 1978. The Physical Examination for Cancer Detection. In *Cancer, A Manual for Practitioners.* 5th ed. Boston: American Cancer Society, Massachusetts Division.

Devey, G., and Wells, P. 1978. Ultrasound in Medical Diagnosis. *Scientific American.* May. 238(5):98–112.

Edelson, E. 1983. Scanning the Body Magnetic. *Science 83.* 60–65.

Elias, J. M. 1982. *Principles and Techniques in Diagnostic Histopathology: Developments in Immunohistochemistry and Enzyme Histochemistry.* Park Ridge, N.J.: Noyes.

Fabricatorian, D., and Gallagher, N. D. 1981. Evaluation of a Commercial Enzyme Radioimmunoassay Kit for Serum Carcinoembryonic Antigen. *Annals of Clinical Biochemistry.* 18(4):248–51.

Fenoglio-Preiser, C., and Hutter, R. V. 1985. Colorectal Polyps: Pathologic Diagnosis and Clinical Significance. *Ca: A Cancer Journal for Clinicians.* 35:322–44.

Foster, M. A. 1983. *Magnetic Resonance in Medicine and Biology.* New York: Pergamon Press.

Friedman, R. J., Rigel, D. S., and Kopf, A. W. 1985. Early Detection of Malignant Melanoma: The Role of Physician Examination and Self-Examination of the Skin. *Ca: A Cancer Journal for Clinicians.* 35:130–50.

Gold, M. 1983. Cancer: When the Chromosome Breaks. *Science 83.* 16–17.

Goldenberg, D., et al. 1980. Radioimmunodetection of Cancer with Radioactive Antibodies to Carcinoembryonic Antigen. *Cancer Research.* 40:2984–92.

Henderson, M. 1976. Validity of Screening. *Cancer.* 37 (1 January Suppl.):573–81.

Jaffee, C. 1982. Medical Imaging. *American Scientist.* 70:576–85.

Kahn, S. 1983. Cancer Diagnosis. In S. Kahn, et al., eds., *Concepts in Cancer Medicine.* New York: Grune & Stratton.

Kennel, S., et al. 1984. Monoclonal Antibodies in Cancer Detection and Therapy. *Bioscience.* 34(3):150–56.

Kennett, R., McKearn, T., and Bechtol, K., eds. 1980. *Monoclonal Antibodies: Hybridomas—A New Dimension in Biological Analyses.* New York: Plenum Press.

Klavins, J. V. 1985. *Tumor Markers.* New York: Alan R. Liss.

Klug, T., et al. 1984. Monoclonal Antibody Immunoradiometric Assay for an Antigenic Determinant (CA 125) Associated with Human Epithelial Ovarian Carcinomas. *Cancer Research.* 44:1048–53.

Kohler, G., and Milstein, C. 1975. Continuous Cultures of Fused Cells Secreting Antibody of Predefined Specificity. *Nature.* 256:495.

Ledley, R., et al. 1984. Computerized Transaxial X-ray Tomography of the Human Body. *Science.* 186:207–12.

Leffall, L. D. 1981. Prevention and Detection of Colorectal Cancer. In J. Fortner and J. Rhoads, eds., *Accomplishments in Cancer Research.* Philadelphia: Lippincott.

Lokich, J. 1977. Leukocyte Alkaline Phosphatase Activity in Patients with Malignant Disease. *Cancer.* 40:1202–05.

Love, R. 1983. Clinical Science of the Early Detection of Cancer. In S. Kahn, et al., eds., *Concepts in Cancer Medicine.* New York: Grune & Stratton.

Lynch, H., and Fusaro, R. 1982. *Cancer-Associated Genodermatoses.* New York: Van Nostrand.

Mackay, B. 1981. *Introduction to Diagnostic Electron Microscopy.* New York: Appleton-Century-Crofts.

Magnani, J., et al. 1983. Identification of the Gastrointestinal and Pancreatic Cancer-Associated Antigen Detected by Monoclonal Antibody 19-9 in the Sera of Patients as a Mucin. *Cancer Research.* 43:5489–92.

Marton, L., et al. 1976. The Relationship of Polyamines in Cerebrospinal Fluid to the Presence of Central Nervous System Tumors. *Cancer Research.* 36:973–77.

McMichael, A., and Fabre, J., eds. 1982. *Monoclonal Antibodies in Clinical Medicine.* New York: Academic Press.

Miller, D. 1976. What Is Early Diagnosis Doing? *Cancer.* 37(January Suppl.):426–32.

Milstein, C. 1980. Monoclonal Antibodies. *Scientific American.* 243(4):66–74.

Milstein, C. 1982. Monoclonal Antibodies. In J. G. Fortner, and J. Rhoads, eds., *Accomplishments in Cancer Research. 1981.* Philadelphia: Lippincott.

National Cancer Institute. 1981. *Questions and Answers About Breast Lumps.* NIH Publication 82-2401. Bethesda, Md.: U.S. Department of Health and Human Services, Public Health Service.

National Cancer Institute. 1982. *Breast Exams: What You Should Know.* NIH Publication 82-2000. Rockville, Md.: U.S. Department of Health and Human Services, Public Health Service.

Nowinski, R., et al. 1983. Monoclonal Antibodies for Diagnosis of Infectious Diseases in Humans. *Science.* 219:637–44.

Olsen, S. J. 1984. *Examinations for Detecting Breast Cancer.* Madison: Cancer Prevention Program, Wisconsin Clinical Cancer Center.

Pykett, I. 1982. NMR Imaging in Medicine. *Scientific American.* May. 246(5): 78–88.

Reivich, M., and Alavi A., eds. 1985. *Positron Emission Tomography.* New York: Alan R. Liss.

Samuel, K. P., et al. 1984. Diagnostic Potential for Human Malignancies of Bacterially Produced HTLV-1 Envelope Protein. *Science.* 226:1094–96.

Schottenfeld, D. 1975. Cancer Detection Programs. In J. F. Fraumeni, Jr., ed., *Persons at High Risk of Cancer.* New York: Academic Press.

Scheinberg, D., Strand, M., and Gansow, O. 1982. Tumor Imaging with Radioactive Metal Chelates Conjugated to Monoclonal Antibodies. *Science.* 215: 1511–13.

Shwartz, M. 1978. An Analysis of the Benefits of Serial Screening for Breast Cancer Based Upon a Mathematical Model of the Disease. *Cancer.* 41:1550–64.

Sikora, K., and Smedley, H. 1984. *Monoclonal Antibodies.* Palo Alto, Calif.: Blackwell.

Stein, R. 1983. *The Clinical Utility of Tumor Markers.* North Chicago: The Tumor Marker Exchange, Abbott Laboratories. [Audio cassette/slide kit.]

Survey of Physicians' Attitudes and Practices in Early Cancer Detection. 1985. *Ca-A Cancer Journal for Clinicians.* 35:197–213.

Vallera, D., et al. 1983. Anti-T-Cell Reagents for Human Bone Marrow Transplantation: Ricin Linked to Three Monoclonal Antibodies. *Science.* 222:512–14.

Waalkes, T. P. 1985. Biological Markers: An Overview. *Laboratory Medicine* 16:276–78. (*Note:* The entire May 1985 issue of *Laboratory Medicine* was devoted to tumor markers.)

Wade, N. 1982. Hybridomas: The Making of a Revolution. *Science.* 215:1073–75.

Weinstein, J., et al. 1982. Monoclonal Antibodies in the Lymphatics: Toward the Diagnosis and Therapy of Tumor Metastases. *Science.* 218:1334–37.

Weinstein, J. N., and Steller, M. A. 1983. Monoclonal Antibodies in the Lymphatics: Selective Delivery to Lymph Node Metastases of a Solid Tumor. *Science.* 222:423–26.

Wepsic, H. T. 1981. Alpha-fetoprotein: Its Quantitation and Relationship to Neoplastic Disease. In A. M. Kirkpatrick, and R. M. Nakamura, eds., *Alpha-fetoprotein, Laboratory Procedures and Clinical Applications.* New York: Masson Publishing USA.

Wilson, G., Rich, M., and Brennan, M. 1980. Evaluation of Bone Scan in Preoperative Clinical Staging of Breast Cancer. *Arch. Surg.* 115:415–19.

Wood, W., and Binder, S. 1978. Biopsy Principles. In *Cancer, A Manual for Practitioners.* 5th ed. Boston: American Cancer Society, Massachusetts Division.

Yallow, R. 1981. Radioimmunoassay and Tumor Diagnosis. In J. Fortner, and J. Rhoads, eds., *Accomplishments in Cancer Research 1980.* Philadelphia: Lippincott.

Yunis, J. J., and Soreng, A. L. 1984. Constitutive Fragile Sites and Cancer. *Science.* 226:1199–203.

Zamora, P. O., et al. 1985. Cancer Radioimmunoimaging and Therapy. *American Biotechnology Laboratory.* Jan/Feb: 50–57.

Our understanding of the biology, physiology, and biochemistry of cancer has improved dramatically during the past three decades. While each new discovery about how cancer cells differ from normal cells may suggest more effective treatments against the cancer cell, it is highly unlikely that the cancer problem will be solved in one fell swoop with a single drug or new treatment. There are no "silver bullets" out there, and probably never will be. But this is not to say that there are no bullets at all! We do, in fact, have weapons against cancer. Many cancers are susceptible to surgery, chemotherapy, radiation therapy, and even immunotherapeutic weapons. The purpose of this chapter is to outline these principal ways of treating cancer.

Obviously, the ideal in cancer treatment is to ensure total and complete removal of all cancer cells. Traditionally, surgery has been the principal modality of cancer management because it accomplishes this objective under many circumstances, and even when it does not, treating cancer may still first require surgical removal of the primary lesion. Surgery alone does not always cure—because of metastases. And it is not appropriate under many circumstances; neoplasms sometimes involve vital organs and tissues that cannot be removed.

During the last several decades, while surgeons were busy improving what they could do for cancer patients, two other forms of treatment were also rapidly developing. Radiation therapy, once used *only* as **palliative treatment** (to relieve certain symptoms), began to be used to help cure cancer. Because radical regional surgery did not consistently "get all" the cancer cells, regional radiation therapy was found to be effective for certain forms of cancer. Radiation beams, being directable, allowed for somewhat selective killing of cancer cells and spared vital organs. During the last 25 years, through the combined and/or selective use of surgery and radiation, a greater percentage of patients were cured. Of course, many patients still succumbed to cancer because of metastases that had developed throughout the body. Anticancer drugs

17

Treatment

S. J. Bertolone, M.D.

provided a way to kill clusters of cancer cells too small to be detected and already growing in other parts of the body.

Surgery, radiation therapy, and chemotherapy amount to a trilogy of increasingly more general and less direct attack strategies. The objective of surgical treatment is to remove cancer. The objective of radiation is to kill cancer cells where they lie, generally in and immediately around discernible masses. Chemotherapy sends cytotoxic drugs throughout the body. Let's look at each of the modes (or **modalities**) of cancer treatment in the order in which they developed.

Surgery

Surgery is the oldest treatment for cancer. As recently as 30 years ago, surgery was the only definitive treatment capable of curing a patient with cancer. Advances in surgical technique, antibiotics, and blood transfusion technology, and an increased understanding of the patterns in which individual cancers spread, have over the last 20 years provided surgeons with the tools and knowledge to allow them to treat more patients successfully. At the same time, the development of chemical and radiation treatment used in combination with surgery has extended the use of surgery into a wide variety of multimodality treatment strategies capable of controlling disseminated as well as localized disease (see later discussion). Improved chemotherapy and radiation therapy techniques have also reduced the extent of surgery done on the average cancer patient. Thus radiation therapy and chemotherapy have in one way increased and in another way decreased the amount of surgery performed on cancer patients. An example of the latter: In children with rhabdomyosarcoma (muscle cancer) of the pelvis, the primary treatment of choice once was radical resection in which the body organs were removed from the lower abdominal cavity. Now, with the combination of radiation and chemotherapy, surgical

treatment amounts to removing most of the primary tumor without any (or minimal) organ removal, followed by a combination of radiation and chemotherapy. With less surgery, we can still achieve cure rates of 75 percent.

Role of Surgery in Preventing Cancer

As discussed in Chapter 11, a variety of underlying conditions and genetic traits are associated with a high risk of cancer. Whenever cancers are practically inevitable in nonvital organs, prophylactic removal of the offending organ makes a certain amount of sense. Cancer cannot develop in an organ that has been removed. Examples of these types of diseases are discussed in Chapters 11 and 16.

The Role of Surgery in Diagnosing Cancer

The role of surgery in the diagnosis of cancer includes surgical staging (for example, laparotomy for Hodgkin's disease or lymph node dissection for breast cancer; see Chapter 5) and biopsy—the acquisition of tissue for exact histologic diagnosis. Biopsy techniques were outlined in Chapter 16.

Surgery as a Treatment Modality

Surgery can be a simple and safe method for the complete cure of patients with some types of solid tumors when the tumor is confined to the site of origin. If every single cancer cell is physically removed from a patient's body, obviously the patient would be cured. Unfortunately, by the time cancer patients come to a physician, 70 percent will already have micrometastases (DeVita, Hellman, and Rosenberg, 1982)—see Chapter 6.

The principal surgical techniques used in cancer are local excision, block dissection, and various special techniques including cryosurgery, electrosurgery, and laser surgery. **Local ex-**

cision means cutting out the neoplasm with a small margin of normal tissue. Local excision is used for neoplasms in which metastasis occurs only rarely, such as basal cell skin cancers. The term **block dissection** or **en bloc dissection** refers to operations that remove the neoplasm and its nearby lymphatic drainage areas. **Electrosurgery** is done by a high-frequency electrode that simultaneously cuts and coagulates. In **cryosurgery**, the neoplasm is actually cold-killed by freezing it with a liquid nitrogen probe. A **laser** is a device that causes the coordinated (coherent) drop of electrons in an excited group of atoms, say of carbon dioxide, from a high energy level to a lower level with the simultaneous emission of photons of visible light. The photons can then be directed as an intense beam of light capable of vaporizing tissue or even metal. Narrow laser beams can be used like a scalpel to cut tissue. The advantages of laser beams over scalpels include: more precision, smaller wounds, less hemorrhage (the laser beam coagulates protein and seals blood vessels and lymphatics as it cuts), and less tissue damage.

The selection of local surgical therapy to be used in cancer treatment varies with the type of cancer and the site of involvement. In many instances, removing the neoplasm together with a sufficient margin of normal tissue is adequate local therapy. An example is the wide excision of a primary skin melanoma that can be cured by surgery alone in approximately 90 percent of all cases.

The surgeon's role in the treatment of cancer patients may actually include (1) definitive surgical treatment for the primary cancer (sometimes in association with localized radiation therapy and/or chemotherapy); (2) surgery to reduce the bulk of an otherwise unremovable neoplasm; (3) surgical resection of metastatic deposits with curative intent; (4) surgery to reduce the direct impact of a neoplastic mass (palliation); and (5) surgery for reconstruction (such as breast) and rehabilitation.

As this list suggests, surgery can indeed sometimes be used to deal effectively with metastatic deposits. Patients with small numbers of metastases in the lung, liver, or brain may also be cured by surgery. This approach is especially effective in combination with anticancer drugs for those cancers that tend to be highly responsive to systemic chemotherapy, such as bony sarcomas in adults and children and/or Wilms' tumor (kidney) in young children. Children or young adults who have Wilms' tumor or osteogenic sarcoma are treated first by surgically removing the tumor, and then by systemic chemotherapy for 6 to 18 months. If patients subsequently develop isolated lung metastases, they may still be cured via surgery to remove these new lesions.

Some emergency situations also require surgery. Surgical emergencies generally include hemorrhages, perforations, abscesses, or the impending destruction of vital organs (see Chapter 12). A complication that sometimes affects surgical emergencies is the fact that the cancer patient is often **neutropenic** (has a low white cell count) and **thrombocytopenic** (low platelet count), which present an enhanced threat of infection or hemorrhage, respectively.

Palliative Surgery

Surgery is often required to relieve pain or functional abnormalities in cancer patients. The palliative use of surgery can do much to improve a cancer patient's quality of life. Palliative surgery may include relieving mechanical obstructions such as intestinal blockages or removing masses that are causing severe pain or disfigurement.

Rehabilitative Surgery

Reconstruction is an important part of cancer treatment, notably for surgical resections involving tissues of the head and neck, and breast cancers. Improvements in surgical techniques permitting patches of skin to be moved from one part of the body to another have greatly extended possibilities for reconstruction. No longer do head and neck cancer patients necessarily have to suffer severe scarring of both skin and feelings because so much tissue is removed. Breast cancer surgery now commonly includes provision for breast reconstruction planned as part of the initial surgery.

Osteogenic sarcoma has been the principal cause of amputations in children. Resection of all or part of a bone can now be followed by implants of titanium, preserving limb function. Recent advances in materials have made prostheses for lower and upper extremities lighter in weight and cosmetically more acceptable.

Other Side Effects and Common Complications of Surgery

Cancer surgery may have side effects other than the anatomical changes requiring physical rehabilitation, reconstruction, and/or plastic surgery. These effects include (1) impaired lymphatic drainage secondary to the removal of lymph nodes and vessels; (2) release of metastases from what appears to be growth suppression by the primary mass, as the primary mass is removed; and (3) various changes in the immune defense system.

Surgery may interfere with lymphatic drainage, and this may result in fluid retention—for example, in an arm after surgical disruption of the lymphatic chain in the armpit as part of breast cancer surgery. The release of metastatic lesions from growth suppression appears to be related to an unexplained growth relationship between primary masses and metastatic deposits. When a primary mass is reduced or removed, residual tumors—including any metastases—sometimes appear to move into a higher growth fraction (greater percentage of cells dividing). This phenomenon gave rise to the popular misunderstanding that cancer surgery can bring the "end" on more quickly because cancers grow faster when "air gets to them".

The effect of surgery on the immune system varies. Sometimes cancer surgery causes increased immune reaction to a neoplasm, apparently through the release of tumor-suppressed cell-mediated and humoral immunity. Sometimes cancer surgery causes the opposite effect; that is, the depression of immune function. Since both surgery and the presence of neoplasms *each* influence the immune system, it is not surprising that cancer surgery causes immune disturbances. The lack of consistency is likewise not surprising in light of the immune system's ambivalence toward cancer and the heterogeneity of metastatic lesions.

Radiation Therapy

Understanding the use of radiation in cancer therapy requires a basic appreciation of the physics of ionizing radiation (already discussed in terms of carcinogenesis in Chapter 9), the nature of cells and tissue (Chapters 2, 4, and 5), and tumor biology (Chapter 6). The types of radiation used, or studied experimentally, in radiation therapy include short wavelength electromagnetic radiation: X-rays and gamma rays, as well as neutrons, alpha and beta particles, and negative pi-mesons. All these forms of radiation share the ability to generate ions in living tissue.

The conversion of radiant energy to biologically overt damage involve a highly complex sequence of events with a time scale of from 10^{-16} seconds to many years. In radiotherapy, the biologic end point of most importance is the loss of cellular reproductive ability. An irradiated cell is considered dead if rendered unable to divide. Thus, irreparable damage to DNA by radiation can be responsible for cell death. Membrane damage by radiation is also important.

There are two possible mechanisms of interaction between radiation and biologically important molecules: (1) the direct effect of radiation on the important target molecule, or (2) the indirect effect of an intermediary radiation product. In either case, the most important target molecule is DNA.

Whatever the critical molecular target, the ultimate effect is a change in its molecular structure. Direct effects are most common for high linear energy transfer radiation (see Chapter 9). Alternatively, radiation may interact with water to produce highly reactive entities called *free radicals*. Although short lived, these in turn can interact with biologically important material, causing the ultimate detrimental effect.

The lifetime of free radicals is so short that their effective range is usually less than 100Å (Å = **angstrom** = 10^{-10} meters). Thus, to produce a radiochemical lesion in DNA, an ionizing event must occur close to a DNA molecule.

A cell so damaged by radiation that it loses its reproductive integrity may divide once or more often before all its progeny are rendered reproductively sterile. This effect is an important consequence of radiation. It means that an irradiated cell may not appear damaged until it faces its first cell division. At the time of reproduction, a number of possible paths open up for this cell. It may die while trying to divide; it may produce unusual forms; it may stay as it is, unable to divide; it may divide, giving rise to one or more generations of daughter cells; or the cell may suffer only minor alterations.

The Oxygen Effect

As early as 1904, researchers noted that interference with the blood supply of irradiated skin reduced radiation skin reactions. However, not until the 1950s was it appreciated that the presence of molecular oxygen at the time of radiation, rather than the metabolic state of cells, determined their radiosensitivity. The most important modifier of the biologic effect of ionizing irradiation is molecular oxygen. Greater doses of radiation are required to achieve the same effect under **hypoxic** (oxygen-poor) conditions. The exact mechanism of the oxygen effect has not been definitively determined, but it is believed that oxygen somehow affects the interaction between the chemical products formed by radiation and key cellular biochemicals.

The clinical importance of the oxygen effect was shown by Tomlinson and Gray, who dem-

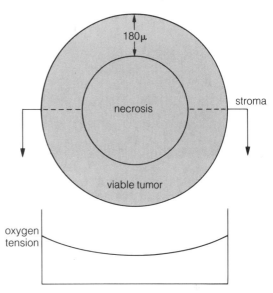

Figure 17.1 Tumor with necrotic (dead, disintegrating) center, a rim of viable, hypoxic tissue, and a normally oxygenated stroma. (Reproduced by permission from Sutow, Wataru W., Fernbach, Donald J., and Vietti, Teresa J.: Clinical Pediatric Oncology, ed. 3, St. Louis, 1984, the C. V. Mosby Co. and Donald J. Fernbach.)

onstrated that human tumors frequently had anoxic regions (Fig. 17.1). Calculations of oxygen diffusion from capillaries and metabolism predicted that in poorly vascularized neoplasms oxygen tension would decrease to zero at about 150 nm. Thus, tumor cells within 100 nm of the capillary blood supply that feeds them are well oxygenated, while those beyond 150 nm tend to be in an oxygen-poor environment. Normal tissue oxygen tension is about 40 mm/Hg. The sensitivity of a cell to radiation damage decreases little until oxygen tension is less than about 20 mm/Hg. At about 4 mm/Hg partial pressure, radiosensitivity is reduced to one-half of its value at full tissue oxygenation (see Fig. 17.2).

Delivering Radiation and Determining Dose

Radiation is delivered to neoplasms in various forms, using various radiation sources and various therapeutic machines. Delivered doses are

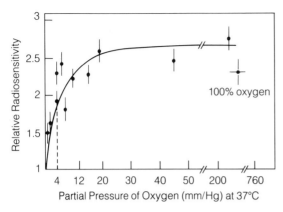

Figure 17.2 Curve relating cellular radiosensitivity to partial pressure of oxygen at the time of irradiation. These particular data were obtained using Ehrlich ascites tumor cells, but very similar curves have been obtained for cell killing of both mammalian cells and bacteria. Note that about half the total sensitization produced by oxygen is seen at a partial pressure of around 4 mm of mercury pressure at 37°C. (Modified from Deschner and Gray, 1959, p. 115.)

measured with calibrated ionization chambers. These ionization chambers have calibration factors that are directly traceable to the National Bureau of Standards (NBS): The instruments are calibrated either at NBS or at a regional calibration laboratory.

There are two general types of radiation therapy techniques: brachytherapy and teletherapy. In **brachytherapy**, a radiation source is placed either within, or close to, the neoplasm. An example is the use of radium implants in the treatment of cervical cancer. Special arrangements can be made for different types of applications based on particular anatomic considerations. **Teletherapy** is provided via machines positioned some distance from the patient. Table 17.1 summarizes the characteristics of various types of teletherapy equipment. The distribution of radiation depends on characteristics of the radiation source, distance from the tumor, and the tissue being irradiated. The radiation

beam may be modified by devices to make isotope distributions best conform to the specific target. Individually designed shields protect vital normal tissue.

Other Aspects of Treatment Planning

Effective radiation therapy requires accurate three-dimensional localization of the target neoplasm and of other dose-limiting *normal* tissue. Such localization requires a physical examination in addition to the use of X-ray films, ultrasound, and other diagnostic procedures (see Chapter 16).

Computerized axial tomography (CAT scans) and nuclear magnetic resonance (NMR) scans have greatly changed the process of tumor localization by allowing much greater accuracy in localizing tumors. Once localization has been completed, the selection of the appropriate treatment plan is made by the clinician, consulting with a radiation dosimetrist. Treatment must take into account the beam distribution, homogeneity of tissue within the target volume, and minimization of the amount of radiation absorbed by the **transient volume**—the normal tissue in the path of the beam. Those tissues whose function does not involve cell renewal, such as muscle and neurologic tissue, are quite resistant to radiation. Both of these types of tissue have blood vessels and other supportive tissues that *do* have cells that may be required to divide, however, and these cells determine the overall sensitivity to radiation. Of course, many tissues of the body engage in *continual* cellular proliferation. Such cell-renewal tissues include skin, gastrointestinal tract, bone marrow, reproductive tissues, and many glands. These tissues typically tolerate comparatively little radiation. Figure 17.3 gives the relative tolerance doses of various organs to radiation.

Dose Fractionation

Radiation therapy is commonly given to patients a little at a time, usually four to five times per

Table 17.1 Characteristics of Radiation Therapy Equipment

	Superficial X-rays	Ortho-voltage	[137]Cs	[60]Co	Betatron[a]	Linear accelerator[a]
Basic components	X-ray tube	X-ray tube	Radioactive source	Radioactive source	Circular accelerating tubes and magnets	Electron gun, klystron, wave guide
Energy	50–140 kv	200–400 kv	0.66 mv	1–2 mv	Variable 18–40 mv	Variable 4–35 mv
Radiation produced	X-rays (photons)	X-rays (photons)	Gamma rays (photons)	Gamma rays (photons)	Photons, electrons*	Photons, electrons*
Size of source or target	5–7 mm	5–7 mm	2–3 cm	1.5–2.5 cm	1–2 mm	1–2 mm
Dose rates (rad/min)	At 20 cm, 50–300, depending on filter	At 80 cm, 50–75, depending on filter	At 50 cm, 50–200, depending on strength of source	At 80 cm, 50–200, depending on strength of source	At 1 m, 50	At 100 cm, 200–1,000
Depth maximum ionization	Skin	Skin	0.2 cm below skin	0.5 cm below skin	4 cm or more below skin	Variable with energy, 0.8 to 5 cm below skin
Clinical use	Skin lesions	Superficial lesions	Deep-seated lesions, moderate doses (5,000–6,000 rad)	Deep-seated lesions, moderate doses (5,000–6,000 rad)	Deep-seated lesions, high doses (6,000–7,000 rad)	Deep-seated lesions, high doses (6,000–7,000 rad)

*Electrons of various energies used for lesions at specific depths (less than 6–8 cm).

Reproduced by permission from Clinical Pediatric Oncology, Third Edition, Pg. 177. Sutow, Wataru W., Fernbach, Donald J., Vietti, Teresa J.; St. Louis, 1984, the C. V. Mosby Co. and Donald J. Fernbach.

week. The rationale for **fractionation** is based on the premise that multiple doses spread over time will allow some repair of lethal radiation damage and that normal cells are better able than cancer cells to repair this damage. It is essential, then, for the radiation therapist to specify not only the total radiation dose and fractions per week but also the dose-time relationship. The total doses that are given to a patient may be divided into two or three series of fractionations (e.g., ten fractions in two weeks with two weeks rest) on the premise that split-dose radiotherapy may enhance the radiation effect by (1) partial regression of the tumor with increased vascularization and *improved oxygenation* (and

thus greater radiosensitivity) of hypoxic cells, and (2) a greater selective impact on cancer cells as a direct consequence of the greater ability of normal cells to repair themselves.

Radiation Modifiers

Recently, interest has been generated in the application of various chemical **radiation sensitizers** to increase, selectively, the effect of ionizing radiation on cancer cells. Multiple animal experiments have shown that tumor cells are killed more readily by radiation in the presence of hypoxic sensitizers (Adams, Fowler, and Wardman, 1978; see also Bump, Yu, and Brown, 1982).

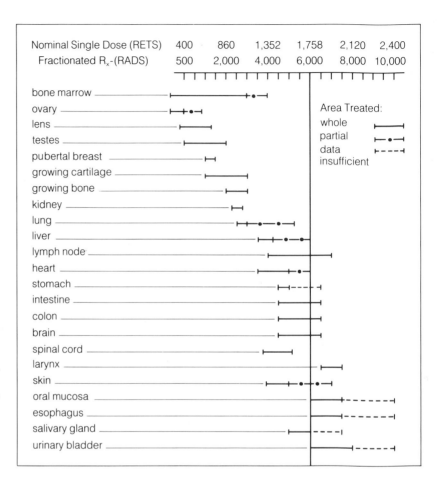

Nominal Single Dose (RETS)	400	860	1,352	1,758	2,120	2,400
Fractionated Rₓ-(RADS)	500	2,000	4,000	6,000	8,000	10,000

Figure 17.3 Graphic representation of tolerance doses of fractionated irradiation for various organs (Modified from Rubin and Casarett, 1972, p. 190. Used by permission of W. B. Saunders, S. Karger AG, Basel, Dr. Phillip Rubin and Dr. John Horton.)

Several compounds, such as metronidazole and misonidazole, have been used to increase this effect. A definite correlation has been found between the concentration of these compounds in the plasma and the radiosensitivity of neoplasms. Therefore, it is important to administer the drugs in the amounts and the times that allow for optimal plasma concentration at the time of irradiation (Wasserman, Stetz, and Phillips, 1981).

Heat enhances radiation killing, and has been shown to have some cancer therapeutic value by itself (Johns and Cunningham, 1974; Hornback, 1984). When tumor temperatures are raised (**hyperthermia**) to between 42.5° and 43.5°C either before, after, or during irradiation, more cells are killed by the radiation (Hahn, 1974). Hyperthermia alone kills cells (exponentially) as a function of time starting at temperature about 44°C. Hyperthermia also selectively kills cells in S phase (see the section "Cell Cycle," Chapter 2) and otherwise radioresistant cells, such as hypoxic tumor cells, while interacting synergistically with ionizing radiation (Nagle, Moss, and Baker, 1982). When heat is combined with radiation, the maximum enhancement occurs if both treatments are delivered simultaneously. Although detailed studies have been performed, the exact mechanism of hyperthermic action on biological systems is as yet unknown. It has marked effects on cell membranes, which influence transport of molecules into the cell and between cell compartments. Nuclear proteins increase acutely after heat exposure (Roti Roti and Winward, 1978) and this results in a large increase in the ratio of nuclear protein to DNA. Although the cause and effect relationship is not known, a correlation has been found in some studies between the extent of cell kill and the level of increased protein demonstrated in the cell after exposure to heat (Roti Roti, Henley, and Winward, 1980).

Side Effects of Radiation Therapy

It is often said that the goal of radiation treatment is to provide the greatest probability of uncomplicated cure. Radiation does have unwanted side effects and the goal is to minimize these. Acute radiation side effects are largely seen in cell renewal tissues (tissues with normally dividing cells); that is, bone, skin or mucosa, small intestine, rectum, bladder, and the vagina. The long-term effects of exposure to radiation are really *the* dose-limiting effects in radiation therapy. These effects include necrosis, fibrosis (scarring), tissue breakdown with fistula formation, nonhealing ulcers, increased risk to other cancers, and damage to specific organs and functions such as the spinal cord and eyes. Chronic exposure to low doses of radiation in a young organism will slow growth and shorten life span (premature aging). There is reason for concern that even low doses of radiation from diagnostic or therapeutic procedures may be carcinogenic and may harm future generations. These effects would result either from damage to the germ cell chromosomes before fertilization or from exposure of the embryo *in utero*.

Combinations of Radiation and Surgery

Radiation and surgery can be combined in many different ways. The rationale for combining surgery and radiation is that the mechanisms of failure for the two techniques are quite different, and they tend to compensate for one another. Radiation *rarely* fails at the periphery of tumors where cells are small in number and well vascularized. When radiation fails, it usually does so in the center of the tumor, where large volumes of tumor cells grow, often under hypoxic conditions. Surgery, in contrast, is often limited by the required preservation of vital normal tissues adjacent to the tumor. In resectable tumors, the gross mass can be removed but the vital normal tissues limit the anatomic extent of the dissection. When surgery fails under these circumstances, the failure is usually caused by tumor cells that are left behind. Thus the mechanism of tumor recurrence for surgery may be quite different from that in radiotherapy. In combining the two techniques, radiation can be given before or after surgery. **Preoperative radiation** has the advantages of sterilizing the cells at the edges of the resection—cells that could perhaps otherwise be dislodged and seeded at the time of surgery—and often reduces tumor size, making surgical removal easier. Also, if surgery is done first, it may interrupt the blood supply, causing the remaining tumor to become more hypoxic and thus more radioresistant.

The use of preoperative radiation has some disadvantages. Pathologic reports may not be as useful if too much time elapses between irradiation and surgery. There may be so much tumor necrosis that the tumor cell type is difficult to define. In contrast, if the tumor is slow growing or if the surgery is done shortly after the irradiation, the radiation effects will not be represented in the pathologic evaluation.

Postoperative radiation has a number of advantages. The subgroup of patients who might be helped by radiation can be very *accurately* defined at surgery and subsequent pathologic review. Unnecessary irradiation to patients *not* likely to benefit can be avoided, and the target volumes can be tailored based on what is found at surgery. Time can be allowed for wound healing so that the radiation will not interfere with this process.

Chemotherapy

The ability to cure cancer depends on a number of variables, most important of which is the presence of viable micro- and/or macrometastases. The need for chemotherapy arises because cancer is often *not* localized at the time of diagnosis and is thus out of curative reach of either surgery or radiation therapy. The objective of chemotherapy under such circumstances is to help cure or to control cancer by snuffing out metastases.

For most types of cancer, chemotherapy is used as an adjuvant to surgery and/or radiation therapy. It is used as the sole method of treatment for only a few types of cancer, the leukemias being the notable examples.

It's amazing the way history does in fact repeat itself. In the early 1900s, Paul Ehrlich devoted much attention to the development of antimicrobial chemotherapeutic agents much in the fashion that is used to identify anticancer drugs today. He stressed the value of using diseased animals to study the effects of these drugs. He coined the word *chemotherapy* for the use of a chemical of known composition in treating parasitic diseases. By the late 1930s, the isolation, purification, and demonstration of the effectiveness of penicillin radically altered the approach to infectious diseases. In later years, resistance to antibiotics by bacteria became a major problem in the successful treatment of these infectious diseases.

There have been many parallels in the development of anticancer drugs. Ehrlich's use of rodent models for infectious diseases led George Clowes in the early 1900s at Roswell Park Cancer Institute to develop inbred rodent lines that could carry transplanted rodent tumors. Such models have since been further developed as the testing ground for potential cancer chemotherapeutic agents (see Fidler and White, 1982). In the 1960s, Skipper and his coworkers laid down the principles of experimental chemotherapy, using the rodent leukemia L-1210 cell line as a model.

Resistance to drugs has also proven to be a problem in cancer chemotherapy. Not all of the cells in a tumor will be equally susceptible to any particular drug. When not all of the cells are killed by drug treatment, the more resistant cells give rise to greater and greater proportions of recurrent cancer, and the cancer becomes increasingly unresponsive to the drug. For the same reason that people with infections are advised to take their antibiotics until they are all gone, dosing is extremely important in cancer chemotherapy. The objective of chemotherapy is to get as close to a total tumor cell kill as possible; even if total cell kill is not achieved, as long as it is closely approximated, the patient's immune system might help eradicate the last malignant cells.

Figure 17.4 shows what might happen in a child with leukemia who had a trillion leukemic cells at the time of diagnosis. After an initial period of treatment, the patient's tumor cell population might be reduced to ten thousand cells, and the patient could be considered to be in complete remission. If therapy were stopped at this point, a relapse might occur and, without further therapy, the patient would die of recurrent disease. If therapy were continued, however, a further reduction in the leukemic cell population to the point of extinction or nearer-extinction might have been possible.

Table 17.2 lists those types of cancer in which a significant fraction of patients with advanced disease can be *cured* with chemotherapy. Table 17.2 also lists advanced cancers in which a significant fraction of the patients *respond* to chemotherapy and improved survival can be demonstrated.

Drug Selection

Most drug therapy is still based on fixed combinations of drugs that have been proven to work against specific cancers. There is much interest now in the strategy of customizing drug therapy for individual patients rather than simply using drugs that have been shown to have some effect on a particular kind of cancer. Individual neoplasms are likely to differ in their respon-

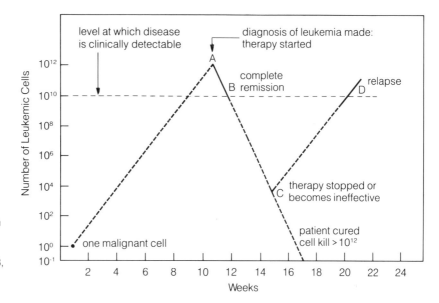

Figure 17.4 The results of therapy in a patient with leukemia. (Reproduced by permission from Sutow, Wataru W., Fernbach, Donald J., and Vietti, Teresa J.: Clinical Pediatric Oncology, ed. 3, St. Louis, 1984, the C. V. Mosby Co. and Donald J. Fernbach.)

siveness to individual drugs. The techniques of finding the right drug are analogous to those used to find the right antibiotic for a particular infection.

A "sensitivity" assay of clonogenic cancer cells has been described by Hamburger and Salmon (1977). A sample of fresh tumor is placed on a plate with growth factors on soft agar. This setup allows tumor colonies to form and grow. The tumor cells are also placed in different plates, each containing a different anticancer drug. After a standard period (approximately three weeks), the number of cells or colonies is determined. The most useful drug allows the smallest number of tumor cells to grow, relative to plates, without added drugs (Salmon et al., 1978). Using this assay, the sensitivity of a particular neoplasm from a particular patient can be determined or at least estimated. A problem is that it is usually difficult to get neoplasms to grow in culture media. Another problem with this assay is that it takes several weeks, and this works against its usefulness for the initial treatment; however, it can identify potentially useful drugs for future treatment. This assay employing certain tumor cell lines in culture is also used to screen new anticancer drug possibilities.

Clinicians generally have two different reasons for giving chemotherapy. The first reason is, to achieve *cure* by completely eradicating residual tumor or metastatic tumor. This goal can be accomplished with anticancer drugs that serve either as the primary treatment or as an adjunct modality (with surgery or radiation therapy). Chemotherapy is also given to achieve palliation, that is, partially eradicating or temporarily controlling tumors to prolong life and to relieve symptoms.

Factors influencing the response of neoplasms to chemotherapeutic agents fall into three main categories: (1) the physiologic status of the patient; (2) the physical, cellular, and biochemical characteristics of the tumor; and (3) the pharmacology and pharmakinetics of the drugs to be used. Within these categories are a number of interrelated factors, shown schematically in Figure 17.5. Each of these factors must be considered in planning the most effective therapeutic regimen for each individual patient.

Physiological Status   The patient's physiological status includes age, nutrition, and metabolism. If severe physiological changes are resulting from the cancer (see Chapter 12) or if

Table 17.2 Response to Chemotherapy

Cancers in Which a Fraction of Patients with
Advanced Disease Can Be Cured with Chemotherapy[a]

Choriocarcinoma	Actue myelogenous leukemia
Acute lymphocytic leukemia in children	Wilms' tumor
Hodgkin's disease	Burkitt's lymphoma
Diffuse histiocytic lymphoma	Embryonal rhabdomyosarcoma
Nodular mixed lymphoma	Ewing's sarcoma
Testicular carcinoma	Small cell cancer of the lung
Ovarian carcinoma	

Advanced Cancers Responding to Chemotherapy[b]

Breast carcinoma	Endometrial carcinoma
Chronic myelogenous leukemia	Adrenal cortical carcinoma
Chronic lymphocytic leukemia	Medulloblastoma
Follicular lymphoma	Neuroblastoma
Multiple myeloma	Polycythemia vera
Small cell carcinoma of the lung	Prostatic carcinoma
Soft tissue sarcomas	Glioblastoma
Gastric carcinoma	Squamous carcinomas of the head and neck
Malignant insulinoma	

[a]A fraction of patients with advanced disease, the remainder often have useful prolongation of life. These 13 cancers accounted for about 75,000 new cases in 1984. About 15,000 of these patients are curable with current chemotherapy. These 13 cancers account for about 10 percent of all cancers per year and about 10 percent of all cancer deaths per year.

[b]Improved survival is demonstrable. The cancers listed account for about 40 percent of all new cancers per year and about 30 percent of all cancer deaths.

Cancer Principles & Practice of Oncology; DeVita, Vincent T., Hellman, Samuel; Rosenberg, Steven A., J. B. Lippincott Co., 1985, Volume 1, Second Edition, p. 282. Used by permission of the publisher.

infection or other intercurrent disease exists, specific supportive measures must be instituted before beginning chemotherapy. If prior therapy has been given, the degree of its toxic effect, the extent of recovery, and degree of residual toxicity must also be taken into account before additional chemotherapy is tried.

Histopathology The type of the tumor and the extent of the disease (stage) at the time of diagnosis are important factors that influence the im-

pact of anticancer drugs and thus survival. These characteristics include histological, cytochemical, and immunological features that are predictive of a particular cancer's potential sensitivity to the chemotherapy to be used. Wilms' tumor in childhood offers a striking example of how histopathology relates to treatment. Two subtypes of Wilms' tumor can be recognized by histopathology. In one type, the cure rate is extremely high (better than 90 percent for Stages I, II, and III). However, there is a small subtype with certain connective tissue elements that has a very unfavorable prognosis, and less than 50 percent of the children with this type of Wilms' tumor do well. In this latter group of patients, increasing the dose of chemotherapeutic agents is likely to be of benefit.

Drug Resistance

As mentioned earlier, a major problem in clinical cancer chemotherapy is the development of drug resistance by cancer cells. This response can arise through a number of mechanisms, all believed to result from evolution of genetic heterogeneity during tumorogenesis (see Chapter 6) and the selective survival of cells that may have (1) undergone modification of the cell membrane so that the drug is not able to move across the membrane, (2) decreased activity or loss of enzymes that convert the parent drug into its effective form(s), (3) increased production or decreased turnover of target macromolecules, (4) increased activity of the enzyme or enzyme systems that break down the anticancer agent, and/or (5) loss of binding proteins or binding sites for the drug.

Functional Types of Antineoplastic Drugs

Two of the most important "vulnerabilities" of proliferating cells are the biochemical sequences involved in chromosomal replication and subsequent cell division. *Most* anticancer agents kill cells by interfering with the synthesis of DNA or with cell division. For many commonly used anticancer agents, the sites of action are illustrated in Figure 17.6. These sites are given in terms of DNA synthesis (replication), the synthesis of RNA from DNA (transcription), and the synthesis of proteins from messenger RNA (translation) (see Chapter 2). Drugs that are effective during the S phase of the cell cycle include arabinosylcytosine, hydroxyurea, 6-mercaptopurine, 6-thioguanine, methotrexate, and 5-fluorouracil. M phase effective drugs include

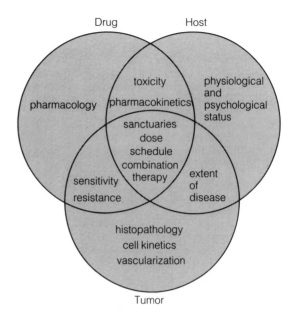

Figure 17.5 Drug, tumor, and host factors and their interactions that influence effectiveness of chemotherapy. (Reproduced by permission from Sutow, Wataru W., Fernbach, Donald J., and Vietti, Teresa J.: Clinical Pediatric Oncology, ed. 3, St. Louis, 1984, the C. V. Mosby Co. and Donald J. Fernbach.)

vincristine and vinblastine. Anticancer drugs that are effective at some specific stage of the cell cycle are called **cell cycle specific agents**. **Cell cycle nonspecific agents** (those whose action is basically the same throughout the cell cycle) include the alkylating drugs, antibiotics, nitrosoureas, and procarbazine. The following section describes some of the classes of anticancer drugs according to their mechanisms of action.

Alkylating Agents   Of the cytotoxic agents that interfere with DNA synthesis, some interfere with the synthesis of precursors of DNA, and some chemically interact with the DNA itself, directly. Most prominent among the latter compounds are drugs known as *alkylating agents* (see Chapter 8). They have the ability to form covalent bonds with nucleic acid. The chemical groups that become attached to the DNA in this reaction interfere with the integrity or function

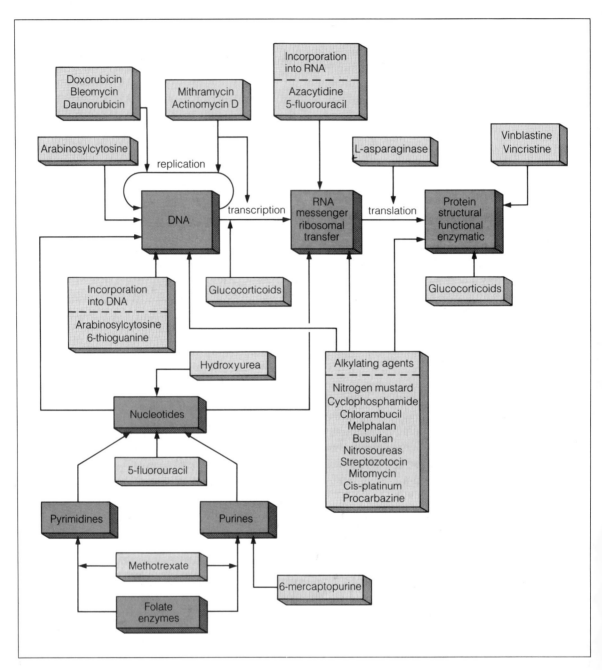

Figure 17.6 Sites of action of antineoplastic agents in relation to synthesis of DNA, RNA, and protein. (Reproduced by permission from Sutow, Wataru W., Fernbach, Donald J., and Vietti, Teresa J.: Clinical Pediatric Oncology, ed. 3, St. Louis, 1984, the C. V. Mosby Co. and Donald J. Fernbach.)

of the DNA, and this prevents cell division. Alkylating agents include the nitrogen mustard derivatives, cyclophosphamide, melphalan (L-PAM), and chlorambucil; alkyl sulfonates (busulfan); and nitrosoureas (e.g., BCNU and CCNU) (see Fig. 17.6).

Antimetabolites Antimetabolites are a group of agents that are structurally similar to *normal* metabolites of cells. They act by interfering with the biosynthesis of proteins, nucleic acids, or other key cellular constituents. As structural analogs of normal metabolites, these agents either bind strongly to an enzyme, thereby inhibiting it, or they are inappropriately incorporated into macromolecules. The substitution of antimetabolites for normal metabolite results in *nonfunctional* macromolecules. Antimetabolites commonly used in cancer therapy include methotrexate, 6-mercaptopurine, 6-thioguanine, arabinosylcytosine, 5-azacytidine, 5-fluorouracil, and hydroxyurea (see Fig. 17.6).

Antitumor Antibiotics Many antibacterial antibiotics are natural products made by fungi. Certain antibiotics made by members of the fungal genus *Streptomyces* have proven to be useful as antitumor agents. Most of these act by inhibiting the synthesis of DNA and RNA. Useful antitumor antibiotics include *mitomycin C, dactinomycin, daunomycin, bleomycin,* and *doxorubicin* (*adriamycin*).

Hormones and Hormone Inhibitors Malignancies originating in tissues normally responsive to hormones, often respond to hormone manipulation (adding hormone or taking it away). Examples of malignancies for which hormonal manipulation is of some palliative value include cancers of the breast, endometrium, and prostate. Within the last decade or so, it has become possible to test tumor tissue for the presence of hormone receptors, enabling the clinician to determine, in advance, the likely hormone responsiveness of a neoplasm. Synthetic hormones have been available for many years; hormone inhibitors (for example the

antiestrogen, *Tomoxifen*) have become available in recent years.

Corticosteriods are a special class of hormonal agent. *Prednisone* (an analog of the hormone cortisone) has been used as an anticancer agent for decades.

Other Agents Various other chemical substances, some natural and some synthetic, fall into *none* of the above classes. Some of the more important of these are the following:

The *vinca alkaloids, vinblastine* (Velban) and *vincristine* (Oncovin) are natural products of the periwinkle plant. These compounds have been found to arrest cell division at mitosis by interfering with microtubules (spindle apparatus) involved in the separation of chromosomes. The vinca alkaloids are used with some success in the treatment of many kinds of cancer.

L-asparaginase is an enzyme product isolated from certain bacteria; it cuts off the exogenous supply of the amino acid, asparagine, to cancer cells that apparently require it. L-asparaginase has proven useful in the treatment of a few types of leukemia.

Hydroxyurea inhibits a particular enzyme involved in the synthesis of DNA; it is used mainly in the treatment of chronic granulocytic leukemia.

Cis-platinum is an inorganic alklyating agent that acts mainly by inhibiting DNA synthesis. Within the last decade cis-platinum has been approved for the treatment of testicular cancer where it is particularly effective, even as a single agent.

Note: The National Cancer Institute publishes a series of information sheets on individual anticancer drugs. Write to Office of Cancer Communications, National Cancer Institute, Building 31, Room 10A18, Bethesda, Maryland, 20892.

Combination Chemotherapy

The fact that all tumors are heterogeneous with respect to drug sensitivity, plus the fact that different chemotherapeutic agents have different kinds of toxicities (that may not be additive in some cases), provides a solid theoretical basis for the expectation that *combinations* of drugs might be effective in treating cancer. Indeed, some of the most important advances in chemotherapy in recent decades have been the definition of effective drug combinations and sequences. It has been found that some drugs interact in such a way tht their cytotoxic effect in combination is greater than the sum of their individual effects. A given drug can, for example, synchronize a population of cancer cells (put most of them in a certain part of the cell cycle), thus setting them up for the action of a second cell-cycle–specific drug. Interestingly, the reasons for the enhanced effect of many drug combinations is not really known; the effects were discovered emperically—by trying them out.

Sanctuaries

Cancer cells can "hide" behind the blood-brain barrier (see Chapter 16) because many drugs cannot get into the sanctuary created by this barrier—while cancer cells *can*. Brain metastases are thus especially problematic in cancer chemotherapy. It has been shown, however, that the relapse of leukemia in the central nervous system can be obviated by injecting chemotherapeutic agents directly into the cerebrospinal fluid and/or by irradiating the head in association with chemotherapy.

Side Effects of Chemotherapy

Anticancer drugs are cytotoxic, and so they kill normal cells along with cancer cells. Both those agents that act at specific points in the cell cycle and those that are effective at any point are most effective against actively dividing cells. This is why anticancer drugs are especially devastating to those normal cells involved in continual cell division. Bone-marrow stem cells, cells that line the gastrointestinal (GI) tract, and cells that give

rise to hair—all divide continuously, and damage to these cells accounts for most of the side effects of chemotherapy. Bone-marrow suppression (**myelosuppression**) leads to anemia, blood coagulation problems, and, most importantly, immune suppression. White cell counts are used to monitor the effect of chemotherapy on bone marrow, and drugs are often given intermittently to allow the bone marrow to recover between doses. Common undesirable side effects resulting from the impact of drugs on the GI epithelium are nausea and vomiting. Hair loss (**alopecia**) is another common side effect of many anticancer drugs. Other organ or tissue-specific toxicities encountered in chemotherapy include neurotoxicity associated with vinca alkaloids. Shock is sometimes associated with L-asparaginase. Kidney toxicity is associated with cis-platinum, and liver toxicity is associated with methotrexate. Certain alkylating agents are carcinogenic (see Chapter 8).

Clinical Trials: Why Does It Take So Long?

The development of anticancer agents encompasses a number of careful steps, and a *long* process separates the inception of a drug and its use in clinical medicine. There are good reasons for this delay, all of which boil down to the directive *Primum non nocere* ("First do no harm"). Let's review the steps in the process of how a new drug is "found."

The steps used in anticancer drug development include acquiring the drugs; screening, producing and formulating; establishing toxicology; Phase I, Phase II, and Phases III-IV clinical trials; and then general medical practice (Fig. 17.7). Inherent in all screening systems is the tenet that biological activity in some experimental animal or cell-culture system must be demonstrated before human testing is performed.

In the early days of drug screening, drugs were selected almost at random to be tested for anticancer activity. In more recent times, knowledge of cell chemistry, biochemistry, cell biology, and pharmacology has been exploited in the identification of what might be called "designer drugs," or drugs *likely* to be effective. Candidate drugs and even incompletely defined extracts are tested in animals bearing cancers of known behavior.

Following the identification of anticancer activity, a candidate anticancer drug must be purified (identified) and formulated as deliverable forms of specific chemicals of known concentrations. The next step is toxicity testing.

Since 1980, a dose response regimen for toxicity testing of new drugs has been established in mice. The lethal dose (LD) in 10, 50, and 90 percent of animals is determined, and the reproducible dose that is lethal in 10 percent of the animals, **LD-10**, becomes the basis for setting the doses to be used in clinical trials. This dose is further tested for toxicity in dogs prior to its use in humans. To maximize safety when administering an unknown compound to humans, 10 percent of the LD-10 dose in rodents is selected for the initial *human* dose. All doses are adjusted on the basis of body surface area, because this adjustment yields *comparable* doses in animals and humans of different sizes.

Antitumor agents then go through four phases of clinical testing (Table 17.3) before they are accepted for general medical practice and marketed or discarded. The average time for discovery of an effective antitumor agent to the marketing of that agent may be anywhere from eight to twelve years. Phase I trials are done on small numbers of patients, usually 15 to 50, and the primary purpose of the study is to identify a maximal tolerated dose in one of several schedules suggested by clinical data. Patients are selected for Phase I studies when they have failed all other standard therapeutic regimens as well as other experimental drugs. Once human-specific toxicity is established in the Phase I trial, the drug is moved forward into a Phase II clinical trial. The only reason not to proceed to a Phase II study would be prohibitive toxicity at the Phase I level. Once a decision is made to proceed with a Phase II testing, trials are begun on a

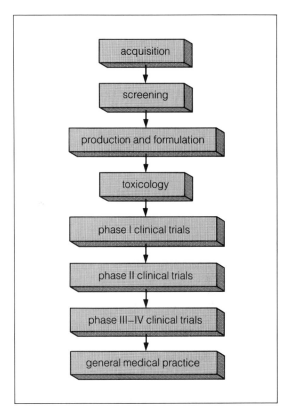

Figure 17.7 Steps in cancer drug development

panel of human neoplasms matching those in the preclinical tumor panel tested on animals. The main problem with Phase II trials is testing agents in a *uniform* way and in a *uniform* population of patients.

Under the best circumstances, a drug that produces *no* antitumor effect in fourteen patients having the same kind of tumor has a greater than 95 percent chance of being *ineffective* against that tumor and could reasonably be dropped from further studies against a specific cancer. One or two responses, however, dictates an expanded trial so as not to miss a drug with a response rate in the 20 percent range.

In general, partial response (tumor shrinks by 50 percent) in 20 percent of patients places an agent in the category of "potential clinical use-

Table 17.3 Clinical Drug Trials

Phase	Purpose
I	Establish maximum dose and toxicity
II	Establish tumor responses
III	Establish benefit of drugs versus other drugs
IV	Standard therapy

fulness." Response rates in the range of 5 to 10 percent are consistent with observer variation in Phase II trials. A few *complete* responses (tumor disappears), even if the overall frequency response is low, normally leads to a decision to proceed with further testing in that disease. At the completion of a Phase II trial, a decision is made to proceed or to discard the agent because of lack of efficacy and/or excessive or intolerable toxicity relative to the observed therapeutic effect.

Since it is not possible to test each new agent against every tumor type, the potential for discarding agents that *might* be useful in rare tumors is significant. If a drug is found effective in Phase II trials, Phase III and IV testing establishes its place in the therapeutic armamentarium. These clinical trials usually require a large number of patients and are all logistically difficult to perform. The basic principle of a clinical trial is to give patients the best known treatment in a preplanned manner that permits reliable conclusions to be drawn that can benefit *future* patients.

For some additional general information about clinical trials, see Nealon (1986).

Informed Consent and Clinical Trials as Good Science

Clinical trials are scientific experiments. As such, whenever two or more treatment regimens are being compared, every precaution must be taken to be sure that "apples are being compared to apples," that except for the treatments being compared, there is as little difference as possible between the groups being compared. Consider the case in which the relative effectiveness of two drugs, say a new one and an old one, against a particular form of cancer was to be determined: After all appropriate determinations of toxicity and dosages have been made, a group of patients should be selected, ideally all having the same histologic type of neoplasm at exactly the same stage; they should all be of the same age, sex, race, socioeconomic status, general health status, etc. In a word, they should all be identical. In practice, this uniformity is never achieved. Even if it were, some unknown factor could always influence the outcome. So it is necessary to select patients as nearly identical as possible and then to randomize—to set up conditions in which the determination of which patient gets which drug is completely random and arbitrary. Such conditions might be constructed, for instance, by drawing an envelope specifying either Treatment A or B from a box—or by having a computer do it. This procedure, of course, raises some interesting dilemmas.

The United States and other countries have adopted the view that treating a patient as part of a clinical trial may create a situation in which a physician scientist may have an interest that conflicts with offering the best available therapy. Regulations and laws have dealt with this potential conflict of interest by requiring that the patient be told that he or she is part of a research study and that the patient be informed of all reasonable possible treatments and their potential side effects.

Informed consent is generally sought before randomization is performed. Consequently, the patient must agree to accept any of the treatments being compared. This provision makes clear to the patient that the physician does not reliably know which treatment is better. This admission may embarrass the physician and unsettle the patient. However, for greatest reliability of conclusions drawn from a randomized study, the randomization should occur before the patient agrees to receive any other treatments. Otherwise, the informed consent process may serve to unconsciously select patients for one treatment or another, based on his or her prognosis. Some clinical trials use prerandomization but then seek informed consent of all patients regardless of the randomization results.

A criticism sometimes voiced about this process is that informed consent is not really informed because many patients have neither the educational background nor the psychological composure to be truly informed (see Fries and Loftus, 1979; Levine, 1986). Research is being conducted on ways of more effectively informing patients about what will be happening and why.

Multimodal Therapy

Surgery, radiation, and chemotherapy have all been individually shown to be effective anticancer treatments. Because local treatment failure is still a too frequent result of these approaches used individually, combinations of all three therapies are used more and more, and the combinations continuously evaluated. The term **multimodal therapy** means the concurrent or sequential use of more than one major method of treatment. At present, four forms of treatment are used clinically: surgery, radiotherapy, chemotherapy, and (to a limited extent) immunotherapy. A multimodal approach to cancer therapy requires that each modality used be at least partially effective *and additive*, given the clinical situation. The objective of any multimodal program should be the strategic combination of measures to obtain the maximum therapeutic effect and at the same time avoid excessive acute and long-term complications. The obvious rationale for combined therapy is to cover situations in which a single method fails to rid the patient of all malignant cells. Although supported by various experimental animal models,

the clinical justification for combined modality therapy in modern cancer treatment rests largely on the results obtained in certain pediatric cancers. A substantial portion of affected children are now able to obtain long-term remission or even cure.

During the last 20 years, Wilms' tumor has served as model for combined modality therapy *and* multidisciplinary evaluation. Most of these recent investigations have been organized by the National Wilms' Tumor Study Group (NWTS), a multi-institutional, multidisciplinary organization that has pioneered the development of cooperative studies. Such cooperative groups have been particularly effective in studying comparatively rare cancers where no single institution, alone, could possibly develop meaningful information. Several NWTS studies have led to the identification of optimal application of improved surgical techniques, improved radiotherapy, and adjuvant combination chemotherapy. For Wilms' tumor, the present drugs of choice are actinomycin-D and vincristine for patients with advanced disease, and it has become recognized that certain histological subgroups require more intensive therapy. The multimodal treatment of Wilms' tumor has resulted in cure rates of better than 92 percent for children who have Stages I, II, or III (already spreading) tumor at the time of diagnosis (D'Angio et al., 1979).

Multidisciplinary Team Management

Most clinical cancer specialists developing and providing treatment to patients, both adults and children, believe that the multimodality team approach is essential for the greatest prospect for success. The disciplines required to diagnose, treat, and support cancer patients include pathology, oncologic surgery, radiation oncology, pediatric or adult hematology and oncology, and diagnostic radiology (tumor imaging). Specialists in oncology nursing, nutrition, clinical pharmacology, and psychosocial evaluation and support (see next chapter) can also make a positive contribution.* Today, surgical oncologists, radiation oncologists, and chemotherapists work closely with one another and with the other disciplines required for the precise histopathologic diagnosis, subclassification, clinical staging, and overall care of patients. The team approach has helped bring about significant improvement in cure rates and quality of life for cancer patients.

Progress in Cancer Treatment

Figure 1.6 shows the improvement in two-year survival rates for the principal tumors of children. From the early 1940s through 1950, surgery was the primary treatment of choice for most childhood cancers. As shown, the two-year survival range had been from approximately 0 to about 20 percent. Radiotherapy was not employed until the mid-1950s and following that, two-year survival rates for Hodgkin's disease and Wilms' tumor showed significant improvement. Clinical trials of cancer chemotherapy and combined chemotherapy did not really begin until the early 1960s and were given initially only to treat recurrence following surgery and radiotherapy. It was later shown that combination chemotherapy was useful earlier in the course of management and combined with surgery and radiotherapy.

Progressing to New Promises

Immunotherapy

As discussed in Chapter 14, being able to vanquish cancer through induced immune reaction is a very appealing idea. It is the most "obvious" "silver bullet" yet imagined. We outlined a

number of *possible* immune enhancement maneuvers in Chapter 15. Here we will reiterate some of the results of what *has* been attempted.

Trials in humans and/or animals fall into one of two general categories: (1) general, nonspecific stimulation of the immune system; and (2) attempted stimulation of immune responses specific to a particular neoplasm.

General stimulants of the immune system are called **immunoadjuvants**. Immunoadjuvants somehow induce the immune system to become more sensitive to *all* antigens.

Interferon (discussed in Chapters 10 and 14) is actually a family of protein substances found in animal cells; the normal function of the interferons appear to be repulsion of viral attacks, and some of them serve as lymphokines able to activate certain elements of the immune system. Some promise still remains that interferon may have some utility (via some kind of general stimulation of the immune system), but this is still being evaluated. The results so far are nowhere near as promising as initially hoped (see Burke, 1977; Sanders, 1981; and Bagliani, 1981).

The best known and most widely explored immunoadjuvant is BCG. BCG stands for Bacille Calmette Guerin, after the two French researchers who made this preparation from bacteria. BCG was developed initially to combat tuberculosis, and has had mixed success against lymphoblastic leukemia and malignant melanoma. Injecting BCG into the bloodstream of leukemic patients has shown some effect (Mathé et al., 1968), although it is not very promising. When BCG has been applied directly to melanomas, however, some dramatic regressions have been reported.

Other immunoadjuvants include **C. parvum**, which has been shown to have some positive antitumor effect when used in conjunction with certain anticancer drugs; and levamisole, which has also been credited with some effectiveness in treating lung cancer.

The reader is referred to Chapter 14 for discussion of current studies of the uses of tumor-necrosis factor and the interleukins.

---

*Nutritional support considerations for patients undergoing cancer treatment are described by Deitel, 1978; Copeland, Van Eys, and Shils, 1978; and National Cancer Institute, 1982a,b,c.

Specific Immune Responses As discussed briefly in Chapter 14, the prospect of specific vaccines for particular kinds of cancer is one of the greatest hopes in the field of cancer medicine. Although interest in this approach has been spurned by the advent of monoclonal antibodies, which has also facilitated searches for tumor-specific antigens (see Chapter 14), little progress has been made thus far. The best prospects appear to be for the development of immunotoxins (Vitetta et al., 1983; Collier and Kaplan, 1984; see also Chapter 14) and the development of vaccines for those cancers linked to viruses (see Chapters 10 and 14).

In Chapter 14 we described some recent advances in **adoptive immunotherapy** (treatment in which immune cells with antitumor activity are injected into the tumor-bearing host). Tumor-sensitized immune cells can be made in a genetically identical organism—other than the tumor-bearing host—by immunizing the second organism with tumor antigens. The sensitized immune cells can then be isolated and transferred to the tumor-bearing organism. This approach, which amounts to getting another organism's immune system to tackle a cancer in a particular host, is not really feasible in humans because genetically identical counterparts are not generally available. But tumor sensitization can also be achieved by isolating a cancer-bearing host's *own* immune cells and activating them using lymphokines (see Chapter 14). In Chapter 14 we described clinical trials being conducted by scientists at the National Cancer Institute in which lymphokine-activated-killer (LAK) cells are being used to treat advanced cancer.

More recently, the same group of scientists reported highly significant cure rates for advanced cancers in mice using a combination of tumor-infiltrating-lymphocytes (TIL), interleukin-2, and immunosuppression (Rosenberg, Spiess, and Lafreniere, 1986). In these more recent studies, TIL cells (apparently a highly tumor-specific subpopulation of lymphocytes) are isolated from tumor tissue. These are made to proliferate in the presence of interleukin-2 and then injected, along with more interleukin-2, back into host animals immunosuppressed with either cyclophosphamide or radiation. The immunosuppression apparently inhibits or eliminates suppressor cells that otherwise inhibit the transferred immune cells. The Rosenberg group reported that the TIL technique is 50 to 100 times more effective than the LAK technique and (because much less interleukin-2 is needed) should involve significantly less severe side effects. TIL cells have already been isolated from several types of human tumors, and this technique was about to be subjected to clinical trial as we went to press.

Treatment Using Differentiation Modifiers

Within the last few years, clinical trials were begun using agents designed to cause cancer cells to change into noncancer cells by inducing their differentiation. This strategy is an appealing one because it would (ideally) circumvent the inadvertent killing of normal cells by drugs designed to kill cancer cells. The strategy is based on the idea that cancer cells are cells stuck at some preterminal stage of differentiation (see Chapters 4 and 11). The most promising of the differentiation inducers thus far is hexamethylene bisacetamide, or HMBA. Several medical centers were involved in trials with HMBA as we went to press.

Cancer Quackery and Unproven Methods

We need to clear up some confusing terminology. An unproven treatment for cancer is just that, unproven. Technically this label applies to new, potentially effective anticancer drugs that have not yet made it all the way through the clinical trial cascade described earlier. It applies to special diets that may or may not do any good, and it applies to completely off-the-wall, fraudulent remedies that may even be *known* to do harm. The phrase *unproven method* is often used as if it were synonymous with cancer quackery.

It is not difficult to imagine why there is such a thing as cancer quackery or even why there are non-quacks who "just know" they really have something and who try to "sell" it before testing is complete. Wherever a demand exists for something expressed in terms of money or some other payoff, someone will inevitably rise up and offer to meet that demand. Consider the especially intense demand for help by an incurably ill patient with money, or by the family member who just has to do *something* after being told that nothing else can be done. And consider the special frustration of someone dying of cancer and aware that a testing program can take more than a decade to certify the effectiveness of a new drug. Consider the power of hope and the desperate *need* for hope—consider the appeal of even a one-in-a-million chance something might work, to a person otherwise stripped of hope. Sometimes people who are not terminally ill also go after the unproven: a grape juice diet might look a lot more appealing than radical surgery and debilitating chemotherapy.

Obviously, we cannot look at all the unproven methods that have been offered over the years and analyze them. Such would be a book in itself. Instead, we will look at just two and refer the reader to the relevant references at the end of the chapter (particularly American Cancer Society (ACS), 1982; Doir and Paxinos, 1978; Burchenal, 1975; and Casileth, 1982).

Laetrile   To date, no substantiated cures have been found in controlled studies using laetrile. Laetrile has been reported to be toxic and has killed some individuals, specifically children who have ingested it by mistake. Laetrile and amygdalin are members of a group of cyanogen glucosides found in the kernels of bitter almonds, apricots, peaches, and plums. Structurally different, the pharmacological actions of these two substances are approximately the same. Morrone (1962) reports that 1 to 10 grams

of amygdalin has been given parenterally to humans, apparently without acute significant toxicity. However, with oral dosing, a toxic potential is evident. Oral laetrile could be 40 times more toxic than parenterally administered doses. Not long ago, a Turkish paper reported nine cases of poisoning, with two fatalities (Sayre and Kaymakcalan, 1964). The deaths and illnesses showed classic signs of cyanide intoxication (vomiting followed by lethargic state, progressing to a comatose moribund condition).

Vitamin C   Linus Pauling has for some time touted vitamin C as an anticancer agent (see Cameron, Pauling, and Leibovitz, 1979). A study done by the Mayo Clinic (Moertel, Fleming, and Creagan, 1985) found, however, that high-dose vitamin C therapy for colon cancer had no benefit in a randomized double-blind study in which 100 patients with advanced colon or rectum cancer were given either high doses of ascorbic acid (10 grams daily) or a placebo. Overall, the patients were in very good general condition and none had received chemotherapy. Vitamin C showed no advantage over placebo therapy in regard either to (1) interval between the beginning of treatment and disease and progression or (2) patient survival.

Unproven methods will be with us as long as there are cancers.

Summary

The three most common forms of cancer treatment are surgery, radiation therapy, and chemotherapy. Each may be used alone, but they are more commonly used in combination. Recently immunotherapy has come into the treatment picture. Surgery is most effective in dealing with primary tumor masses but fails to deal with distant metastases at all, and sometimes neoplasms become inoperable because they become fixed to vital tissues or for other reasons. Radiation therapy is best applied to inoperable primary neoplasms and when applied to the region around a tumor as an *adjuvant* to surgery. Radiation is most effective against rapidly dividing, well-oxygenated cells at the periphery of neoplasms. Chemotherapy is a "broadcast" or "shotgun" approach to cancer. Ideally, it kills cancer cells wherever they may be and leaves normal cells alone. Surgery, radiation, and chemotherapy *all* have unwanted side effects. Surgery's side effects are mostly structural, although cancer surgery can apparently modify the immune system and stimulate the growth of mestastases. The side effects of radiation and chemotherapy derive from the sensitivity of normal dividing cells to these modalities. Immunotherapy, which is really a special kind of chemotherapy, still offers more *promise* than it does actual help. Advances in immunotherapy await better definition of tumor-specific antigens, among other improvements. Even though the application of surgery, radiation, and chemotherapy alone and in combination have brought about some remarkable gains, the fact is these weapons fall woefully short. More cancer patients have to deal with the failure of treatment than with the sequels to success.

References and Further Reading

Adams, G. E., Fowler, J. F., and Wardman, P., eds. 1978. Hypoxic Cell Sensitizers in Radiobiology and Radiotherapy. Section 9: Clinical Studies with Radiosensitizers. *British Journal of Cancer.* 37(Suppl. 3):264–321.

American Cancer Society. 1982. *Unproven Methods of Cancer Management.* New York: American Cancer Society.

Anonymous. 1980. Interferon Nomenclature. *Nature.* 286:110.

Aur, R. J., et al. 1972. A Comparative Study of Central Nervous System Irradiation and Intensive Chemotherapy Early in Remission of Childhood Acute Lymphocytic Leukemia. *Cancer.* 29:381–91.

Baglioni, C. 1981. The Action of Interferon at the Molecular Level. *American Scientist.* 69:392–399.

Becker, F. F., ed. 1977. *Cancer: A Comprehensive Treatise.* Vol. 5, Chemotherapy. New York: Plenum Press.

Beckwith, J. B., and Palmer, N. F. 1978. Histopathology and Prognosis of Wilms' Tumor: *Cancer.* 41: 1937–48.

Bennett, A. H. Classics in Oncology—History. *Medico-Chirurgical Transactions.* Vol. 68. London: Adlard, 1885. 68:243–76.

Bump, E. A., Yu, N. Y., and Brown, J. M. 1982. Radiosensitization of Hypoxic Tumor Cells by Depletion of Intracellular Glutathione. *Science.* 217:544–45.

Burchenal, J. N. H. 1975. From Wild Fowl to Stalking Horses: Alchemy in Chemotherapy. *Cancer.* 35: 1121–35.

Burke, D. C. 1977. The Status of Interferon. *Scientific American.* 236(4):42–50.

Butler, F. 1955. *Cancer Through the Ages, The Evolution of Hope.* Fairfax, Va.: Virginia Press.

Cairns, J. 1985. The Treatment of Diseases and the War Against Cancer. *Scientific American.* 253(5):51–59.

Cameron, E., Pauling, L., and Leibovitz, B. 1979. Ascorbic Acid and Cancer: A Review. *Cancer Res.* 39: 663–81.

Casileth, B. R. 1982. After Laetrile, What? *Cancer News.* 36(3):2–3.

Coleman, M. S. 1983. Selective Enzyme-Inhibitors as Anti-Leukemic Agents. *Bioscience.* 33(11):707–11.

Coli, B. W. 1981. Contributions to the Knowledge of Sarcoma. *Annals of Surgery.* 14:199–220.

Collier, R. J., and Kaplan, D. A. 1984. Immunotoxins. *Scientific American.* July. 251(1):56–64.

Comstock, G. W., Martinez, I., and Livesay, V. T. 1975. Efficacy of BCG Vaccination and Prevention of Cancer. *Journal of the National Cancer Institute.* 54:835–39.

Copeland, E. M., Van Eys, I., and Shils, M. 1978. *Nutrition and Cancer.* New York: American Cancer Society.

Crooke, S. T., and Prestayko, A. W. 1981. *Cancer and Chemotherapy.* Vol. 3: *Antineoplastic Agents.* New York: Academic Press.

D'Angio, G. J., et al. 1979. Results of the Second National Wilms' Tumor Study (NWTS-2). *American Society of Clinical Oncology Abstract C-74.* P. 309.

Deitel, M. 1978. Specialized Nutritional Support in the Cancer Patient: Is It Worthwhile? *Cancer.* 41(6): 2359–63.

Deschner, E. E., and Gray, L. H. 1959. Influence of Oxygen Tension on X-Ray Induced Chromosomal Damage in Ehrlich Ascites Tumor Cells Irradiated In Vitro and In Vivo. *Radiation Research.* 11:115–46.

DeVita, V. 1980, *Cancer Treatment.* Bethesda Md.: National Cancer Institute.

DeVita, V. T., Hellman, S., and Rosenberg, S. T., eds. 1982. *Cancer, Principles and Practices of Oncology.* Philadelphia: Lippincott.

DiPalma, J. R., and McMichael, R. 1979. The Interaction of Vitamins with Cancer Chemotherapy. *Ca-A Cancer Journal for Clinicians.* 29(5):280–86.

Doir, R. T., and Paxinos, J. 1978. The Current Status of Laetrile. *Annals of Internal Medicine.* 89:389–97.

Fidler, I., and White, R. J. 1982. *Design of Models for Testing Cancer Therapeutic Agents.* New York: Van Nostrand.

Frei, E., III. 1982. The National Cancer Chemotherapy Program. *Science.* 216:600–06.

Frei, E. 1985. Curative Cancer Chemotherapy. *Cancer Research.* 12:6523–37.

Fries, J. F., and Loftus, E. F. 1979. Informed Consent: Right or Rite? *Ca-A Cancer Journal for Clinicians.* 29(5):316–18.

Gilman, A. G., Goodman, L. S., and Gilman, A. 1980. *Goodman and Gilman's The Pharmacological Basis of Therapeutics,* 6th ed. Riverside, N.J.: Macmillan.

Greaves, M. F., et al. 1975. Antisera to Acute Lymphoblastic Leukemia Cells. *Immunology-Immunopathology.* 4:67–84.

Hahn, G. M. 1974. Metabolic Aspects of the Role of Hyperthermia in the Mammalian Cell in Inactivation and the Possible Relevance to the Cancer Treatment. *Cancer Research.* 34:3117–23.

Halpern, B. N., et al. 1959. Effet de la Stimulation du Systeme Reticulo Endothelial par l'Innoculation du Bacille de Calmette-Guerin sur le Development de l'E-pihelione Atypique T-S de Guerin Chez la Rat. [Effect of Stimulation of the Reticuloendothelial System by Inoculation of the Calmette-Guerin Bacillus on the Development of the Atypical Guerin T-S Epithelioma in the Rat.] *Compt. Rend. Sos. Biol.* 153:919–23.

Hamburger, A. W., and Salmon, S. E. 1977. Primary Bioassay of Human Tumor Stem Cells. *Science.* 197:461–63.

Hanna, M. G., and Key, M. E. 1982. Immunotherapy of Metastases Enhances Subsequent Chemotherapy. *Science.* 217:367–69.

Haskell, C. M., ed. 1985. *Cancer Treatment.* 2nd ed. Philadelphia: Saunders.

Heyn, R., et al. 1975. ECG in the Treatment of Acute Lymphocytic Leukemia. *Blood.* 46:431–42.

Hornback, N. B. 1984. *Hyperthermia and Cancer: Human Clinical Trial Experience.* Vols. 1 and 2. Boca Raton, Fla.: CRC Press.

Huggins, C. 1967. Endocrine-Induced Regression of Cancers. *Science.* 156:1050–54.

Johns, H. E., and Cunningham, J. R., eds. 1974. *The Physics of Radiology.* Springfield, Ill.: Thomas.

Kolata, G. 1986. Why Do Cancer Cells Resist Drugs? *Science.* 231:220–21.

Krakoff, I. H. 1981. *Cancer Chemotherapeutic Agents.* American Cancer Society Professional Education Publication, Vol. 31, No. 3: pp. 130–40.

Levine, A., et al. 1981. Interferon Induction Cytotoxicity in Clinical Efficacy in Leukemia, Lymphoma, Solid Tumors, Myeloma, and Papillomatosis. In E. M. Hersh, M. A. Chirigos, and M. Mastrangelo, eds., *Augmenting Agents in Cancer Therapy.* (Progress in Cancer Research Therapy, Vol. 16.) New York: Raven Press.

Levine, R. J. 1986. Referral of Patients with Cancer for Participation in Randomized Clinical Trials: Ethical Considerations. *Ca: A Cancer Journal for Clinicians.* 36(2):95–99.

Lindenmann, J., Burke, D. C., and Isaacs, A. 1957. Studies on the Production Mode of Action and Properties of Interferon. *British Journal of Experimental Pathology.* 38:551–62.

Mathé, G., et al. 1968. Demonstration de l'Efficacite de l'Immunotherapie Active dans la Leukemie Aigue Lymphoblastique Humaine. *Rev. Franc. d'et Clin. Biol.* 13:454–.

Mathé, G., et al. 1969. Active Immunotherapy for Acute Lymphoblastic Leukemia. *Lancet.* 1:697–99.

Marx, J. L. 1979. Interferon (I): On the Threshold of Clinical Application. *Science.* 204:1183–86.

Marx, J. L. 1979. Interferon (II): Learning About How It Works. *Science.* 204:1293–95.

Moertel, C. G., Fleming, T. R., and Creagan, E. T. 1985. High Dose Vitamin C Versus Placebo in the Treatment of Patients with Advanced Cancer Who Have Had No Prior Chemotherapy. *New England J. Med.* 312:137–41.

Moore, C. 1985. Multidisciplinary Pretreatment Cancer Planning. *J. Surg. Oncology.* 28:79–86.

Morrone, J. A. 1962. Chemotherapy of Inoperable Cancer. *Experimental Medicine and Surgery.* 20:299–308.

Morton, D. L., et al. 1971. Immunologic Aspects of Neoplasia: A Rational Basis for Immunotherapy. *Annals of Internal Medicine.* 74:587–604.

Mulvilhil, J. J. 1980. Cancer Control Through the Genetics. In F. E. Avignhi, P. N. Rao, and E. Stubblefield, eds., *Genes, Chromosomes and Neoplasia.* New York: Rabur Press.

Nagle, W. A., Moss, A. J., and Baker, M. L. 1982. Increased Lethality from Hyperthermia at 42° Centigrade for Hypoxic Chinese Hamster Cells Heated Under Conditions of Energy Deprivation. *Cancer Therapy by Hyperthermia, Drugs and Radiation.* Pp. 107–10. NCI Monograph No. 61. Washington, D.C.: U.S. Government Printing Office.

National Cancer Institute. 1981. *Cancer Treatment: An Annotated Bibliography of Patient Education Materials.* Bethesda, Md.

National Cancer Institute. 1982a. *Eating Hints: Recipes and Tips for Better Nutrition During Cancer Treatment.* Bethesda, Md.

National Cancer Institute. 1982b. *Nutrition and the Cancer Patient,* 2nd ed. Bethesda, Md.

National Cancer Institute. 1982c. *Diet and Nutrition: A Resource for Parents of Children with Cancer.* Bethesda, Md.

National Cancer Institute. 1985a. *Chemotherapy and You: A Guide to Self-Help During Treatment.* Bethesda, Md.

National Cancer Institute. 1985b. *Radiation Therapy and You: A Guide to Self-Help During Treatment.* Bethesda, Md.

Nealon, E. 1986. *What Are Clinical Trials All About?* Bethesda, Md.: National Cancer Institute.

Oldham, R. K. 1983. Monoclonal Antibodies and Cancer Therapy. *J. Clin. Oncology.* 1:582–90.

Oldham, R. K., et al. 1984a. Lymphokines, Monoclonal Antibodies and Other Biological Response Modifiers in the Treatment of Cancer. *Cancer.* 54:2795–806.

Oldham, R. K., et al. 1984b. Monoclonal Antibody Therapy of Malignant Melanoma(s); In Vivo Localization in Cutaneous Metastasis After Intravenous Administration. *J. Clin. Oncology.* 2:1235–44.

Poplack, D. G., et al. 1978. Treatment of Acute Lymphocytic Leukemia with Chemotherapy Alone and Chemotherapy Plus Immunotherapy. In W. D. Terry and D. Windhorst, eds., *Immunotherapy of Cancer, Present Status of Trials in Man.* New York: Raven Press.

Prehn, L. M. 1981. Role of Immunity in Cancer Remains a Puzzle. *Bioscience.* 31(6):449–52.

Reisfeld, R. A. and Sell, S., eds. 1985. *Monoclonal Antibodies and Cancer Therapy.* New York: Alan R. Liss.

Rider, W. D. 1963. Radiation Damage to the Brain—A New Syndrome. *Journal of the Canadian Association of Radiology.* 14:67–69.

Robinson, R. A., et al. 1976. A Phase I–II Trial of Multiple Dose Polyriboinosinic-Polyribocytidylic Acid in Patients with Leukemia or Solids Tumors. *Journal of the National Cancer Institute.* 57:599–602.

Rosenberg, S. A., Spiess, P., and Lafreniere, R. 1986. A New Approach to the Adoptive Immunotherapy of Cancer with Tumor-Infiltrating Lymphocytes. *Science.* 233:1318–21.

Roti Roti, J. L., Henley, K. J., and Winward, R. 1980. The Kinetics of Increase in Chromatin Protein Content in Heated Cells: A Possible Way of Cell Killing. *Radiation Research.* 84:504–13.

Roti Roti, J. L., and Winward, R. 1978. The Effects of Hyperthermia on the Protein-to-DNA Ratio of Isolated HeLa Cell Chromatin. *Radiation Research.* 74:159–69.

Rubin, P., and Casarett, G. 1972. A Direction for Clinical Radiation Pathology: The Tolerance Dose. In J. M. Vaeth, ed., *Radiation Effect and Tolerance, Normal Tissue; Frontiers of Radiation Therapy and Oncology.* Vol. 6. Basel: Karger.

Salmon, S. E., et al. 1978. Quantitation of Differential Sensitivity of Human Tumor Stem Cells to Anticancer Drugs. *New England J. Med.* 298:1321–27.

Sanders, F. K. 1981. *Interferons: An Example of Communication.* Burlington, N.C.: Scientific Publications Division, Carolina Biological Supply Company.

Sayre, J. W., and Kaymakcalan, S. 1964. Cyanide Poisoning from Apricot Seeds Among Children in Central Turkey. *New England J. Med.* 270:1113–15.

Sherman, C. 1983. Principles of Surgical Oncology. In S. B. Kahn, et al., eds., *Concepts In Cancer Medicine.* New York: Grune & Stratton.

Simpson-Herren, L., Sanford, A. H., and Holmquist, J. P. 1974. Cell Population Kinetics of Transplanted and Metastic Lewis Lung Carcinoma. *Cell Tissue Kinetics.* 7:349–61.

Skipper, H. E., et al. 1950. Implications of Biologic Cytokinetic Pharmacologic and Toxicologic Relationship in the Design of Optimal Therapeutics Schedules. *Cancer Chemotherapy Reports.* 54:431–50.

Sugahara, T., ed. 1984. *Modification of Radiosensitivity in Cancer Treatment.* Orlando, Fla.: Academic Press.

Sun, M. 1981. Laetrile Brush Fire Is Out, Scientists Hope. *Science.* 212:758–59.

Sunkara, P. S., ed. 1984. Novel Approaches to Cancer Chemotherapy. Orlando, Fla.: Academic Press.

Takasugi, M., Mickey, M. R., and Terasaki, T. I. 1973. The Activity of Lymphocytes from Normal Process on Cultured Tumor Cells. *Cancer Research.* 33:2898–902.

Tukey, J. W. 1977. Some Thoughts on Clinical Trials, Especially Problems of Multiplicity. *Science.* 198:679–84.

Vitetta, E. S., et al., 1983. Immunotoxins: A New Approach to Cancer Therapy. *Science.* 219:644–50.

Volger, L. G., et al. 1978. Pre-B Cell Leukemia, A New Hemo Type of Childhood Lymphoblastic Leukemia. *New England J. Med.* 198:872–78.

Wagner, D. J., et al., eds. 1985. *Primary Chemotherapy in Cancer Medicine.* New York: Alan R. Liss.

Wang, A. M., et al., 1985. Molecular Cloning of the Complementary DNA for Human Tumor Necrosis Factor. *Science.* 228:149–54.

Wasserman, T. H., Stetz, J., and Phillips, J. L. 1981. Clinical Trials of Misonidazo 1. In the United States. *Cancer Clinical Trials.* 4:7–16.

Weiss, R. B., and Jacobs, E. M. 1979. The National Cancer Institute Cooperative Clinical Trials Program. *Ca- A Cancer Journal for Clinicians.* 29(5):287–90.

This chapter summarizes the salient features of the most important types of cancer. Included in each summary are U.S. incidence and mortality figures, mortality trends, survival patterns, risk factors, primary prevention strategies, warning signs and symptoms, tests for early detection, common forms of treatment, and a description of some of the major subtypes. The summaries are brief and are intended only to permit some basic comparisons and to put the most commonly encountered cancers in the United States into general perspective. The bibliography at the end of this chapter and others offer many good starting points from which the reader might further study any particular kind of cancer—including those not included in this summary. The National Cancer Institute, the American Cancer Society and the other organizations listed in Chapter 19 are good ongoing sources of information about particular cancers.

Some types of cancer are deadlier than others, and the top ten cancers in terms of incidence are not necessarily among the top ten leading killers. Incidence and mortality patterns are different for men and women. These facts were considered in selecting the cancers featured in this chapter. Figure 1.2 shows the incidence and mortality rankings for the ten leading cancers by sex.

Nearly all the data presented in this chapter come from the National Cancer Institute's Cancer Surveillance, Epidemiology, and End Results (SEER) program (see Chapter 13). The data were gleaned from a number of different National Cancer Institute and American Cancer Society sources, all of which are identified in the bibliography at the end of the chapter. The order of the presentations was derived from the combined impact of each cancer in terms of both incidence and mortality.

18

Synopsis of Common Cancers

Lung Cancer

Incidence   Approximately 144,000 new cases of lung cancer are diagnosed each year. Lung can-small cell   squamous cell

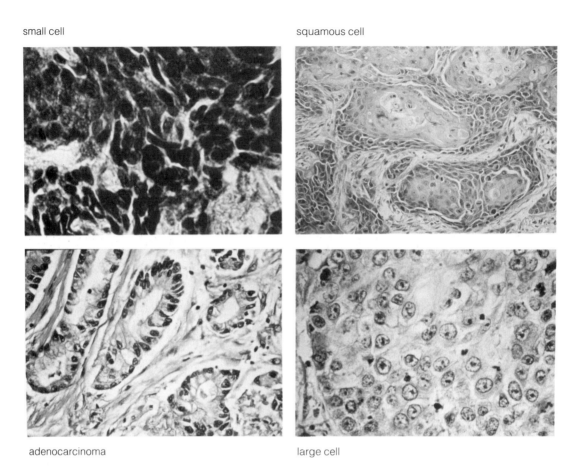

adenocarcinoma   large cell

Figure 18.1 Lung cancer: Some of the most common types as they look under the microscope. (Photos courtesy of Dr. John Minna and Dr. Adi Gazdar of the National Cancer Institute.)

cer incidence (new cases per 100,000 people) has risen dramatically over the past half century. In very recent years, there has been a particularly dramatic increase in lung cancer in women.

Mortality Approximately 125,000 people die of lung cancer each year. Lung cancer age-adjusted mortality rates (deaths per 100,000 people after adjusting for differences in age structure) have increased dramatically since the late 1940s (see Fig. 1.5). Between 1950 and 1979, lung cancer death rates rose 116 percent in white

males, 185 percent in nonwhite males, 199 percent in white females, and 188 percent in nonwhite females (National Cancer Institute, 1984b). In the last few years, lung cancer surpassed breast cancer as the leading cancer killer of females.

Survival The odds of living five years or more after the diagnosis of lung cancer are about 1 in 8, or 13 percent (National Cancer Institute, 1984a). Five-year survival rates have improved only slightly in the last two decades.

Risk Factors Cigarette smoking is the biggest single risk factor for lung cancer. Other risk factors include occupational exposure to various substances such as asbestos (see Chapter 13 and the Epilog to Part III).

Prevention Strategies Don't smoke. Don't work unprotected in occupational environments where there are known or suspect carcinogens. Eat a balanced diet.

Warning Signs and Symptoms Persistent cough; wheezing; shortness of breath; chest pains; blood-streaked sputum; persistent pneumonia or bronchitis; loss of appetite; unexplained weight loss; hormone disruptions that have no apparent connection to the lung (see Chapter 12).

Early Detection Tests It is very difficult to detect lung cancer early; it can eventually be detected by X-rays, sputum cytology, and bronchoscopy (see Chapter 16).

Treatment Depending upon the type of lung cancer and its stage, surgery, radiation therapy, and chemotherapy are all used. Surgery tends to be the "first choice" for early stages of epidermoid carcinoma, adenocarcinoma, and large-cell carcinoma. Radiation is used for inoperable lung cancers and often in combination with surgery. Drugs are used to treat widespread lung cancer, but none has yet been found to be very effective.

Types of Lung Cancer The World Health Organization recognizes 13 different types of lung cancer; 4 of these (see Fig. 18.1) make up 90 percent of all cases (National Cancer Institute, 1980d). Epidermoid carcinoma (synonym: *squamous cell carcinoma*) is the most common (35 percent of total). It tends to remain localized longer than the other common types. Adenocarcinoma (20 percent of total) of the lung can be identified under the microscope by its glandular appearance; large-cell carcinoma (28 percent of total) is

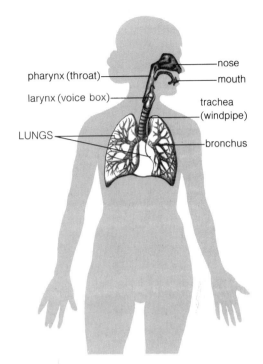

Figure 18.2 The lungs (respiratory system)

recognized by the large size of individual cancer cells. Small-cell carcinoma (synonym: *oat cell carcinoma*), 14 percent of total, is an aggressive type of lung cancer—it spreads very early and less than 1 percent of patients with this form of cancer are alive five years after diagnosis. Oat cell carcinoma is the type most highly correlated with cigarette smoking, although all types show correlation with smoking.

Cancer of the Colon and Rectum

Incidence Approximately 138,000 new cases of cancer of the colon or rectum (Fig. 18.3) are now diagnosed each year. Incidence rates have generally been steady over the past half century.

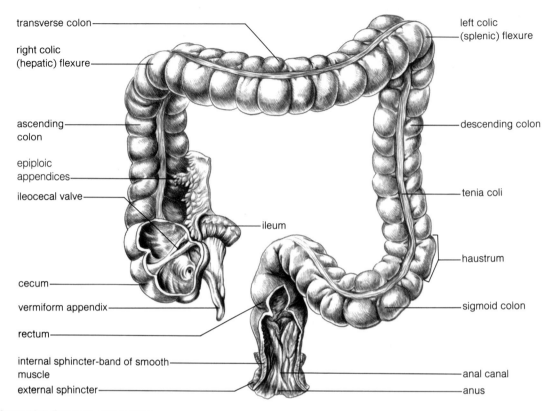

transverse colon

right colic (hepatic) flexure

ascending colon

epiploic appendices

ileocecal valve

cecum

vermiform appendix

rectum

internal sphincter-band of smooth muscle

external sphincter

left colic (splenic) flexure

descending colon

tenia coli

ileum

haustrum

sigmoid colon

anal canal

anus

Figure 18.3 The colon and rectum

Mortality Approximately 59,900 colon or rectal cancer deaths (8,300 of which are rectal) are reported each year. Colon cancer death rates have increased 17 percent in white males, 61 percent in nonwhite males, and 24 percent in nonwhite females; they have dropped 9 percent in white females since 1950 (National Cancer Institute, 1984b). Rectal cancer death rates dropped in all four groups during the same period.

Survival The overall odds of living five years or more after the diagnosis of colon or rectal cancer are 50:50. For individual cases of these types of cancer, survival odds depend heavily on the stage at diagnosis. For localized cancer of the colon for example, the odds of living five years are very good—about 9 in 10. Five-year survival

has improved slightly but statistically significantly for colon cancer since the early 1970s (National Cancer Institute, 1984a).

Risk Factors Family history of colon cancer is a risk factor, as are diet and ethnic background (Czechs high, Japanese in Japan low); personal or family history of inflammatory bowel diseases or polyps. Age is a risk factor in a sense—the risk of dying of colon cancer increases 1,000 times between ages 20 and 80 (Cairns, 1975).

Prevention Strategies Some findings indicate that high-fiber, low-fat diets may help prevent colon cancer.

Warning Signs and Symptoms Signals of trouble include changes in bowel habits, blood in stool, anemia, rectal bleeding, abdominal pain, unexplained weight loss, and fatigue.

Early Detection Tests   The large intestine is another cancer site that spells difficulty in early detection. The American Cancer Society recommends a digital rectal exam as part of every annual checkup after age 40, an annual test for occult blood in the stool after age 50; and a proctoscopic exam every three to five years (depending on risk and other indications) after age 50 (American Cancer Society, 1985).

Treatment   Depending on type, site, and stage of the cancer and on the general health of the patient, surgery, radiation therapy, and/or chemotherapy may be used. Most commonly surgery is used—alone or in combination with radiation.

Types of Colon Cancer   Data from the SEER program for 1950–1973 indicate that of the half dozen different types of colon cancer, adenocarcinoma is by far the most common amounting to more than 90 percent of all cases—if the mucus-producing variety (roughly 8 percent of the total) is included (Prorok, 1978).

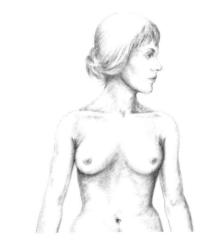

Figure 18.4   The mammary glands (breasts)

Breast Cancer

Incidence   Approximately 119,900 new cases of breast cancer are diagnosed each year. If present trends continue, 1 in 10 women will eventually get breast cancer; the incidence rate has increased slightly over the past half century.

Mortality   Approximately 38,700 women die of breast cancer each year. Breast cancer mortality rates have been constant since the 1930s. Breast cancer is feared even more than cancers that kill more people, partly because it may strike young women. It kills more women aged 40 to 44 than any other disease (National Cancer Institute, 1980a).

Survival   The overall odds of living five years or more after the diagnosis of breast cancer are about 6 in 8, up from 6 in 10 in the early 1960s (American Cancer Society, 1985).

Risk Factors   The following factors raise risk: age; obesity; family history of breast cancer; childlessness; late child bearing (after 35; some data indicate even after 30); late menopause; early onset of menstruation; benign breast disease; and socioeconomic status—high status = high risk (Page and Asire, 1985).

Prevention Strategies   A low-fat diet may help prevent breast cancer. Avoid becoming or staying overweight.

Warning Signs and Symptoms   Any changes in the breasts, including lumps (more than 80 percent will *not* be cancerous), thickening, swelling, dimpling, distortion, retraction of nipple, discharge from a nipple, pain, tenderness, and irritation.

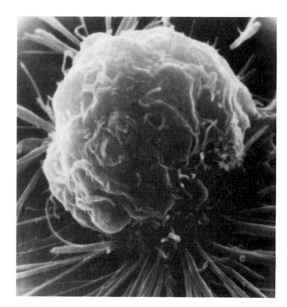

Figure 18.5 Scanning electron micrograph of a cultured breast cancer cell (HBT-3) multiplied 2,500 times. (*Source*: Bruce Wetzel, Ph.D., National Cancer Institute)

Early Detection Tests Self-examination is the most effective overall; it should be a monthly routine for women over 20. The American Cancer Society recommends annual mammograms (Chapter 16) for women past 50 and for younger women at high risk. Any lump, or other finding on a mammogram, thought by an expert to be suspicious (something other than normal lumpiness) should be evaluated by a biopsy. At the time of biopsy, confirmed cancer tissue may be tested for the presence of female hormone receptors. If present, these receptors indicate that the cancer will be able to interact with hormones and that the patient may benefit from hormone therapy.

Treatment As with other cancers, treatment depends on type of breast cancer, its potential responsiveness to hormone manipulation, its stage, and other factors. Surgery, radiation therapy, and chemotherapy are all used, often in combination.

Types of Breast Cancer There are seven major histological types of breast cancer. Based on SEER program data for 1950–1973, the most common type is ductal adenocarcinoma, not otherwise specified (52 percent), followed by otherwise unspecified carcinoma (26 percent), and nonductal adenocarcinoma (15 percent). Lobular carcinomas, mucin-producing adenocarcinomas, medullary carcinomas, and inflammatory carcinomas each make up 2 percent or less. Overall five-year survival rates (all stages) are highest for mucin-producing adenocarcinomas (85 percent in white women) and lowest for inflammatory carcinoma (14 percent). See Asire and Shambaugh (1981).

Prostate Cancer

The prostate gland is a male organ (Fig. 18.6) about the size of two walnuts, located below the bladder and actually surrounds the canal (urethra) through which urine passes on its way out of the body. The prostate's normal function is to secrete a fluid that helps transport sperm.

Incidence Approximately 86,000 new cases of prostatic cancer are diagnosed each year. It is predominantly a disease of older men, being rare in men younger than 55; the average age at diagnosis is 70. The incidence of prostatic cancer in black males is 66 percent higher than it is among whites.

Mortality Approximately 25,500 men die of prostate cancer each year; prostate cancer is the second leading cause of cancer deaths in men. Prostatic cancer mortality in nonwhite males increased 30 percent between 1950 and 1979, but the rate dropped 2 percent in whites (National Cancer Institute, 1984a).

Survival The odds of living five years or more after the diagnosis of prostate cancer are 7 in 10, up from 50:50 in the late 1960s.

prostate and include difficulty urinating, frequent urination (**polyuria**), painful or burning urination, and dribbling after urination.

Early Detection Tests Digital rectal exam with each annual physical for all men after age 40. Also, elevation in serum levels of prostatic acid phosphatase may indicate the presence of prostatic cancer.

Treatment As with every type of cancer, treatment varies with the patient's medical history, general health, age, and the stage of the cancer. **Prostatectomy**, the surgical removal of the prostate, is usually very effective treatment for localized disease. The location of the prostate allows a variety of surgical approaches. The approach used depends on the surgeon, the patient's physical condition, and the size of the tumor (National Cancer Institute, 1981c). Impotence is a common complication of prostatectomy; urinary incontinence is a relatively rare complication. Radiation therapy and hormone manipulation are also used in treating prostatic cancer.

Types of Prostate Cancer According to Moore (1970), practically all prostatic cancers are adenocarcinomas. The small-cell subtype grows more rapidly and invades and metastasizes earlier than the other, well-differentiated subtype. Rarely, leiomyosarcomas, rhabdomyosarcomas, and lymphomas appear in the prostate.

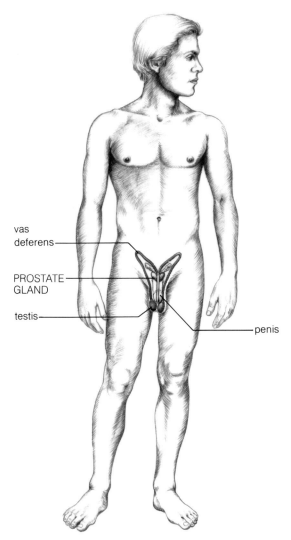

Figure 18.6 The prostate gland (male reproductive system)

vas deferens

PROSTATE GLAND

testis

penis

Risk Factors None (save a possible connection to obesity) have been identified; the cause or causes of prostate cancer are unknown.

Prevention Strategies Avoid obesity.

Warning Signs and Symptoms The symptoms are similar to those of benign enlargement of the

The Lymphomas

The term *lymphoma* applies generally to cancers that develop from lymphoid tissue (Fig. 18.7) (see Chapters 3, 6, and 14). Lymphoid tissues (lymph nodes, spleen, thymus, and parts of other tissues such as the tonsils, the intestines, and the skin) make up part of the body's lymphatic system, which also includes the lymphatic vessels that transport lymph. Hodgkin's disease (after Thomas Hodgkin, who first de-

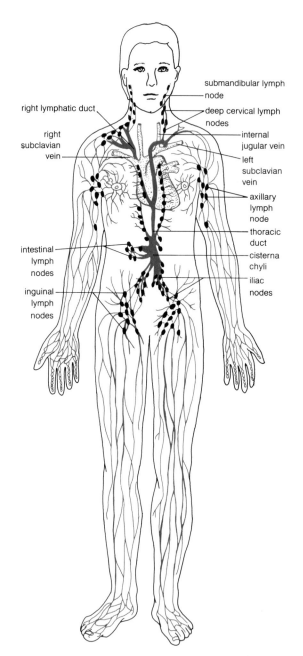

Figure 18.7 The lymphatic system

Labels in figure:
- right lymphatic duct
- right subclavian vein
- intestinal lymph nodes
- inguinal lymph nodes
- submandibular lymph node
- deep cervical lymph nodes
- internal jugular vein
- left subclavian vein
- axillary lymph node
- thoracic duct
- cisterna chyli
- iliac nodes

scribed the disease in 1832) is the most common lymphoma. Although there are several other types of lymphoma, it is common to speak of Hodgkin's disease and non-Hodgkin's lymphomas—as if there were only two basic types.

Incidence   Approximately 43,300 new lymphomas are diagnosed each year.

Mortality   Approximately 22,300 people die from lymphoma each year.

Survival   The overall odds of living five years or more after the diagnosis of Hodgkin's disease are roughly 3 in 4; the odds for non-Hodgkin's lymphomas are roughly 50:50 (National Cancer Institute, 1984a). Five-year survival rates have increased considerably since the early 1960s, when the odds for Hodgkin's disease were 2 in 5 and the odds for non-Hodgkin's lymphomas were 3 in 10.

Risk Factors   None known. Lymphomas do not run in families although they do tend to afflict those past 50; and they are more likely to occur in men and in city dwellers.

Prevention Strategies   None known.

Warning Signs and Symptoms   Signals include painless swelling of lymph nodes in the neck or other places—the same sort of swelling that occurs with an infection; abdominal swelling, small lumps in the skin, rashes, enlarged tonsils, fever, weakness, and loss of appetite. Hodgkin's disease is also marked by itching and night sweats (National Cancer Institute, 1980c, 1981d, 1982).

Early Detection Tests   Lymphoma can be detected by palpation of swollen lymph glands or other lymphoid organs, followed by X-rays, blood tests for certain organ function markers, scans, and lymphangiograms.

Treatment Usually radiation (if the lymphoma is confined to lymph nodes) and/or chemotherapy are used to treat lymphomas.

Types of Lymphomas There are two basic types: Hodgkin's disease and non-Hodgkin's lymphomas. Hodgkin's disease is distinguished by its appearance under the microscope, specifically by the presence of Reed-Sternberg cells—large cells having polylobular nuclei or multiple nuclei. The principal types of non-Hodgkin's lymphomas are lymphocytic lymphoma (or lymphosarcoma), histiocytic lymphoma (or reticulum cell sarcoma), and mixed cell lymphoma. Burkitt's lymphoma is a type of non-Hodgkin's lymphoma rare in the United States, common in Africa.

Cancer of the Uterus

The uterus is a pear-shaped organ (Fig. 18.8) also called the *womb*, that carries the fetus during pregnancy. The narrow end of the uterus, which opens into the vagina is called the **cervix**. The upper portion is called the **corpus** or *body* of the uterus; the lining of the body of the uterus is called the **endometrium**.

Incidence Approximately 52,000 new cases of uterine cancer are diagnosed each year. This figure includes both cancer of the uterine cervix (15,000) and the uterine corpus (37,000), but does not include carcinoma *in situ*. The incidence trend for invasive cancer of the uterus has been notably downward over the past half century; carcinoma *in situ* incidence rates have risen, however.

Mortality Approximately 6,800 cervical cancer deaths and 2,900 deaths attributable to cancer of the uterine body occur each year. Uterine cancer deaths have sharply declined since the 1930s. From 1950 through the 1970s, endometrial cancer death rates dropped 46 percent in white fe-

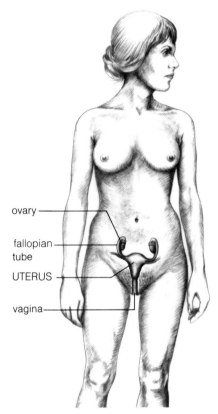

Figure 18.8 The uterus (female reproductive system)

males and 57 percent in nonwhite females; similar decreases have appeared in cervical cancer death rates (National Cancer Institute, 1984b).

Survival The odds of living five years or more after the diagnosis of cervical cancer or cancer of the uterine corpus are 7 in 10 and nearly 9 in 10, respectively—up about one person in 10 in both categories in the past 20 to 25 years (although survival for endometrial cancer declined slightly from the early 1970s to the early 1980s).

Risk Factors For cervical cancer, the risk factors are beginning intercourse early and/or having multiple sex partners. For cancer of the uterine corpus, they are obesity, prolonged estrogen therapy, and a history of infertility.

Prevention Strategies Begin intercourse after puberty, avoid promiscuity, avoid unnecessarily prolonged estrogen therapy, and avoid obesity.

Warning Signs and Symptoms Be alert for unusual vaginal discharge, bleeding between normal menstrual periods, postmenopausal bleeding.

Early Detection Tests The Pap test is recommended by the American Cancer Society once every three years following two negative tests one year apart, beginning at age 21.

Treatment Surgery and/or radiation, often some combination of the two. Precancerous conditions can be treated by cryosurgery (destroying aberrant tissue with extreme cold) or by any of several other methods of local ablation.

Types of Uterine Cancer Epidermoid or squamous cell carcinoma is by far the most predominant type of cervical cancer, comprising 85 percent or more of the total. Adenocarcinomas (not otherwise specified) make up roughly 70 percent of all cancers of the uterine corpus. Other endometrial cancers include papillary carcinomas, adenoacanthomas, leiomyosarcomas, carcinomas (not otherwise specified), mixed mullerian tumors, and carcinosarcomas (Asire, Shambaugh, and Heise, 1981).

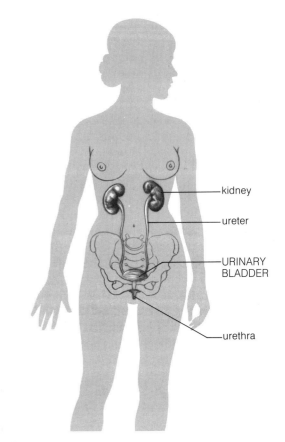

Figure 18.9 The bladder (urinary system)

Bladder Cancer

The bladder is a muscular, expandable, sac (Fig. 18.9) that serves to store, between urinations, urine produced by the kidney. Each kidney is connected to the bladder via a tube called a *ureter*; the bladder empties to the outside via a single tube called the *urethra*.

Incidence Approximately 40,000 new cases of bladder cancer are diagnosed each year.

Mortality Approximately 10,800 people die of bladder cancer each year. Bladder cancer death rates have decreased noticeably in women since 1950—27 percent in whites and 14 percent in nonwhites (National Cancer Institute, 1984b).

Survival The odds of living five years or more after the diagnosis of bladder cancer are 3 in 4 overall, up from 50:50 in the early 1960s.

Risk Factors Risk is raised by being male (males have three times the risk women have); smoking; and working with aromatic amines and their derivatives.

Prevention Strategies Avoid certain unprotected occupational situations (see Chapter 8); don't smoke.

Warning Signs and Symptoms Bloody urine is the primary sign.

Early Detection Tests After the confirmation of blood in the urine, urine cytology (looking at urine sediment under the microscope for cancer cells) is usually the next step—along with a pelvic exam; this may be followed by a test called an IVP (intervenous pyelogram) that makes possible the X-ray visualization of the bladder and/or cystoscopy (looking into the bladder via a lighted tube inserted through the urethra).

Treatment Treatment depends on many factors but most often includes surgery.

Types of Bladder Cancer Sampling done as part of the SEER program (Axtell and Lourie, 1978) indicates that almost all bladder cancers are papillary or transitional cell carcinomas (88 percent of the total).

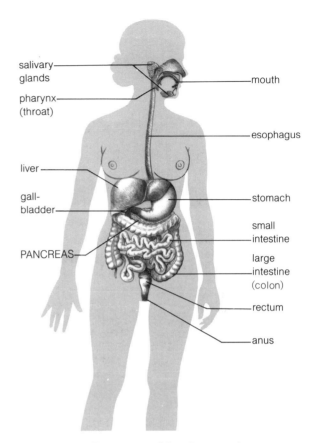

Figure 18.10 The pancreas (digestive system)

Pancreatic Cancer

Incidence Approximately 25,200 new cases of pancreatic cancer are diagnosed each year.

Mortality Approximately 24,200 people die of pancreatic cancer each year. Pancreatic cancer rates have increased steadily since the 1930s—up 30 percent since 1950; the increase reflects increased incidence, the cause of which is unknown.

Survival The prospect of living five years or more after the diagnosis of pancreatic cancer is among the worst of any cancer. Roughly 2 percent are still alive after five years (National Cancer Institute, 1984a).

Risk Factors Cigarette smoking and being male raise risk.

Prevention Strategies Don't smoke.

Warning Signs and Symptoms A person may feel vague upper abdominal pain, nausea, loss of appetite, unexplained weight loss, jaundice (if the cancer blocks the common bile duct), irregularities in blood sugar levels (if the cancer interferes with normal insulin production).

Early Detection Tests No good methods exist for detecting pancreatic cancer early. Eventually,

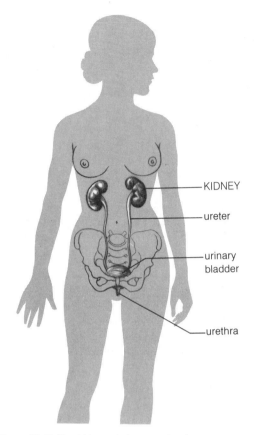

KIDNEY

ureter

urinary
bladder

urethra

Figure 18.11 The kidneys (urinary system)

pancreatic neoplasms may be detected by X-rays (that show distortions of the GI tract caused by pancreatic masses [see Fig. 18.10]), ultrasound, and various types of scans.

Treatment It is best when the entire neoplastic mass can be removed by surgery. Usually this is not possible, but surgery is sometimes still used to relieve symptoms or to relieve discomfort. Radiation and/or anticancer drugs are also used when the cancer cannot be removed surgically.

Types of Pancreatic Cancer Five or six types make up 98 percent of pancreatic cancers. Adenocarcinomas (mostly of duct cell origin) are the most common (Moore, 1970).

Kidney Cancer

The human body has two kidneys, one on each side of the body, just inside the upper part of the small of the back (Fig. 18.11). The normal function of the kidneys is to filter the blood and remove water, salts, and nitrogenous waste products so that these things stay roughly constant in the blood and tissues.

Incidence Approximately 19,700 new cases of kidney cancer and associated urinary tract cancers other than bladder (see earlier section) are diagnosed each year. The average age at diagnosis is 55 (National Cancer Institute, 1981b).

Mortality Approximately 8,900 people die of kidney-urinary tract cancer each year. The trend with respect to mortality rates has been upward in men and steady in women since the 1930s.

Survival The odds of living five years or more after the diagnosis of kidney cancer are 50:50—about the same as it has been for several decades.

Risk Factors Kidney cancer risk increases with smoking pipes, cigars, and cigarettes; working around coke ovens; Wilms' tumor or the tendency to develop it may be hereditary.

Prevention Strategies Don't smoke anything; don't work unprotected around coke ovens.

Warning Signs and Symptoms Blood in urine, abdominal pain, and abdominal lumps are the most common symptoms. Other symptoms include high blood pressure (related to the fact that the kidney helps regulate blood pressure), fever, weight loss, anemia.

Early Detection Tests Detection is via X-rays (including the IVP) followed by ultrasound, arteriograms, CAT scanning, etc.

Treatment   The principal therapy is surgical removal of the affected kidney (**nephrectomy**); radiation therapy with high-energy X-rays is effective in Wilms' tumor. Multiple drug combinations have also proven to be effective in treating widespread Wilms' tumor.

Types of Kidney Cancer   According to the National Cancer Institute (1981b), five different types of kidney cancer occur. The four types of renal cell cancer all occur almost entirely in adults. Wilms' tumor occurs only in children. Of the renal cell cancers, renal cell adenocarcinoma accounts for more than 80 percent of the total; it is three times more common in men than in women. Only 500 cases of Wilms' tumor occur in the United States each year but this amounts to 90 percent of all childhood kidney cancers and makes Wilms' tumor the fifth most common childhood cancer.

Leukemia

The term *leukemia* applies to the entire class of cancers that can generally be described as uncontrolled multiplication and accumulation of abnormal white blood cells (Fig. 18.12).

Incidence   Approximately 24,600 new cases of leukemia are diagnosed each year. Roughly half are acute leukemias, and roughly half are chronic (see below). Leukemias are the most common form of childhood cancer, but leukemias are found with much greater frequency in adults.

Mortality   Approximately 17,200 deaths are attributed to leukemia each year. The trend with respect to mortality rates has been fairly steady since the 1930s; an upward trend beginning in 1950 has since leveled off.

Survival   In the aggregate, the odds of living five years or more after the diagnosis of leuke-

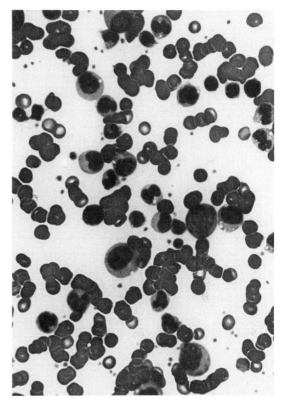

Figure 18.12   Leukemic blood smear. (Photo courtesy of Per H.B. Carstens, M.D., and Alvin W. Martin, M.D., Department of Pathology, University of Louisville School of Medicine.)

mia are just a little better than 1 in 3. Survival rates for some types of leukemia are very low (see section on granulocytic leukemia, below). Improvement in survival of patients with acute lymphocytic leukemia has been one of the most remarkable success stories in cancer. Just fifteen years ago, only one in 20 acute lymphocytic leukemia patients was alive five years later; today, 3 of 4 patients treated in some centers are alive and well five years after diagnosis.

Risk Factors   Disposing factors are Down's syndrome, radiation exposure, and exposure to certain chemicals such as benzene.

Prevention Strategies Avoid unnecessary exposure to radiation and to chemicals linked to leukemia.

Warning Signs and Symptoms Chronic leukemias give little if any warning; acute leukemias at first resemble colds and other common diseases but are subsequently marked by enlarged lymph nodes and spleen, fatigue, pallor, weight loss, repeated infections, easy bruising, and nosebleeds. Ultimately the same array of symptoms develop in chronic leukemia as well. The symptoms of leukemia result from the fact that the leukemic process interferes with the production of normal blood cells and thus interferes with both blood clotting (platelets—see Chapter 3) and immune defense. Hemorrhage and infection are the principal causes of death in leukemia patients.

Early Detection Tests Blood and bone-marrow examinations are used to detect; each show abnormally high numbers of white blood cells (see Figs. 16.4, 16.5 and 18.12).

Treatment Chemotherapy is the most effective treatment. Although some dramatic gains have been made in treating the acute leukemias with drug combinations, as of yet little progress has been made in increasing life expectancy for the chronic leukemias. A general problem in treating leukemias with drugs is that leukemia cells can "hide out" in the brain behind the blood-brain barrier, where drugs cannot get at them. Much research is directed at solving this problem. Because the drugs that kill leukemic cells also kill the cells that give rise to normal cellular elements of the blood, leukemic patients under treatment may need considerable supportive care in the form of transfusions and protection from infection.

Types of Leukemia There are two general classes: acute and chronic. The two predominant acute types are acute lymphoblastic leukemia (ALL) and acute myelocytic leukemia (AML). ALL (synonyms: *acute lymphatic leukemia, acute lymphoblastic leukemia*) is the predominant childhood type. The cells "gone wrong" in this type most closely resemble normal lymphocytes. AML (synonyms: *acute granulocytic leukemia, myelogenous leukemia*) is apparently derived from neutrophils. Chronic myelocytic leukemia (synonyms: *chronic granulocytic leukemia, chronic myeloid leukemia, chronic myelogenous leukemia, chronic myelosis*) and chronic lymphocytic leukemia (National Cancer Institute, 1981a) are the predominant chronic forms.

Stomach Cancer

Incidence Approximately 24,700 new cases of stomach cancer are diagnosed each year. The incidence trend has generally been downward over the past half century.

Mortality Approximately 14,300 people die of stomach cancer each year. There has been a remarkable, unexplained decline in stomach cancer mortality since the 1930s—rates are now one-sixth of what they were then. Between 1950 and 1980 alone, stomach cancer death rates fell 56 percent in white males and 60 percent in white females. In nonwhites, the declines were 12 percentage points less than those of the white counterparts during the same period (National Cancer Institute, 1984b).

Survival In the aggregate, the probability of living five years or more after the diagnosis of stomach cancer is 16 percent. For localized cancer, the odds are 40 percent. Survival has not significantly changed for several decades.

Risk Factors There is some suggestion, if not proof, that excessive alcohol consumption, chronic exposure to very hot or very cold liquids, and chewing tobacco may be risk factors for stomach cancer. Family history (although this correlation may reflect shared diet rather than genetics) and consumption of smoke-cured foods may also be risk factors, along with other unknown dietary factors.

Prevention Strategies   Avoid salt-cured, smoked, and nitrite-cured foods. Eat fresh fruits and vegetables. Don't smoke or chew tobacco.

Warning Signs and Symptoms   Signals include vomiting, weight loss, "heartburn," persistent indigestion, blood in the stools, and stomach pain. There is no systematic practical way of detecting stomach cancer early.

Early Detection Tests   Only 10 percent of stomach cancer cases are found before invasion and metastasis have taken place. Eventually, stomach cancers can be visualized by barium X-ray, gastroscopy, and in other ways.

Treatment   Surgery is the most common form of treatment because so far at least, it is the only successful form of treatment.

Types of Stomach Cancer   Adenocarcinomas make up more than three quarters of stomach cancer cases; other types include carcinomas (16 percent), reticulum cell sarcomas (3 percent), lymphomas (2 percent), and leiomyosarcomas (1 percent). See Prorok (1978).

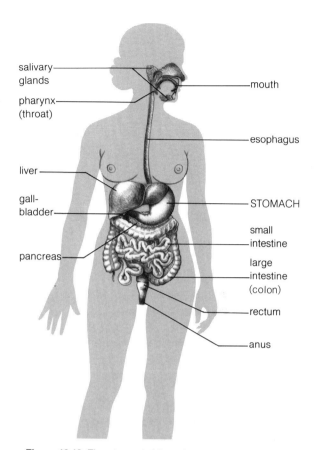

Figure 18.13   The stomach (digestive system)

Oral Cancer

Incidence   Approximately 28,000 new cases of oral (lip, tongue, mouth, pharynx) cancer are diagnosed each year.

Mortality   About 9,500 people die of oral cancer each year. The trend with respect to mortality rates has been steady since the 1930s.

Survival   Hankey (1978) indicates that the odds of living five years or more after diagnosis are about 85 percent for all stages of lip cancer; 32

and 44 percent for tongue cancer in males and females respectively; 42 and 47 percent for cancers of the mouth floor, in men and in women, respectively; and 21 and 30 percent, respectively, for cancer of the pharynx. Five-year survival rates for cancer of the lip, tongue, and mouth have not changed since 1950.

Risk Factors   The most risky behaviors are smoking *anything*, especially in combination with heavy alcohol consumption; and chewing snuff or other forms of tobacco. Sunlight is a risk factor for lip cancer.

Prevention Strategies   Don't smoke cigarettes, pipes, cigars; don't use smokeless tobacco;

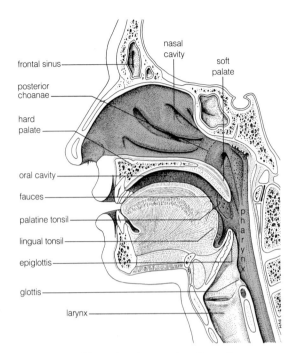

frontal sinus

posterior choanae

hard palate

oral cavity

fauces

palatine tonsil

lingual tonsil

epiglottis

glottis

larynx

nasal cavity

soft palate

pharynx

Figure 18.14 The oral cavity, nasal cavity, and the pharynx

avoid excessive alcohol consumption, especially if you smoke. Use lip sunscreen.

Warning Signs and Symptoms   Watch for growths, swellings, changes in color—persistent red, brown, black, or white patches, sores that do not heal, tingling, burning, numbness, difficulty swallowing, or talking.

Early Detection Tests   Visual confirmation is followed by biopsy.

Treatment   Choice of surgery or radiation therapy depends on location and size of the neoplasm, age, and general condition of the patient. Inoperable neoplasms are treated with radiation. Drugs may also be used with both surgery and radiation.

Types of Oral Cancer   The most common sites of oral cancer are floor of the mouth, pharynx,

lips, and tongue. The most frequent histologic type of pharyngeal cancer is squamous cell carcinoma (85 percent).

Ovarian Cancer

The ovaries are paired organs (Fig. 18.15) that produce eggs and secrete female hormones, including estrogen.

Incidence   Approximately 18,500 new cases of ovarian cancer are diagnosed each year.

Mortality   About 11,600 women die of ovarian cancer each year. The trend in ovarian cancer mortality rates has been fairly steady; between 1950 and 1980, the rates increased 3 percent in white females and 6 percent in nonwhites (National Cancer Institute, 1984a).

Survival   The odds of living five years or more after the diagnosis of ovarian cancer are 4 in 10. This statistic has changed little in the last several decades.

Risk Factors   Ovarian cancer shows some tendency to run in families and some indication of a relationship to obesity.

Prevention Strategies   None known.

Warning Signs and Symptoms   The most frequent initial symptom is enlargement of the abdomen, secondary either to fluid accumulation or to the growth of the neoplasm itself.

Early Detection Tests   An annual pelvic exam is the best way to detect ovarian cancer. Ultrasound is used to confirm and define any masses detected in the physical exam; X-rays can be used to visualize distortion of normal abdominal architecture caused by tumor-induced displacement.

Treatment Usually surgery is followed by radiation therapy or drug therapy.

Types of Ovarian Cancer Histologic types of ovarian cancer and their approximate proportions as reported by Asire, Shambaugh, and Heise (1981) include cystadenocarcinoma (25 percent), papillary carcinoma (23 percent), adenocarcinoma (19 percent), mucinous cystadenocarcinoma (11 percent), and otherwise unspecified carcinoma (8 percent).

Skin Cancer

Incidence Skin cancer is the most common form of cancer—this is at least partly related to the facts that the skin is the body's largest organ and the organ in most direct contact with the outside environment. More than 300,000 cases will be diagnosed this year alone; approximately 20,000 of these will be melanomas.

Mortality Approximately 7,400 people die of skin cancer each year, more than half from melanoma. Mortality rates for most types of skin cancer have held steady since the late 1940s. Melanoma mortality, however, has increased 88 percent among white males, 51 percent among white females, 49 percent among nonwhite males, and 15 percent among nonwhite females (National Cancer Institute, 1984a).

Survival The odds of surviving five years after the diagnosis of nonmelanoma skin cancer exceed 95 percent and could be 100 percent. The odds of living five years or more after the diagnosis of malignant melanoma are 8 in 10.

Risk Factors Fair skin and exposure to sunlight are risk factors.

Prevention Strategies Avoid prolonged exposure to direct sunlight.

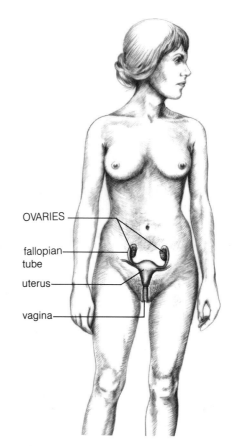

OVARIES

fallopian tube

uterus

vagina

Figure 18.15 The ovaries (female reproductive system)

Warning Signs and Symptoms Watch for sores that do not heal, and any change in a wart or mole.

Early Detection Tests Visual inspection is followed directly by a biopsy.

Treatment Surgery—sometimes cryosurgery or electrosurgery—and radiation therapy are all effective. In some instances, where melanoma recurs, immunotherapy has helped.

Types of Skin Cancer The two most common forms of nonmelanoma skin cancer are basal

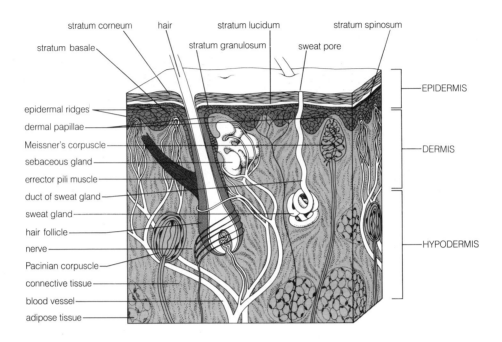

Labels on figure:
stratum corneum, hair, stratum lucidum, stratum spinosum
stratum basale, stratum granulosum, sweat pore
epidermal ridges, dermal papillae, Meissner's corpuscle, sebaceous gland, errector pili muscle, duct of sweat gland, sweat gland, hair follicle, nerve, Pacinian corpuscle, connective tissue, blood vessel, adipose tissue
EPIDERMIS, DERMIS, HYPODERMIS

Figure 18.16 The skin

cell carcinoma and squamous cell carcinomas. The former rarely metastasizes; the latter often does, but is rarer. Both types can appear anywhere on the body but are more common on exposed body parts. Malignant melanomas are not strictly skin cancers but they do arise from skin—from melanocytes, to be specific, and most often from melanocytes in preexisting moles. Malignant melanomas metastasize quickly and can involve many different organs.

References and Further Readings

American Cancer Society. 1985. *Cancer Facts and Figures 1985*. New York: American Cancer Society.

Asire, A., and Shambaugh, E. 1981. *Survival for Cancer of the Breast*. NIH Publication No. 81-1542. Bethesda, Md.: National Institutes of Health.

Asire, A., Shambaugh, E., and Heise, H. 1981. *Survival for Cancers of the Genital Organs*. NIH Publication No. 81-1543. Bethesda, Md.: National Institutes of Health.

Axtell, L., and Lourie, W. 1978. *Survival for Cancers of the Urinary Organs*. NIH Publication NO. 78-1554. Bethesda, Md.: National Institutes of Health.

Barber, H. R. 1986. Ovarian Cancer. *Ca: A Cancer Journal for Clinicians*. 36:149–84.

Bassil, B., Dosoretz, D., and Prout, G. R. 1985. Classification and Staging of Renal Cell Carcinoma. *Ca-A Cancer Journal for Clinicians*. 35:152–63.

Bryan, G., ed. 1983. *The Pathology of Bladder Cancer*. Vols. 1, 2. Boca Raton, Fla.: CRC Press.

Cairns, J. 1975. The Cancer Problem. *Scientific American*. 233:64–79.

Cubilla, A. L., and Fitzgerald, P. J. 1985. Cancer of the

Exocrine Pancreas: The Pathologic Aspects. *Ca-A Cancer Journal for Clinicians*. 35:2–18.

Davis, N., et al. 1976. Primary Cutaneous Melanoma: A Report from the Queensland Melanoma Project. *Ca-A Cancer Journal for Clinicians*. 26(2)80–107.

Elsebai, I., ed. 1983. *Bladder Cancer*. Vol. 1: *General Review*. Boca Raton, Fla.: CRC Press.

Friedman, R. J., Rigel, D. S., and Kopf, A. W. 1985. Early Detection of Malignant Melanoma: The Role of Physician Examination and Self-Examination of the Skin. *Ca-A Cancer Journal for Clinicians*. 35:130–51.

Gale, R. P., and Golde, D. W., eds. 1985. *Leukemia: Recent Advances in Biology and Treatment*. New York: Alan R. Liss.

Graham, S. D., ed. 1986. *Urologic Oncology*. New York: Raven Press.

Green, S. 1978. *Survival for Lymphomas and Leukemias*. NIH Publication No. 78-1546. Bethesda, Md.: National Institutes of Health.

Hankey, B. 1978. *Survival for Cancers of the Buccal Cavity and Pharynx*. NIH Publication No. 78-1539. Bethesda, Md.: National Institutes of Health.

Holland, J., and Frei, E. 1982. *Cancer Medicine*. 2nd ed. Philadelphia, Pa.: Lea & Febiger.

Hoogstraten, B., ed. 1981. *Breast Cancer*. Boca Raton, Fla.: CRC Press.

Ingall, J. R., and Mastromarino, A. J., eds. 1985. *Carcinoma of the Large Bowel and Its Precursors*. New York: Alan R. Liss.

Kahn, S., et al., eds. 1983. *Concepts in Cancer Medicine*. New York: Grune & Stratton.

Kelsey, J., and Hildreth, N. 1983. *Breast and Gynecologic Cancer Epidemiology*. Boca Raton, Fla.: CRC Press.

Khoury, S., et al., eds. 1985. *Testicular Cancer*. New York: Alan R. Liss.

Lacher, M. 1985. Hodgkin's Disease: Historical Perspective, Current Status, and Future Directions. *Ca: A Cancer Journal for Clinicians*. 35:95–115.

Lacher, M. J. 1985. Hodgkin's Disease: Historical Perspective, Current Status and Future Directions. *Ca-A Cancer Journal for Clinicians*. 35:88–94.

Leffall, L. 1974. Early Diagnosis of Colorectal Cancer. *Ca-A Cancer Journal for Clinicians*. May. 24:152–59.

Levin, D., and Baranovsky, A. 1982. *Survival for Melanoma of the Skin and Cancers of the Eye, Brain and Cranial Meninges, Thyroid, Bone, and Connective Tissue*. NIH Publication No. 82-1545. Bethesda, Md.: National Institutes of Health.

Moore, C. 1970. *Synopsis of Clinical Cancer*. 2nd ed. St. Louis: Mosby.

National Cancer Institute. Bethesda, Md.

1980a. *The Breast Cancer Digest*. NIH Publication No. 80-1691. Office of Cancer Communications.

1980b. *Oral Cancer Education*. Selected Annotations. NIH Publication No. 81–1514.

1980c. *Progress Against Hodgkin's Disease*. NIH Publication No. 81-172.

1980d. *Research Report: Cancer of the Lung*. NIH Publication No. 81-526.

1981a. *Progress Against Leukemia*. NIH Publication No. 81-367.

1981b. *Research Report: Cancer of the Kidney*. NIH Publication No. 81-2342.

1981c. *Research Report: Cancer of the Prostate*. NIH Publication No. 81-528.

1981d. *What You Need to Know About Hodgkin's Disease*. NIH Publication No. 81-1555.

1982. *What You Need to Know About Non-Hodgkin's Lymphoma*. NIH Publication No. 82-1567.

1984a. *Cancer Patient Survival Statistics*. Update. November 26.

1984b. *New Publication: Trends for Cancer Deaths by County*. Update. February.

Nelson, J., Averette, H., and Richart, R. 1979. Detection, Diagnostic Evaluation and Treatment of Dysplasia, Carcinoma in Situ and Early Invasive Cervical Carcinoma. *Ca-A Cancer Journal for Clinicians*. 29(3):174–92.

Page, H. S., and Asire, A. J. 1985. *Cancer Rates and Risks*. 3rd ed. NIH Publication No. 85-691. Bethesda, Md.: National Institutes of Health.

Prorok, P. 1978. *Survival for Cancers of the Digestive System*. Publication No. 78-1541. Bethesda, Md.: National Institutes of Health.

Silverman, D. 1982. Reprinted from 1976. *Survival for Cancers of the Respiratory System*. Publication No. 82-1540. Bethesda, Md.: National Institutes of Health.

Ultman, J. E., and Jacobs, R. H. 1985. The Non-Hodgkin's Lymphomas. *Ca-A Cancer Journal for Clinicians*. 35:66–87.

Appendix 18.1
Publications Available from
the National Cancer Institute

The following are available free of charge from Office of Cancer Communications, National Cancer Institute, Building 31–Room 10A18, Bethesda, MD 20205. The most recent versions are described in the *Publications List*, available from the same source.

Breast Cancer: We're Making Progress Every Day. Publication No. 83-2409. Revised September 1983. This pamphlet summarizes current information about breast cancer, including risks and signs of the disease; mammography, biopsy, and treatment options; breast reconstruction; and rehabilitation. Includes illustrated guide for breast self-examination.

Progress Against . . . (series). This series of pamphlets contains information on causes, symptoms, diagnosis, treatment, and research for various cancer sites, e.g., *Cancer of the Larynx* (Publication No. 83-448), *Cancer of the Skin* (84-310), *Cancer of the Mouth* (84-118).

Questions and Answers About Breast Lumps. Publication No. 84-2401. Revised September 1983. This pamphlet describes some of the most common noncancerous breast lumps and what can be done about them. Includes instructions for breast self-examination and a glossary of terms. 14 pages.

Research Reports (series). These in-depth reports cover current research on the cause and prevention, symptoms, detection and diagnosis, and treatment of various types of cancer:

> *Bone Cancers and Other Sarcomas.* Publication No. 84-721. 14 pages.
>
> *Cancer of the Bladder.* Publication No. 83-722. 12 pages.
>
> *Cancer of the Colon and Rectum.* Publication No. 84-95. 11 pages.
>
> *Cancer of the Kidney.* Publication No. 84-2342. 10 pages.
>
> *Cancer of the Lung.* Publication No. 82-526. 13 pages.
>
> *Cancer of the Prostate.* Publication No. 82-528. 14 pages.
>
> *Cancer of the Uterus.* Publication No. 84-171. 14 pages.
>
> *Hodgkin's Disease and the Non-Hodgkin's Lymphomas.* Publication No. 84-172. 15 pages.

> *Leukemia.* Publication No. 84-329. 25 pages.
>
> *Progress in Treatment of Testicular Cancer.* Publication No. 84-654. 14 pages.

What Black Americans Should Know About Cancer. Publication No. 82-2635. Revised April 1982. This pamphlet explains the rates and risks of cancer among blacks and answers the most often asked questions on cancer—its causes, detection, prevention, treatment, rehabilitation, and common misconceptions. Includes instructions for breast self-examination. 28 pages.

Mastectomy: A Treatment for Breast Cancer. Publication No. 84-658. This booklet presents information about the different types of breast surgery, what to expect in the hospital and during the recovery period, and coping with having breast surgery. 24 pages.

Breast Cancer: Understanding Treatment Options. Publication No. 85-2675. This booklet summarizes the biopsy procedure, types of breast surgery (giving advantages and disadvantages for each), radiation therapy as primary treatment, and making treatment decisions. 20 pages.

Radiation Therapy: A Treatment for Early Stage Breast Cancer. Publication No. 84-659. This booklet discusses the treatment steps (lymph node surgery and radiation therapy), possible side effects, precautions to take after treatment, and emotional adjustments to having breast cancer. 20 pages.

What You Need to Know About Cancer . . . (series). This series of pamphlets designed for cancer patients discusses symptoms, diagnosis and rehabilitation, emotional issues, and questions to ask the doctor. Includes glossary of terms and Cancer Information Service telephone numbers. (Publication numbers are listed in parentheses. An asterisk * indicates the publication is also available in Spanish.)

> Cancer (General) (83-1566)
>
> Bladder (84-1559)
>
> Bone (84-1571)
>
> Brain and Spinal Cord (84-1558)
>
> Breast (84-1556)
>
> *Colon and Rectum (84-1552)
>
> *Dysplasia, Very Early Cancer and Invasive Cancer of the Cervix (84-2047)
>
> Esophagus (82-1557)
>
> Hodgkin's Disease (83-1555)
>
> Kidney (83-1569)

Larynx (82-1568)

Adult Leukemia (84-1572)

Childhood Leukemia (84-1573)

*Lung (83-1553)

Melanoma (83-1563)

*Mouth (83-1574)

Multiple Myeloma (83-1575)

Non-Hodgkin's Lymphoma (82-1567)

Ovary (84-1561)

Pancreas (84-1560)

*Prostate (84-1576)

Skin (84-1564)

*Stomach (83-1554)

Testis (83-1565)

*Uterus (83-1562)

Wilms' Tumor (83-1570)

National Cancer Institute Publications for Health Professionals

Incidence of Nonmelanoma Skin Cancer in the United States. Publication No. 83-2433. This booklet provides the data obtained from a special National Cancer Institute survey of nonmelanoma skin cancer in eight geographic locations with varying solar ultraviolet (UV) intensities. 113 pages.

Cancer Patient Survival: Report Number 5. Publication No. 81-992. This paperback book provides survival statistics covering the period 1950 to 1973 for 39 forms of cancer. 315 pages. Certain individual chapters are available as reprints.

Note: Similar publications are also available from other sources. See listing of individual divisions of American Cancer Society and other sources at the end of the next chapter.

19

After Cancer

Cancer has a tremendous emotional impact. Waiting for the pathology report, dealing with the diagnosis, coping with treatment and its side effects and after-effects, living with the fear of recurrence or the spectre of imminent death— all exact an enormous emotional toll on cancer patients and the people around them. In a study of cancer patients at three major cancer centers (see Roberts, 1984) 47 percent of cancer patients were found to be distressed enough by their disease to have recognizable psychiatric disorders. Most of these suffered from transient, severe, reactive depression and anxiety; 13 percent evidenced more severe major depression.

Thus, cancer patients need help that goes well beyond the provision of basic treatment. This chapter suggests some good resources, summarized in Table 19.1 and in the appendices at the end of the chapter.

Sources of Stress and Distress in Cancer Patients

The Diagnosis

Although a lump or other symptom may have already raised some anxiety, hearing the words "You have a cancer" must be indescribably devastating. It is normal not to be able to accept or absorb a diagnosis of cancer at first. Cancer patients report a mixture of bewilderment, disbelief, anger, anxiety, hope, fear, despair, acceptance, and resolve. It takes a while for the conflicting emotions to be sorted and put into perspective. This process can be overwhelming, more than the switchboard of the brain can handle well. After the acute stress and surge of anxiety accompanying the announced diagnosis subside, lower-level chronic stress takes their place.

Cancer patients need emotional support, but they often do not receive it because anxiety, fear, disbelief, and anger can also have a devastating impact on family members. Even physicians, nurses, and clergy members react to cancer in ways that diminish the support they give to cancer patients.

Consider the difficulty of a typical cancer specialist. Several times a day, he or she may have to deliver what are for all practical purposes death notices. He or she may have to continue to give bad news as the disease runs its course. Cancer specialists often must stand by helplessly and watch people die—people in whom they have invested both personal interest and the best they had to offer as professionals. Is it any wonder that physicians and other health professionals sometimes have trouble helping—why they sometimes erect barriers to their emotions? Is it any wonder that some of them cope by remaining detached? Barriers and detachment on the part of health-care professionals can be damaging sources of additional stress on the cancer patients and their families.

Problems Associated with Treatment

We reviewed the side effects of cancer treatment in Chapter 17. Many of the side effects of treatment (see Gralla, 1983)—infections that result from suppressed immunity, nausea and vomiting, and treatment-related nutritional problems—are stressful and must be taken into account in the supportive care of the cancer patient. But even when treatment is completed and has otherwise been successful, it often leaves problems that must continue to be endured.

Treatment for some kinds of cancer causes disfigurement and functional impairment. Some examples of such treatments are: radical head and neck or breast surgery, bowel or bladder surgery that make it necessary to "replumb" the urinary and fecal passages to bring waste materials out of the body through artificial openings (ostomies), and surgery that leads to impaired sexual function. Radical surgery of the oral cavity can leave the patient with problems swallowing or speaking, as well as with disfigurement.

Laryngectomees lose their vocal cords. Removal of the larynx (**laryngectomy**) makes normal speech impossible. A laryngectomee can learn to speak again using esophageal speech—by learning to swallow air and releasing it in a controlled burp; esophageal speech takes considerable patience and practice. Artificial electronic voice devices are also available. These handheld devices produce a monotone vibration when pressed against muscles in the throat and tilted a certain way. Forming words in something close to the usual way causes muscles to modulate the vibration to resemble normal speech. An even more successful restorative method has been developed in which an opening is made to allow air to pass into the throat; this allows guttural but "real" speech.

Some breast cancer patients treated by radical surgery face lymphatic drainage problems in arms from which axillary lymph nodes have been removed; these patients must learn to do without pectoralis muscles. (However, modern breast cancer management seldom involves these defects.) People with ostomies must learn to live with disposable plastic bags affixed outside their body walls. Patients with bone cancers sometimes lose a limb. All these problems can be alleviated by physical restoration, training, and other forms of rehabilitation.

Some forms of reconstructive surgery—breast reconstruction, for example (see National Cancer Institute, 1984)—have been available for some time. New reconstructive surgical techniques are becoming available all the time. These range from using skin from various parts of the body to rebuild portions of the mouth and throat, to using intestinal segments to rebuild parts of the esophagus and throat. A whole science is devoted to the development of biocompatible artificial materials that can be used, for example, to replace the bone in a jaw. Skilled maxillofacial prosthodontists are able to fashion artificial materials into ears and other replacement parts of the head and neck.

Although many improvements in reconstructive surgery and other forms of rehabilita-

Table 19.1   Some Organizations and Programs Offering Services to the Cancer Patient and the Family

	General Description	Psychological and Emotional Support; Education	Medical, Physical, Logistical Support	Financial and Employment Assistance
National organizations and affiliates				
American Cancer Society 777 Third Ave. New York, NY 10017	Voluntary organization offering programs of cancer research, education, and patient service and rehabilitation	Programs to support psychological and physical rehabilitation of patients Patient education and information	Equipment loans for care of homebound, blood programs, surgical dressings, medication Transportation to and from treatment, e.g., volunteer drivers or taxi fare reimbursement	Financial counseling Assistance with employment problems
CanSurmount	Composed of patient, family member, trained volunteer (also a cancer patient), health professional Volunteers visit hospitals and homes.	Patient and family education and information	. . .	. . .
I Can Cope	Addresses the educational and psychological needs of people with cancer	Educational program to provide information and psychological support	. . .	. . .
International Association of Laryngectomees	Voluntary umbrella organization of 225 local clubs (varying names) that promote and support total rehabilitation program Volunteers visit hospitals.	Support and education programs for persons who have had laryngectomees	. . .	Program to inform employees about reemployability of laryngectomees
Reach to Recovery (Breast cancer)	Provides rehabilitation support for women who have had mastectomies Volunteers visit hospitals.	Information on rehabilitative exercises Psychological support	Demonstrate rehabilitative exercises Provide temporary prosthesis	. . .
Cancer Information Service (see Appendix 19-2)	Telephone information and referral service, supplemented by printed materials	Information on local and regional resources and programs	Information on local and regional resources and programs	Information on local and regional resources and programs
The Concern for Dying 250 W. 57th St. New York, NY 10019	Nonprofit educational organization distributes the living will, a document that records patient wishes concerning treatment	Provides copies of living will and referral to local sources of same	. . .	. . .
Leukemia Society of America 211 E. 43rd St. New York, NY 10017	Offers financial assistance and consultation services for referrals to other means of local support to cancer patients with leukemia and allied disorders	. . .	. . .	Financial assistance to outpatients for drugs, laboratory costs associated with blood transfusions, transportation, and radiation therapy

	General Description	Psychological and Emotional Support; Education	Medical, Physical, Logistical Support	Financial and Employment Assistance
Make Today Count P.O. Box 303 Burlington, IA 52601	More than 200 chapters comprising patients and family members, with the general goal of living each day as fully and completely as possible	Peer emotional support	. . .	. . .
The National Hospice Organization 1311A Dolly Madison Blvd. McLean, VA 22101	Membership organization consisting of groups providing or preparing to provide hospice care; institutions concerned with care of the terminally ill and their families	Literature, information, and referral to local and regional resources	Literature, information, and referral to local and regional resources	. . .
United Cancer Council, Inc. 1803 N. Meridian St. Indianapolis, IN 46202	Federation of voluntary cancer agencies that seek the control of cancer through a three-point program of service, education, and research Agencies are funded by the United Way of Giving.	Health promotion and education programs and therapy groups	Screening, nursing, homemaking, medication, prostheses	. . .
United Ostomy Association 1111 Wilshire Blvd. Los Angeles, CA 90017	Nonprofit organization with more than 500 chapters in United States and Canada. General goal is to provide ostomy patients with mutual aid, moral support, and education. Members visit hospitals.	Publish ostomy information Peer support	Encourage development of better equipment and supplies Promote better management techniques	Insurance programs for members include hospital income plan and major medical plan

Regional organizations and programs

	General Description	Psychological and Emotional Support; Education	Medical, Physical, Logistical Support	Financial and Employment Assistance
Cancer Call PAC (People Against Cancer) American Cancer Society 37 S. Wabash Ave. Chicago, IL 60603	Emotional support telephone service; volunteers are recovered cancer patients and family members	Trained volunteers provide emotional support, information, and appropriate referrals	. . .	. . .

Source: Blumberg and Flaherty, 1980, p. 1716. Used by permission of the National Cancer Institute, Bethesda, MD and Barbara D. Blumberg

tion have been made in recent years, all of them still fall short of "good as new."

Sex

A satisfying sexual relationship has an important place in the emotional well-being of most of us. Because of this, sex sometimes poses special emotional problems for cancer patients. Many things about cancer conspire to cause potential problems with sex after diagnosis and treatment (see Donahue and Bennett, 1978). First of all, certain treatments for cancers of the rectum or prostate in men and cancers of the vagina or uterus in women can impair or destroy normal sexual function. Other kinds of problems stem from the basic incompatibility between sex and stress or between sex and anxiety. Disfiguring treatment (see below) and an irrational fear that cancer is contagious have been reported among other contributing factors.

But My Work?

Having a satisfying place in the grand scheme of the world of work also fulfills an important emotional need in most of us. Hospitalization and treatment schedules are inconvenient and, to say the least, cancer can disrupt one's life's work or budding career. The stress associated with the threat of losing part of one's identity and the feeling of helplessness in the face of work to be done can be significant.

Social Problems

Cancer sometimes brings social problems involving the world at large, beyond the family. Among these are financial problems that result from medical costs and the inability to work; problems with employers, some of whom tend not to want to employ cancer patients; and problems with personal associations derived from

"not knowing what to say to," or general discomfort around someone who has had cancer and who may or may not die soon. All these things are added sources of stress for cancer patients.

Self-Image Disfiguring surgery, hair loss, physical impairment, and the like have an impact on body-image or self-image, apart from the exacerbation of problems with sex and social relationships, and this is a source of stress for the cancer patient, too. At least one in five mastectomy patients develop body-image problems, and in half of these, the problem is severe (Maguire, 1985).

Isolation Social stresses often lead to increasing isolation—which is also stressful. Patients with self-image problems can easily become withdrawn. Also, some people stay away from cancer patients because they are uncomfortable around people who are sick or stressed. All of this conspires to deprive patients of the support of friends and family when they need it most.

The Cost of Cancer The costs of cancer care are considerable. Medical bills for cancer patients average just over $20,000 and can go well beyond that. In one study (by Cancer Care, Inc. of the National Cancer Foundation) of 115 families involving advanced cancer, total costs of illness (hospital, doctor, and burial expenses) ranged from $5,000 to more than $50,000, with an average of $21,718 (see National Cancer Institute, 1980c).

Discrimination on the Job Problems with employment are important for many reasons. Beyond the dollars lost (Page and Asire, 1985, estimated the earnings lost due to cancer and benign tumors to be $26.4 billion in 1977) because of the inability to work or the inability to find work, are the problems that arise from work being an important source of self-esteem. Work is a means of directing energy outward, restoring purpose and normalcy. Job discrimination is sometimes a problem even for cancer patients who have been cured, because employers are reluctant to invest training in someone who "may not be around much longer." Discrimination against cancer patients in the work place was made illegal by the Federal Rehabilitation Act of 1973, but this didn't end all problems. The key, as pointed out by Mellette (1985), is to have more employers and potential employers realize that cancer is a spectrum of diseases—that functional impairment in cancer patients ranges from severe disability to no problem at all. Employers and the public at large need to be made aware of this and of the improved prognosis for many kinds of cancer in recent years.

Life and Health Insurance Cancer patients, even those with a high degree of probability of having been cured, generally have a hard time buying life insurance: "Come back and see us in five years and we will reconsider!" Medical insurance is also problematic. Loss of insurability compounds work/career problems because cancer patients have to consider very carefully the possible loss of insurance benefits if they change jobs.

The Fear of Recurrence

Perhaps the number one long-running emotional problem for the patient who has been treated for cancer is the fear of recurrence. Therapists can never be sure they "got it all." Often, the best a cancer patient can hope for is a long period of uncertainty during which every ache or pain is worrisome. Although the likelihood of cure increases with the passage of time following treatment, cancer patients never know when or if they are really free of cancer.

Pain

Cancer-related pain is a problem for 50 to 80 percent of patients with metastatic cancer (Ahles,

1985) (the causes of pain associated with cancer were described in Chapter 12). Approximately one patient in three suffers pain to a degree that it significantly diminishes the quality of life (Cleeland, 1985). Nearly 10,000 cancer deaths this year will be associated with almost unbearable pain. Progress has been made in treating pain, but this problem is by no means solved. Some of the treatments are addicting (heroin and morphine), and the effectiveness of some is short-lived; nearly all have undesirable side effects. Varying degrees of success have been reported using psychological approaches to treatment, but these need more evaluation of their effectiveness and practicality. It appears that cancer-associated pain will continue to be a primary treatment priority for patients in the last stages of their illness.

Affective Disorders

Within the first year and a half after surgery, 20 percent of the women who have a mastectomy develop an anxiety state, depressive illness, or both (Maguire, 1985). Cancers with a poor prognosis such as lung cancer lead to severe depression in a "substantial minority" of patients, but even cancers with a relatively favorable prognosis generate considerable psychological problems (Maguire, 1985). Goldberg and Cullen (1985) note that certain specific cancer sites tend to be associated with psycho-social problems and that for some of these, specific organic cause-and-effect relationships have been proposed. They also note that certain chemotherapeutic agents are now recognized as the cause of psychiatric symptoms in some patients.

Overall, acute stress with depression or anxiety is the most common psychiatric syndrome associated with cancer, and the most important treatment is the development of a trusting relationship with the extended treatment team that includes family and friends, which serves as a source of reassurance, good information about treatment, and acknowledgement of the problem (Massie, 1983). Often, depression and anxiety also require psychiatric intervention, including the use of drugs. A study at the Memorial Sloan-Kettering Cancer Institute found that 24 percent of hospitalized cancer patients required psychiatric help, including antidepressant drugs. In another study of more than 1,500 patients, 51 percent were given at least one psychotropic drug (Massie, 1983).

The Importance of a Positive Outlook?

Some suggest or imply that a positive mental attitude about one's cancer actually influences outcome (see Simonton, Matthews-Simonton, and Creighton, 1978). Indeed, there is even some evidence for a positive correlation between positive outlook and the length of survival. But correlation (even if it does hold up), is a far cry from proof of cause-and-effect. It could legitimately be argued that if indeed there is a correlation between attitude and outcome, it may be the result of more-or-less fixed prospects for survival being somehow perceived by cancer patients and this having an influence on mental attitude. There is some evidence that social or psychological factors individually or in combinations do not influence survival or the course of malignant disease (Cassileth et al., 1985). In 1985, the American Cancer Society approved the following statement on the "Effect of Emotions on Cancer:"

> The American Cancer Society recognizes that a positive mental attitude, psychosocial techniques and support are important for improving the quality of life for cancer patients. At the present time available evidence does not support the theory that the use of techniques for reducing stress can change the risk of developing cancer or the duration of survival in humans. The Society recognizes the need for continuing research in this area. However, the use of psychosocial interventions which claim to alter tumor growth or spread cannot be recommended at this time. (quoted by Monaco, 1986; p. 2)

Imaging of Another Kind

There are those who claim that if a cancer patient pictures the cells of his or her immune system attacking and killing cancer cells, this can have a positive effect on cures and/or survival. Although such *imaging* may have some value in helping patients feel better and less helpless, its effects on cancer's outcome are totally conjectural; there has been no research to support this idea.

Death and Dying

The study of death and dying is called *thanatology*. The need for this discipline stems from the fact that few if any of us are able to see death as an inevitable part of life and living. Problems in dealing with death and dying—for both those doing the dying and those having to experience the loss of a loved one—stem from the shock of having to surrender the false sense of physical immortality that seems to be built into all of us. The deaths of those around us chip away at the illusion, but usually not until death gets very close does the reality—that separation from this life is an inevitable part of living—really sink in. It doesn't sink in easily.

Those who study death and dying say that there is a pattern. First there is *denial:* "It can't be happening to me." Denial melts away gradually, perhaps as part of a mechanism that lets reality sink in slowly. Denial helps us deal with "it" by allowing us not to have to deal with "it"—for a while. *Anger* often follows denial. Anger is a substitute emotion for anxiety and despair. It lets us accept our ultimate fate with another cushion. Some people die angry; others graduate from anger and move through phases of *depression*, then *acceptance* (see Kubler-Ross, 1974; Feifel, 1977; Miller et al., 1979). For some people, religious conviction serves as a cushion that makes the transition to acceptance less difficult.

Hospice

It's hard to die. It's also hard to be around when someone close is dying. It is little comfort to know that death is part of the natural order: that dying has been going on forever, that we will all die eventually. Even a belief in a better afterlife doesn't seem to blunt the impact very much. Each death is a new, traumatic experience. For the most part, our health-care systems and our approach to death as humans are based on the idea that it isn't over till it's over: that a miracle may turn things around; that measures with curative intent, however heroic, should be used until the end. A concept called **hospice** is based on the idea that when death is inevitable, the patient and the patient's family need help making the last days as comfortable as possible.

The term *hospice*, as it applies to cancer, came from Britain, where it refers to institutions designed to relieve both the emotional and physical suffering of the terminally ill. Although St. Christopher's Hospice in London is the prototype, hospice programs today come in various forms, all having in common the following (see Markel and Sinon, 1978; Consumer Reports, 1986):

Coordinated in-patient and out-patient services for the terminally ill and their families

Physician-directed narcotic and nonnarcotic pain control

Interdisciplinary psychological, medical, spiritual, and sociological services involving physicians, nurses, psychologists, pastors, occupational therapists, physical therapists, and social workers

Twenty-four–hour, seven-days-a-week service extending through the bereavement period

Hospice organizations have sprung up all over the United States and Europe. They are typically run by religious groups, community groups, or hospitals. The help provided by these organizations is usually provided in the patient's own home. Of the 1,700 hospice organizations in the United States, about 800 are sponsored by hospitals, 300 are associated with home health-care agencies, and the remainder are independent (Consumer Reports, 1986). The most common mode of operation of hospices is to help the family; they typically do not take over the care of the dying. Although home nursing care is available through hospices around the clock, for example, it more often involves periodic nursing visits and/or nurses and other health professionals available for emergencies.

Medicare has provided some hospice benefits since 1983, although this provision was up for reconsideration as this was being written. Some private insurance companies also provide some benefits. The names of hospice organizations and more information about hospices can be obtained from the following sources:

The National Hospice Organization (Suite 902, 1901 North Fort Myer Drive, Arlington, Va. 22209)

The National Cancer Institute (call 800-4-CANCER)

Cancer Centers (see Appendix 19.1)

The American Cancer Society (see Appendix 19.3)

Physicians, local hospitals, and churches can also supply names of hospices.

A Summary

There are many sources of stress and distress that besiege cancer patients. The stresses include the side effects and after effects of treatment, the high cost of care, job discrimination, social stigmas, and the fear of recurrence. Most of the time, cancer patients somehow cope with these stresses, and emotional support is a big factor in enabling them to do so. Sometimes the stresses lead to significant psychiatric disorders that require psychiatric intervention. Psychosocial problems related to cancer are an important part of the overall problem of cancer; they deserve as much attention as the search for improved methods of detection and treatment.

A Resource Guide

The first and foremost resource available to a cancer patient is a knowledgeable physician. Patients rarely use this resource to any great extent, which poses a problem for patients and thus for the medical profession. Patients tend to be intimidated by physicians and the ambience of medicine in general. They fail to ask important questions, and unasked/unanswered questions mean unnecessarily unrelieved anxiety.

Cancer is too important for a patient to rely on a single physician. Medicine is too vast and complex a field for any individual to keep up with even a fraction of the entire field. Ideally, a patient should be seen by a cancer expert. This is the age of specialization precisely because specialists give better results. Specialists armed with the latest knowledge, the most up-to-date equipment, and the most complete array of support services are most likely to be found in a Comprehensive Cancer Center (see Appendix 19.1). In addition, the American College of Surgeons reviews and approves the cancer treatment and patient support programs of hundreds of hospitals and medical centers throughout the United States. An up-to-date listing of approved programs can be obtained from the American College of Surgeons, 55 East Erie Street, Chicago, IL 60611.

Although it is best to treat cancer as soon after the diagnosis is confirmed as possible, it is far more important to be sure that the diagnosis is correct and that the treatment is appropriate. Almost always, it is best to get a second opinion. A confirming diagnosis and a recommendation regarding treatment should come from a physician certified in the subspecialty of oncology or otherwise recognized (by other physicians) as an expert.

Organizational Resources

Cancer is too big a burden to bear alone or even as a member of a small group. Cancer patients need their families for support, and together with their families they can benefit greatly from the help available from numerous well-established, creditable organizations and groups. Some of the largest organizations are described below and in Table 19.1 (see also Moen, Roover, and Stonberg, 1978; American Cancer Society, 1980; Blumberg and Flaherty, 1980; National Cancer Institute, 1980b, 1980c).

The National Institutes of Health (NIH) The National Institutes of Health is a division of the Public Health Service, which is part of the U. S. Department of Health and Human Services. It is the principal, though certainly not the only, research arm of the U. S. government. The purpose of the NIH is "to improve the health of the Nation by increasing our understanding of the processes underlying human health and by acquiring new knowledge to help prevent, detect, diagnose, and treat disease." (National Institutes of Health, 1980). The NIH provides money (90 percent of its total budget) for research support in universities, hospitals, and research centers throughout the United States and abroad. The NIH also has its own clinics and research laboratories in Bethesda, Maryland, where some 14,000 physicians, dentists, veterinarians, research scientists, and support personnel engage in some 2,600 research projects at any one time (National Institutes of Health, 1980). All together, the NIH supports more than 40 percent of the more than $6 billion annual national investment in health research. The NIH encompasses 11 individual research institutes, each with its own clinical and laboratory research programs. One of these is the National Cancer Institute.

The National Cancer Institute (NCI) The National Cancer Institute is the division of the NIH that focuses on cancer. The NCI supports cancer research directly throughout the world and has its own programs of clinical cancer research and laboratory research in Bethesda and Frederick, Maryland. The NCI's Office of Cancer Communications provides a wide range of information services to the public and to health-care professionals. For a list of available materials write or call:

The Cancer Information Clearinghouse
Office of Cancer Communications
National Cancer Institute
7910 Woodmont Avenue
Suite 1320
Bethesda, MD 20014
(301) 496-4070

One of the services of the Office of Cancer Communications is the Cancer Information Service, a national system of toll-free telephone numbers through which trained lay and professional volunteers are available to answer questions about cancer. A list of **Cancer Information Service** offices and their telephone numbers is given in Appendix 19.2 at the end of the chapter. A national hot-line number, 1(800)638-6694, is answered every day from 8 A.M. to midnight.

The American Cancer Society The American Cancer Society (ACS) is one of the oldest and largest voluntary health organizations in the United States. Founded for the purpose of educating the public and the medical profession about cancer, the ACS raises well over $100 million each year to support cancer research, train cancer specialists, and educate the public and members of various health professions.

The ACS headquarters is in New York City, with separate divisions (see Appendix 19.3) in each of the 50 states and in Puerto Rico. Most of the 58 divisions are state divisions, which in turn are organized into "units" (roughly 3,100) organized by county. Every year, more than 2 million ACS volunteers are mobilized for a fund-raising campaign. Of the contributions not otherwise restricted, 60 percent remains in the division where the money was raised and goes to support local cancer control programs; 25 percent goes to the ACS's national research program.

The remainder goes to the national headquarters to support programs for training, cancer control, and professional and public education throughout the country. Locally, the ACS's Information and Guidance Service provides information and direct help to cancer patients all across the spectrum of emotional, economic, and physical problems that cancer brings. A loan and gift service provides dressings, sickroom supplies and equipment, and other items needed by cancer patients. The ACS also provides a transportation service for patients in need of such. The ACS offers rehabilitation programs for patients who have had laryngectomies, mastectomies, and ostomies. For more information about the ACS, see Table 19.1 (also American Cancer Society, 1980); write to the division headquarters listed in Appendix 19.3.

References and Further Reading

Ahles, T. A. 1985. Psychological Approaches to the Management of Cancer-Related Pain. *Semin. Oncol. Nurs.* 1:141–46.

American Cancer Society. 1974. *The Psychological Impact of Cancer.* A series of articles originally appearing in *Cancer.* New York: American Cancer Society.

American Cancer Society. 1980. *The American Cancer Society: A Factbook for the Medical and Related Professions.* New York: American Cancer Society.

American Cancer Society. 1982. *Professional Education Materials Catalog.* New York: American Cancer Society. Describes publications, films, fliers, and audiotapes on all aspects of cancer (including rehabilitation and emotional impacts) available to physicians and nurses—too many to list here. (126 pages)

Anonymous. 1982. *Sourcebook on Death and Dying.* Chicago: Marquis Who's Who.

Baltrusch, H. J., and Waltz, M. 1985. Cancer from a Biobehavioural and Social Epidemiological Perspective. *Soc. Sci. Med.* 20:789–94.

Blues, A., and Zerwekh, J. 1984. *Hospice and Palliative Nursing Care.* Orlando, Fla.: Grune & Stratton (Harcourt Brace Jovanovich).

Blumberg, B., and Flaherty, M. 1980. Services Available to Persons with Cancer. *JAMA.* 244(15):1715–17.

Cassileth, B., ed. 1979. *The Cancer Patient: Social and Medical Aspects of Care.* Philadelphia, Pa.: Lea & Febiger.

Cassileth, B., and Cassileth, P., eds. 1982. *Clinical Care of the Terminal Cancer Patient.* Philadelphia, Pa.: Lea & Febiger.

Cassileth, B. R., et al. 1985. Psychosocial Correlates of Survival in Advanced Malignant Disease? *N. Eng. J. Med.* 312:1551–55.

Cleeland, C. S. 1985. Measurement and Prevalence of Pain in Cancer. *Semin. Oncol. Nurs.* 1:87–92.

Consumer Reports. 1986. Hospices: Not to Cure but to Help. January:24–26.

Costello, A. 1979. Supporting the Patient with Problems Related to Body Image. In L. Kruse, J. Reese, and L. Hart, eds., *Cancer: Pathophysiology, Etiology, and Management.* St. Louis: Mosby.

Craven, J., and Wald, F. 1979. Hospice Care for Dying Patients. In L. Kruse, J. Reese, and L. Hart, eds., *Cancer: Pathophysiology, Etiology, and Management.* St. Louis: Mosby.

Donahue, V., and Bennett, A. 1978. Sexual Dysfunction in Cancer. In *Cancer: A Manual for Practitioners.* 5th ed. Boston. American Cancer Society, Massachusetts Division.

Feifel, H. 1977. *New Meaning of Death.* New York: McGraw-Hill.

Gates, C. 1978. *Psychological Issues in Cancer.* In *Cancer: A Manual for Practitioners.* 5th ed. Boston: American Cancer Society, Massachusetts Division.

Giacquinta, B. 1979. Helping Families Face the Crisis of Cancer. In L. Kruse, J. Reese, and L. Hart, eds., *Cancer: Pathophysiology, Etiology, and Management.* St. Louis: Mosby.

Goldberg, R. J., and Cullen, L. O. 1985. Factors Important to Psychosocial Adjustment to Cancer: A Review of the Evidence. *Soc. Sci. Med.* 20:803–7.

Gralla, R. J. 1983. *Supportive Care of the Cancer Patient.* New York: Biomedical Information Corporation.

Harker, B. 1979. Cancer and Communication Problems: A Personal Experience. In L. Kruse, J. Reese, and L. Hart, eds., *Cancer: Pathophysiology, Etiology, and Management.* St. Louis: Mosby.

Hill, G. S. 1984. *Management of Pain in the Cancer Patient (Selected Abstracts).* International Cancer Research Data Bank. Bethesda Md.: National Cancer Institute.

Holland, J. (Interview.) 1980. Understanding the Cancer Patient. *Ca-A Cancer Journal for Clinicians.* 30(2): 103–12.

Institute of Medicine, National Research Council, Committee on the Health Consequences of the Stress of Bereavement. 1984. *Bereavement: Reactions, Consequences, and Care.* Washington, D.C.: National Academy Press.

Kahn, S., et al., eds. 1983. *Concepts in Cancer Medicine.* New York: Grune & Stratton.

Kassakian, M., et al. 1979. A Revival of an Old Custom: Home Care of the Dying. In L. Kruse, J. Reese, and L. Hart, eds., *Cancer, Pathophysiology, Etiology, and Management.* St. Louis: Mosby.

Kruse, L., Reese, J., and Hart, L., eds. 1979. *Cancer: Pathophysiology, Etiology, and Management.* St. Louis: Mosby.

Kubler-Ross, E. 1969. *On Death and Dying.* New York: Macmillan.

Kubler-Ross, E. 1974. *Questions and Answers on Death and Dying.* New York: Macmillan.

Kutscher, A. H., et al., eds. 1983. *Hospice, U.S.A.* New York: Columbia University Press.

Maguire, P. 1985. The Psychological Impact of Cancer. *Br. J. Hospital Med.* 34:100–3.

Markel, W., and Sinon, V. 1978. The Hospice Concept. *Ca-A Cancer Journal for Clinicians.* 28(45):225–37.

Massie, M. J. 1983. Psychopharmacologic Management of Psychiatric Syndromes in Cancer Patients. In R. J. Gralla, *Supportive Care of the Cancer Patient.* New York: Biomedical Information Corporation.

McCorkle, R. 1979. The Advanced Cancer Patient: How He Will Live—and Die. In L. Kruse, J. Reese, and L. Hart, eds., *Cancer: Physiopathology, Etiology, and Management.* St. Louis: Mosby.

Mellette, S. J. 1985. The Cancer Patient at Work. *Ca: A Cancer Journal for Clinicians.* 35:360–73.

Miller, C. L., Denner, P. R., and Richardson, V. E. 1979. Assisting the Psychological Problems of Cancer Patients: A Review of Current Research. In L. Kruse, J. Reese, and L. Hart, eds., *Cancer: Physiopathology, Etiology, and Management.* St. Louis: Mosby.

Moen, J., Roover, J., and Stonberg, M. 1978. Resources and Rehabilitation. In *Cancer: A Manual for Practitioners*. 5th ed. Boston: American Cancer Society, Massachusetts Division.

Monaco, G. P. 1986. Psychosomatic Oncology Problems. *Oncology Times*. April, p. 2.

Mora, M., and Potts, E., 1980. *Choices: Realistic Alternatives in Cancer Treatment*. New York: Avon Books.

Morris, T., Buckley, M., and Blake, S. M. 1985. Defining Psychological Responses to a Diagnosis of Cancer. In M. Watson and T. Morris, eds., *Psychological Aspects of Cancer*. New York: Pergamon Press.

National Cancer Institute. 1984. *Advanced Cancer: Living Each Day*. Bethesda, Md.

National Cancer Institute, Office of Cancer Communications, Bethesda, Md. (Publication numbers in parentheses follow titles.)

1980a. *The Breast Cancer Digest*. (80-1691)

1980b. *Coping with Cancer*. An annotated bibliography of public, patient, and professional information and education materials. (80-2129)

1980c. *Coping with Cancer*. A resource for the health professional. (80-2080)

1981. *Patient and Professional Education Materials for Ostomates*. Selected annotations. (81-1512)

1982a. *If You've Had Breast Cancer*. (82-2400)

1982b. *Taking Time*. Support for people with cancer and the people who care about them. (82-2059)

1984. *Breast Reconstruction: A Matter of Choice*. (84-2151)

National Cancer Institute. The following are available free of charge from Office of Cancer Communication, National Cancer Institute, Building 31, Room 10A18, Bethesda, MD 20205. The most recent versions will be described in the "Publication List" available from the same source. (Publication numbers in parentheses follow titles.)

Breast Biopsy: What You Should Know. (84-657)

After Breast Cancer: A Guide to Followup Care. (84-2400)

Breast Reconstruction: A Matter of Choice. (84-2151)

Services Available to Persons with Cancer. Reprint from *JAMA*. 244: (Oct. 10, 1980) 1715.

Taking Time: Support for People with Cancer and the People Who Care About Them. (83-2059)

When Cancer Recurs: Meeting the Challenge Again. (85-2709)

The Breast Cancer Digest: A Guide to Medical Care, Emotional Support, Educational Programs and Resources. 2nd ed., revised April 1984. (84-1691)

Coping with Cancer—A Resource for the Health Professional. (82-2080)

Students with Cancer: A Resource for the Educator. (84-2086)

Decade of Discovery: Advances in Cancer Research 1971–1981. (81-2323)

National Cancer Institute Fact Book. (Updated yearly)

National Institutes of Health. 1980. *The National Institutes of Health*. NIH Publication No. 80-1. Washington, D.C.: NIH.

Page, H. S., and Asire, A. J. 1985. *Cancer Rates and Risks*. 3rd ed. NIH Publication No. 85-691. Bethesda, Md.: National Institutes of Health.

Pearse, M. 1979. The Child with Cancer: Impact on the Family. In L. Kruse, J. Reese, and L. Hart, eds., *Cancer: Physiopathology, Etiology, and Management*. St. Louis: Mosby.

Pettingale, K. W. 1985. A Review of Psychobiological Interactions in Cancer Patients. In M. Watson and T. Morris, eds. *Psychological Aspects of Cancer*. New York: Pergamon Press.

Ray, C., and Baum, M. 1985. *Psychological Aspects of Early Breast Cancer*. New York: Springer-Verlag.

Reeves, R. 1979. What Do We Mean By Hope? In L. Kruse, J. Reese, and L. Hart, eds., *Cancer: Physiopathology, Etiology, and Management*. St. Louis: Mosby.

Renneker, M., and Leib, S. 1979. *Understanding Cancer*. Palo Alto, Calif.: Bull.

Richards, V. 1978. *Cancer: The Wayward Cell*. 2nd ed. Berkeley: University of California Press.

Roberts, L. 1984. *Cancer Today*. Washington, D.C.: National Academy Press.

Scotto, J., and Chiazze, L. 1977. Cancer Prevalence and Hospital Payments. *Journal of the National Cancer Institute*. 59(2):345–49.

Sherman, C. 1983. Coping with Cancer. In S. Kahn et al., eds., *Concepts in Cancer Medicine*. New York: Grune & Stratton.

Simonton, O. C., Matthews-Simonton, S., and Creighton, J. L. 1978. *Getting Well Again*. New York: Bantam Books.

Stoll, B. A. 1985. Psychoendocrine Pathways and Cancer Prognosis. In M. Watson and T. Morris, eds., *Psychological Aspects of Cancer*. New York: Pergamon Press.

Watson, M., and Morris, T., eds. 1985. *Psychological Aspects of Cancer*. New York: Pergamon Press.

Appendix 19.1
Comprehensive Cancer Centers

The institutions listed have been identified as Comprehensive Cancer Centers by the National Cancer Institute.

Alabama
University of Alabama in Birmingham Comprehensive Cancer Center
Lurleen Wallace Tumor Institute
1824 6th Avenue South
Birmingham, Alabama 35294
Phone: (205) 934-5077

California
University of Southern California Comprehensive Cancer Center
1441 Eastlake Avenue
Los Angeles, California 90033-0804
Phone: (213) 224-6416

UCLA-Jonsson Comprehensive Cancer Center
Louis Factor Health Sciences Bldg.
10833 LeConte Avenue
Los Angeles, California 90024
Phone: (213) 825-5268

Connecticut
Yale Comprehensive Cancer Center
Yale University School of Medicine
333 Cedar Street
New Haven, Connecticut 06510
Phone: (203) 785-4095

District of Columbia
Georgetown University/Howard University Comprehensive Cancer Center
—Vincent T. Lombardi Cancer Research Center
 Georgetown University Medical Center
 3800 Reservoir Road, N.W.
 Washington, D.C. 20007
 Phone: (202) 625-7721
—Howard University Cancer Research Center
 College of Medicine

Department of Oncology
2041 Georgia Avenue, N.W.
Washington, D.C. 20060
Phone: (202) 636-7697

Florida
Comprehensive Cancer Center for the State of Florida
University of Miami School of Medicine
1475 N.W. 12th Avenue
Miami, Florida 33101
Phone: (305) 545-7707

Illinois
Illinois Cancer Council
36 South Wabash Avenue, Suite 700
Chicago, Illinois 60603
Phone: (312) 346-9813
—Northwestern University Cancer Center
 303 East Chicago Avenue
 Chicago, Illinois 60611
 Phone: (312) 266-5250
—University of Chicago Cancer Research Center
 950 East 59th Street
 Chicago, Illinois 60637
 Phone: (312) 962-6180
—University of Illinois
 Department of Surgery (Oncology)
 840 South Wood Street
 Chicago, Illinois 60612
 Phone: (312) 996-6666
—Rush Cancer Center
 Suite 820
 1725 West Harrison Street
 Chicago, Illinois 60612
 Phone: (312) 942-6028

Maryland
Johns Hopkins Oncology Center
600 North Wolfe Street
Baltimore, Maryland 21205
Phone: (301) 955-8822

Massachusetts
Dana-Farber Cancer Institute
44 Binney Street
Boston, Massachusetts 02115
Phone: (617) 732-3555

Michigan
Michigan Cancer Foundation
Meyer L. Prentis Cancer Center
110 East Warren Avenue
Detroit, Michigan 48201
Phone: (313) 833-0710

Minnesota
Mayo Clinic
200 First Street, S.W.
Rochester, Minnesota 55905
Phone: (507) 284-8964

New York
Columbia University Cancer Research Center
701 West 168th Street, Rm. 1208
New York, New York 10032
Phone: (212) 694-3647

Memorial Sloan-Kettering Cancer Center
1275 York Avenue
New York, New York 10021
Phone: (212) 794-6561

Roswell Park Memorial Institute
666 Elm Street
Buffalo, New York 14263
Phone: (716) 845-5770

North Carolina
Duke Comprehensive Cancer Center
P.O. Box 3814
Duke University Medical Center
Durham, North Carolina 27710
Phone: (919) 684-2282

Ohio
Ohio State University Comprehensive Cancer Center
Suite 302
410 West 12th Avenue
Columbus, Ohio 43210
Phone: (614) 422-5022

Pennsylvania
Fox Chase/University of Pennsylvania Cancer Center
—The Fox Chase Cancer Center
    7701 Burholme Avenue
    Philadelphia, Pennsylvania 19111
    Phone: (215) 728-2781
—University of Pennsylvania Cancer Center
    3400 Spruce Street
    7th Floor, Silverstein Pavilion
    Philadelphia, Pennsylvania 19104
    Phone: (215) 662-3910

Texas
The University of Texas System Cancer Center
M.D. Anderson Hospital and Tumor Institute
6723 Bertner Avenue
Houston, Texas 77030
Phone: (713) 792-6000

Washington
Fred Hutchinson Cancer Research Center
1124 Columbia Street
Seattle, Washington 98104
Phone: (206) 292-2930 or 292-7545

Wisconsin
Wisconsin Clinical Cancer Center
University of Wisconsin
Department of Human Oncology
600 Highland Avenue
Madison, Wisconsin 53792
Phone: (608) 263-8610

Source: Courtesy American Cancer Society.

Appendix 19.2
Telephone Information Services

The Cancer Information Service (CIS) is a toll-free telephone inquiry system that supplies information about cancer and cancer-related resources to the general public, cancer patients and their families, and health professionals. CIS is administered by the National Cancer Institute, and most CIS offices are associated with Comprehensive Cancer Centers.

A list of CIS offices by state with regional toll-free numbers follows:

Alabama   1-800-292-6201
Alaska   1-800-638-6070
California from (213, 714, and 805)
    1-800-252-9066
Colorado   1-800-332-1850
Connecticut   1-800-922-0824
Delaware   1-800-523-3586
District of Columbia (Includes suburban
    Maryland and northern Virginia)
    (202) 636-5700
Florida   1-800-432-5953
Georgia   1-800-327-7332
Hawaii Oahu   524-1234 (Neighboring islands,
    ask operator for Enterprise 6702)
Illinois   800-972-0586
Kentucky   800-432-9321
Maine   1-800-225-7034

Maryland   800-492-1444
Massachusetts   1-800-952-7420
Minnesota   1-800-582-5262
Montana   1-800-525-0231
New Hampshire   1-800-225-7034
New Jersey (Northern)   800-223-1000
New Jersey (Southern)   800-523-3586
New Mexico   1-800-525-0231
New York City   (212) 794-7982
New York State   1-800-462-7255
North Carolina   1-800-672-0943
North Dakota   1-800-328-5188

Ohio   1-800-282-6522
Pennsylvania   1-800-822-3963
South Dakota   1-800-328-5188
Texas   1-800-392-2040
Vermont   1-800-225-7034
Washington   1-800-552-7212
Wisconsin   1-800-362-8038
Wyoming   1-800-525-0231
ALL OTHER AREAS   800-638-6694

Source: Courtesy American Cancer Society.

Appendix 19.3
Chartered Divisions of the American
Cancer Society, Inc.

NATIONAL HEADQUARTERS
American Cancer Society, Inc.
90 Park Avenue
New York, NY 10016

Alabama Division, Inc.
402 Office Park Drive
Suite 300
Birmingham, Alabama 35223
(205) 879-2242

Alaska Division, Inc.
1343 G Street
Anchorage, Alaska 99501
(907) 277-8696

Arizona Division, Inc.
634 West Indian School Road
P.O. Box 33187
Phoenix, Arizona 85067
(602) 234-3266

Arkansas Division, Inc.
5520 West Markham Street
P.O. Box 3822
Little Rock, Arkansas 72203
(501) 664-3480-1-2

California Division, Inc.
1710 Webster Street
P.O. Box 2061
Oakland, California 94604
(415) 893-7900

Colorado Division, Inc.
2255 South Oneida
P.O. Box 24669
Denver, Colorado 80224
(303) 758-2030

Connecticut Division, Inc.
Barnes Park South
14 Village Lane
P.O. Box 410
Wallingford, Connecticut 06492
(203) 265-7161

Delaware Division, Inc.
1708 Lovering Avenue
Suite 202
Wilmington, Delaware 19806
(302) 654-6267

District of Columbia Division, Inc.
Universal Building, South
1825 Connecticut Avenue, N.W.
Washington, D.C. 20009
(202) 483-2600

Florida Division, Inc.
1001 South MacDill Avenue
Tampa, Florida 33609
(813) 253-0541

Georgia Division, Inc.
1422 W. Peachtree Street, N.W.
Atlanta, Georgia 30309
(404) 892-0026

Hawaii Pacific Division, Inc.
Community Services Center Bldg.
200 North Vineyard Boulevard
Honolulu, Hawaii 96817
(808) 531-1662-3-4-5

Idaho Division, Inc.
1609 Abbs Street
P.O. Box 5386
Boise, Idaho 83705
(208) 343-4609

Illinois Division, Inc.
37 South Wabash Avenue
Chicago, Illinois 60603
(312) 372-0472

Indiana Division, Inc.
9575 N. Valparaiso
Indianapolis, Indiana 46268
(317) 872-4432

Iowa Division, Inc.
Highway #18 West
P.O. Box 980
Mason City, Iowa 50401
(515) 423-0712

Kansas Division, Inc.
3003 Van Buren Street
Topeka, Kansas 66611
(913) 267-0131

Kentucky Division, Inc.
Medical Arts Bldg.
1169 Eastern Parkway
Louisville, Kentucky 40217
(502) 459-1867

Louisiana Division, Inc.
Masonic Temple Bldg., 7th Floor
333 St. Charles Avenue
New Orleans, Louisiana 70130
(504) 523-2029

Maine Division, Inc.
Federal and Green Streets
Brunswick, Maine 04011
(207) 729-3339

Maryland Division, Inc.
1840 York Rd., Suite K–M
P. O. Box 544
Timonium, Maryland 21093
(301) 561-4790

Massachusetts Division, Inc.
247 Commonwealth Avenue
Boston, Massachusetts 02116
(617) 267-2650

Michigan Division, Inc.
1205 East Saginaw Street
Lansing, Michigan 48906
(517) 371-2920

Minnesota Division, Inc.
3316 West 66th Street
Minneapolis, Minnesota 55435
(612) 925-2772

Mississippi Division, Inc.
345 North Mart Plaza
Jackson, Mississippi 39206
(601) 362-8874

Missouri Division, Inc.
3322 American Avenue
P. O. Box 1066
Jefferson City, Missouri 65102
(314) 893-4800

Montana Division, Inc.
2820 First Avenue South
Billings, Montana 59101
(406) 252-7111

Nebraska Division, Inc.
8502 West Center Road
Omaha, Nebraska 68124
(402) 393-5800

Nevada Division, Inc.
1325 East Harmon
Las Vegas, Nevada 89109
(702) 798-6877

New Hampshire Division, Inc.
686 Mast Road
Manchester, New Hampshire 03102
(603) 669-3270

New Jersey Division, Inc.
CN2201, 2600 Route 1
North Brunswick, New Jersey 08902
(201) 297-8000

New Mexico Division, Inc.
5800 Lomas Blvd., N.E.
Albuquerque, New Mexico 87110
(505) 262-2336

New York State Division, Inc.
6725 Lyons Street, P. O. Box 7
East Syracuse, New York 13057
(315) 437-7025
—*Long Island Division, Inc.*
  535 Broad Hollow Road
  (Route 110)
  Melville, New York 11747
  (516) 420-1111
—*New York City Division, Inc.*
  19 West 56th Street
  New York, New York 10019
  (212) 586-8700
—*Queens Division, Inc.*
  112-25 Queens Boulevard
  Forest Hills, New York 11375
  (212) 263-2224
—*Westchester Division, Inc.*
  901 North Broadway
  White Plains, New York 10603
  (914) 949-4800

North Carolina Division, Inc.
11 South Boylan Avenue
Suite 221
Raleigh, North Carolina 27603
(919) 834-8463

North Dakota Division, Inc.
Hotel Graver Annex Bldg.
115 Roberts Street
P.O. Box 426
Fargo, North Dakota 58102
(701) 232-1385

Ohio Division, Inc.
1375 Euclid Avenue
Suite 312
Cleveland, Ohio 44115
(216) 771-6700

Oklahoma Division, Inc.
3800 North Cromwell
Oklahoma City, Oklahoma 73112
(405) 946-5000

Oregon Division, Inc.
0330 S.W. Curry
Portland, Oregon 97201
(503) 295-6422

Pennsylvania Division, Inc.
Route 422 & Sipe Avenue
P.O. Box 416
Hershey, Pennsylvania 17033
(717) 533-6144

—*Philadelphia Division, Inc.*
  1422 Chestnut Street
  Philadelphia, Pennsylvania 19102
  (215) 665-2900

Puerto Rico Division, Inc.
(Avenue Domenech 273
Hato Rey, P.R.)
GPO Box 6004
San Juan, Puerto Rico 00936
(809) 764-2295

Rhode Island Division, Inc.
345 Blackstone Blvd.
Providence, Rhode Island 02906
(401) 831-6970

South Carolina Division, Inc.
2442 Devine Street
Columbia, South Carolina 29205
(803) 256-0245

South Dakota Division, Inc.
1025 North Minnesota Avenue
Hillcrest Plaza
Sioux Falls, South Dakota 57104
(605) 336-0897

Tennessee Division, Inc.
713 Melpark Drive
Nashville, Tennessee 37204
(615) 383-1710

Texas Division, Inc.
3834 Spicewood Springs Road
P.O. Box 9863
Austin, Texas 78766
(512) 345-4560

Utah Division, Inc.
610 East South Temple
Salt Lake City, Utah 84102
(801) 322-0431

Vermont Division, Inc.
13 Loomis Street, Drawer C
Montpelier, Vermont 05602
(802) 223-2348

Virginia Division, Inc.
4240 Park Place Court
P.O. Box 1547
Glen Allen, Virginia 23060
(804) 270-0142

Washington Division, Inc.
2120 First Avenue North
Seattle, Washington 98109
(206) 283-1152

West Virginia Division, Inc.
Suite 100
240 Capitol Street
Charleston, West Virginia 25301
(304) 344-3611

Wisconsin Division, Inc.
615 North Sherman Avenue
P.O. Box 8370
Madison, Wisconsin 53708
(608) 249-0487
—*Milwaukee Division, Inc.*
  11401 West Watertown Plank Road
  Wauwatosa, Wisconsin 53226
  (414) 453-4500

Wyoming Division, Inc.
Indian Hills Center
506 Shoshoni
Cheyenne, Wyoming 82009
(307) 638-3331

Source: Courtesy American Cancer Society.

boldface indicates page on which a definition can be found
i indicates an illustration

Index

boldface indicates page on which a definition can be found
i indicates an illustration

boldface indicates page on which a definition can be found
i indicates an illustration

boldface indicates page on which a definition can be found
i indicates an illustration

promoter (carcinogenesis), **123**, 131, 132–134
  in human cancer, 134*i*
  mechanism of action, 133–134
promoter gene, 35
promotion (see promoter)
prophase (of mitosis), **36**
prospective epidemiological study, 221*i*
prostaglandins, **289**
prostatic acid phosphatase, **288**
prostatic cancer, 7*i*, 8*i*, 328–329
proteases, and the cancer cell surface, **60**
protein kinase, **116**
protein kinase C, 239
proteins, **18***i*
proto-oncogenes, 106*i*, **107**, **109**–120, 182–183
  activation of, 112–115
pyrogen, **211**

Q

quackery/unproven methods (treatment), 317–318

R

radiation (see ionizing radiation)
radiation sensitizers, 303
radiation therapy, 300–305
  side effects/complications, 305
radioactive decay, 148*i*
radioactive isotope (see radioisotope)
radioactive nuclide (see radionuclide)
radioactive waste, 154–155
radioimmunoassay, **289**–290
radioisotope, **146**
radionuclide, **146**
  bone-seeking, 150*i*
radium, **146**
rad (radiation absorbed dose), **146**, 151*i*
Ramazzini, Bernardino, 124
Reach to Recovery, 346*i*
recessive genes, **185**
rectal cancer, 7*i*, 8*i*, 325–327
registeries, cancer, 232
regulator gene, 34*i*
relative biological effectiveness (RBE), **147**

relative risk, **221**
rem (rad-equivalent mammal), **147**
repressible enzyme systems, 35
repressor (of gene transcription), 34*i*, 35
reproductive system, 329, 331
respiration, cellular, 26–28
respiratory system, 325*i*
retinoblastoma, 107, **186**, 187*i*–189*i*
retinoids, 262
retrospective epidemiological study, **220**–221
ribose, 19*i*
ribosomal RNA (see RNA)
ribosomes, 16*i*, 17*i*, 21, 22–23
RNA (ribonucleic acid), **18***i*
  messenger RNA (mRNA), **32**, 34*i*–36
  polymerase, 32
  ribosomal RNA (rRNA), **32**
  transfer RNA (tRNA), **32**
Roentgen (R), **147**
rough endoplasmic reticulum, 16*i*, 22*i*
Rous, Peyton, 132, 165

S

saccharin, 258, 268
Safe Drinking Water Act, 268–269*i*
sarcoma, **75**
screening (people for cancer), 279–282
secondary prevention, **254**, 279
SEER Program (National Cancer Institute), 270
sensitivity (of cancer tests), 281*i*
septicemia in cancer patients, **214**
seven warning signs of cancer, 3, 278–279
sex and cancer, 348
skin, 340*i*
skin cancer, 7*i*, 154*i*, 339–340
skin changes in cancer patients, 212
smokeless tobacco, 260
smoker death rates, 6*i*
smoking and cancer (see cancer, smoking and)
smooth endoplasmic reticulum, 16*i*, 22i
specificity (of cancer tests), 281*i*
S phase (see cell, cycle)
squamous cell carcinoma, **75**

staging (of neoplasms), **76**–77
  purposes of, 77
steroids, 18*i*, 19*i*
stomach cancer, 8*i*, 336–337
stress and cancer, 261
strontium 90, 150
structural gene, **30**
sunlight and cancer, 260–61
supressor genes, 185
supressor T-cell, **238**–239*i*
Surgeon General's warnings, 265*i*
surgery, 298–300, 305, 315
  side effects/complications, 300
  types of, 298–300
surgical staging, **76**
survival patterns in cancer patients, 232
synergy, positive, **259**

T

T-cells, 237*i*, 240*i*, 242
Telephone Information Service, 357–358
teletherapy, **302**
telophase (of mitosis), 36
temperature sensitive mutants, 52
teratocarcinomas, mouse, **183**, 184*i*
tertiary prevention, **254**
thermography, 286
Three Mile Island, 155
thrombocytopenia, **209**
thromboses (see blood-clotting abnormalities)
tight junctions (between cells), **62**
tissue, **39**
  areolar connective, **41**
  connective, **40**–41
  epithelial, **39**–40
  types of, 39–41
TNM system of staging, **76**
Toxic Substances Control Act, 268–269*i*
transcription (of DNA), **32**
transfer factor, 247
transfer RNA (see RNA)
transient volume, **302**
translation (of DNA), **32**, 36
trigger protein, 65
tumor, **70**
tumor-associated antigens, 62, **245**, 286
tumorigenesis, 67, 277
tumor-infiltrating lymphocytes, 317
tumor marker, **287**–288
tumor necrosis factor (TNF), **242**, 243, 247

boldface indicates page on which a definition can be found
i indicates an illustration

boldface indicates page on which a definition can be found
i indicates an illustration